# Interventional Management of Ventricular Arrhythmias

*Editors*

AURAS R. ATREYA
CALAMBUR NARASIMHAN

# CARDIAC ELECTROPHYSIOLOGY CLINICS

www.cardiacEP.theclinics.com

*Consulting Editors*
JORDAN M. PRUTKIN
EMILY P. ZEITLER

December 2022 • Volume 14 • Number 4

**ELSEVIER**

1600 John F. Kennedy Boulevard • Suite 1800 • Philadelphia, Pennsylvania, 19103-2899

http://www.theclinics.com

**CARDIAC ELECTROPHYSIOLOGY CLINICS Volume 14, Number 4**
**December 2022 ISSN 1877-9182, ISBN-13: 978-0-323-98797-4**

Editor: Joanna Collett
Developmental Editor: Hannah Almira Lopez

*Cardiac Electrophysiology Clinics* (ISSN 1877-9182) is published quarterly by Elsevier Inc., 360 Park Avenue South, New York, NY 10010-1710. Months of issue are March, June, September, and December. Subscription prices are $247.00 per year for US individuals, $525.00 per year for US institutions, $259.00 per year for Canadian individuals, $549.00 per year for Canadian institutions, $315.00 per year for international individuals, $549.00 per year for international institutions and $100.00 per year for US, Canadian and international students/residents. To receive student/resident rate, orders must be accompanied by name of affilliated institution, date of term, and the signature of program/residency coordinator on institution letterhead. Orders will be billed at individual rate until proof of status is received. Foreign air speed delivery is included in all Clinics subscription prices. All prices are subject to change without notice. **POST-MASTER:** Send address changes to Cardiac Electrophysiology Clinics, Elsevier Health Sciences Division, Subscription Customer Service, 3251 Riverport Lane, Maryland Heights, MO 63043. **Customer Service: 1-800-654-2452 (US and Canada). From outside of the US and Canada, call 314-477-8871. Fax: 314-447-8029. E-mail: JournalsCustomerService-usa@elsevier.com (for print support); JournalsOnlineSupport-usa@elsevier.com (for online support).**

*Reprints.* For copies of 100 or more of articles in this publication, please contact the Commercial Reprints Department, Elsevier Inc., 360 Park Avenue South, New York, NY 10010-1710. Tel.: 212-633-3874; Fax: 212-633-3820; E-mail: reprints@elsevier.com.

*Cardiac Electrophysiology Clinics* is covered in *MEDLINE/PubMed (Index Medicus).*

# Contributors

## CONSULTING EDITORS

**JORDAN M. PRUTKIN, MD, MHS**
Professor of Medicine, University of Washington, Division of Cardiology, Seattle, Washington, USA

**EMILY P. ZEITLER, MD, MHS**
Dartmouth Health, The Dartmouth Institute, Lebanon, New Hampshire, USA; Assistant Professor of Medicine, The Geisel School of Medicine at Dartmouth, Hanover, New Hampshire, USA

## EDITORS

**AURAS R. ATREYA, MD, MPH, FACC, FHRS**
Consultant, Cardiologist and Electrophysiologist, Interventional Cardiology, Electrophysiology Section, AIG Hospitals Institute of Cardiac Sciences and Research, Hyderabad, Telangana, India; Assistant Professor, Division of Cardiovascular Medicine, Electrophysiology Section, University of Arkansas for Medical Sciences, Little Rock, Arkansas, USA

**CALAMBUR NARASIMHAN, MD, DM**
Head of Electrophysiology, Senior Consultant Cardiology, AIG Hospitals Institute of Cardiac Sciences and Research, Gachibowli, Hyderabad, Telangana, India

## AUTHORS

**YOSHIMORI AN, MD**
Department of Cardiovascular Medicine, Cleveland Clinic, Cleveland, Ohio, USA

**SAMUEL J. ASIRVATHAM, MD**
Department of Cardiovascular Medicine, Mayo Clinic, Professor of Medicine and Pediatrics, Mayo Clinic College of Medicine, Rochester, Minnesota, USA

**AURAS R. ATREYA, MD, MPH, FACC, FHRS**
Consultant, Cardiologist and Electrophysiologist, Interventional Cardiology, Electrophysiology Section, AIG Hospitals Institute of Cardiac Sciences and Research, Hyderabad, Telangana, India; Assistant Professor, Division of Cardiovascular Medicine, Electrophysiology Section, University of Arkansas for Medical Sciences, Little Rock, Arkansas, USA

**FRANK BOGUN, MD**
Professor of Medicine, Division of Cardiovascular Medicine, University of Michigan, Ann Arbor, Michigan, USA

**JASON S. BRADFIELD, MD**
UCLA Cardiac Arrhythmia Center, David Geffen School of Medicine at UCLA, Los Angeles, California, USA

**QUIM CASTELLVI, PhD**
Department of Information and Communications Technologies, Pompeu Fabra University, Barcelona, Spain

**RONPICHAI CHOKESUWATTANASKUL, MD**
Department of Medicine, Center of Excellence in Arrhythmia Research Chulalongkorn University, Bangkok, Thailand

**JOHN-ROSS CLARKE, MD**
Harvard Thorndike Electrophysiology Institute
and Arrhythmia Service, Beth Israel Deaconess
Medical Center, Harvard Medical School,
Boston, Massachusetts, USA

**JAKUB CVEK, MD, Ing, PhD**
Department of Oncology, University Hospital
Ostrava and Ostrava University Medical
School, Ostrava, Czech Republic

**ANDRE D'AVILA, MD, PhD**
Harvard Thorndike Electrophysiology Institute
and Arrhythmia Service, Beth Israel Deaconess
Medical Center, Harvard Medical School,
Boston, Massachusetts, USA

**ASHLEY M. DARLINGTON, MD**
Department of Cardiovascular Medicine, Mayo
Clinic, Rochester, Minnesota, USA

**CHRISTOPHER V. DESIMONE, MD, PhD**
Department of Cardiovascular Medicine, Mayo
Clinic, Rochester, Minnesota, USA

**FATIMA M. EZZEDDINE, MD**
Department of Cardiovascular Medicine, Mayo
Clinic, Rochester, Minnesota, USA

**THOMAS FLAUTT, DO**
Division of Cardiac Electrophysiology,
Department of Cardiology, Houston Methodist
DeBakey Heart and Vascular Center, Houston
Methodist Hospital, Houston, Texas, USA

**ALESSIO GASPERETTI, MD**
ARVC Program, Division of Cardiology, Johns
Hopkins School of Medicine, Baltimore,
Maryland, USA

**MICHAEL GHANNAM, MD**
Assistant Professor of Medicine, Division of
Cardiovascular Medicine, University of
Michigan, Ann Arbor, Michigan, USA

**TETSUYA HARUNA, MD, PhD**
Department of Cardiology, Kitano Hospital,
Osaka, Japan

**JANA HASKOVA, MD**
Department of Cardiology, IKEM, Prague,
Czech Republic

**JUSTIN HAYASE, MD**
UCLA Cardiac Arrhythmia Center, David
Geffen School of Medicine at UCLA, Los
Angeles, California, USA

**AYMAN A. HUSSEIN, MD**
Department of Cardiovascular Medicine,
Cleveland Clinic, Cleveland, Ohio, USA

**ATSUSHI IKEDA, MD, PhD**
Department of Medicine, Nihon University
School of Medicine, Tokyo, Japan

**JOSEF KAUTZNER, MD, PhD**
Department of Cardiology, IKEM, Prague,
Czech Republic; Palacky University Medical
School, Olomouc, Czech Republic

**YOSHITAKA KIMURA, MD, PhD**
Department of Cardiology, Heart Lung Center,
Leiden University Medical Center, Leiden, the
Netherlands; Center for Congenital Heart
Disease Amsterdam-Leiden (CAHAL), the
Netherlands; Willem Einthoven Center of
Arrhythmia Research and Management

**JACKSON J. LIANG, DO**
Electrophysiology Section, Division of
Cardiology, University of Michigan, Frankel
Cardiovascular Center, Ann Arbor, Michigan,
USA

**TIMOTHY MAHER, MD**
Harvard Thorndike Electrophysiology Institute
and Arrhythmia Service, Beth Israel Deaconess
Medical Center, Harvard Medical School,
Boston, Massachusetts, USA

**DANIELE MUSER, MD**
Cardiothoracic Department, Udine University
Hospital, Udine, Italy; Electrophysiology
Section, Division of Cardiology, Hospital of the
University of Pennsylvania, Philadelphia,
Pennsylvania, USA

**KOONLAWEE NADEMANEE, MD**
Professor, Department of Medicine, Center of
Excellence in Arrhythmia Research
Chulalongkorn University, Bumrungrad
Hospital, Bangkok and Pacific Rim
Electrophysiology Research Institute,
Bangkok, Thailand; Las Vegas, Nevada, USA

**HIROSHI NAKAGAWA, MD, PhD**
Department of Cardiovascular Medicine,
Cleveland Clinic, Cleveland, Ohio, USA

**CALAMBUR NARASIMHAN, MD, DM**
Head of Electrophysiology, Senior Consultant
Cardiology, AIG Hospitals Institute of Cardiac
Sciences and Research, Gachibowli,
Hyderabad, Telangana, India

**SACHIN NAYYAR, MBBS, MD, DM, PhD, FRACP, CCDS, CCEP**
Associate Professor, Townsville University Hospital, James Cook University, Townsville, Queensland, Australia

**TAKASHI NITTA, MD, PhD**
Emeritus Professor, Chief Consultant of Cardiology, Hanyu General Hospital, Hanyu City, Saitama, Japan; Nippon Medical School, Tokyo, Japan

**AKIHIKO NOGAMI, MD, PhD**
Department of Cardiology, Faculty of Medicine, University of Tsukuba, Ibaraki, Japan

**WIPAT PHANTHAWIMOL, MD**
Department of Cardiology, Faculty of Medicine, University of Tsukuba, Ibaraki, Japan

**VICKRAM VIGNESH RANGASWAMY, MD, DM**
Electrophysiology Section, AIG Hospitals Institute of Cardiac Sciences and Research, Hyderabad, India

**DALJEET KAUR SAGGU, MD, DM**
Electrophysiology Section, AIG Hospitals Institute of Cardiac Sciences and Research, Gachibowli, Hyderabad, India

**WALID I. SALIBA, MD**
Department of Cardiovascular Medicine, Cleveland Clinic, Cleveland, Ohio, USA

**PASQUALE SANTANGELI, MD, PhD**
Electrophysiology Section, Division of Cardiology, Hospital of the University of Pennsylvania, Philadelphia, Pennsylvania, USA

**MAREK SRAMKO, MD, PhD**
Department of Cardiology, IKEM, Prague, Czech Republic

**MUTHIAH SUBRAMANIAN, MD, DM**
Electrophysiology Section, AIG Hospitals Institute of Cardiac Sciences and Research, Gachibowli, Hyderabad, India

**HARIKRISHNA TANDRI, MD**
ARVC Program, Division of Cardiology, Johns Hopkins School of Medicine, Baltimore, Maryland, USA

**MIGUEL VALDERRÁBANO, MD**
Director, Division of Cardiac Electrophysiology, Department of Cardiology, Houston Methodist DeBakey Heart and Vascular Center, Houston Methodist Hospital, Houston, Texas, USA

**P. VIJAY SHEKAR, MD, DM**
Electrophysiology Section, AIG Hospitals Institute of Cardiac Sciences and Research, Gachibowli, Hyderabad, India

**ZAIN VIRK, MD**
Harvard Medical School, Boston, Massachusetts, USA; Department of Medicine, Vanderbilt University Medical Center, Nashville, Tennessee, USA

**JUSTIN WALLET, MD**
Department of Cardiology, Heart Lung Center, Leiden University Medical Center, Leiden, the Netherlands; Center for Congenital Heart Disease Amsterdam-Leiden (CAHAL), the Netherlands; Willem Einthoven Center of Arrhythmia Research and Management

**OUSSAMA M. WAZNI, MD**
Department of Cardiovascular Medicine, Cleveland Clinic, Cleveland, Ohio, USA

**SACHIN D. YALAGUDRI, MD, DM**
Electrophysiology Section, AIG Hospitals Institute of Cardiac Sciences and Research, Gachibowli, Hyderabad, India

**TAKUMI YAMADA, MD, PhD**
Cardiovascular Division, University of Minnesota, Minneapolis, Minnesota, USA

**KATSUAKI YOKOYAMA, MD**
Department of Medicine, Nihon University School of Medicine, Tokyo, Japan

**KATJA ZEPPENFELD, MD, PhD**
Department of Cardiology, Heart Lung Center, Leiden University Medical Center, Leiden, the Netherlands; Center for Congenital Heart Disease Amsterdam-Leiden (CAHAL), the Netherlands; Willem Einthoven Center of Arrhythmia Research and Management

# Contents

Ventricular arrhythmias present with a wide spectrum of clinical manifestations, from mildly symptomatic frequent premature ventricular contractions to life-threatening events. Pathophysiologically, idiopathic ventricular arrhythmias occur in the absence of structural heart disease or ion channelopathies. Ventricular arrhythmias in the context of structural heart disease are usually determined by scar-related reentry and are associated with increased mortality. Catheter ablation is safe and highly effective in treating ventricular arrhythmias. The proper characterization of the arrhythmogenic substrate is essential for accurate procedural planning. We provide an overview on the main mechanisms of ventricular arrhythmias and their implications for catheter ablation.

The pathogenesis of ventricular tachycardia (VT) in most patients with a prior myocardial scarring is reentry involving compartmentalized muscle fibers protected within the scar. Often the 12-lead ECG morphology of the VT itself is not available when treated with a defibrillator. Consequently, VT ablation takes on an interesting challenge of finding critical targets in sinus rhythm. High-density recordings are essential to evaluate a substrate based on whole electrogram voltage and activation delay, supplemented with substrate perturbation through alternate site pacing or introducing an extra stimulation. In this article, we discuss contemporary intracardiac electrogram targets for VT ablation, with explanation on each of their specific fundamental physiology.

Techniques for catheter ablation have evolved to effectively treat a range of ventricular arrhythmias. Pre-operative electrocardiographic and cardiac imaging data are very useful in understanding the arrhythmogenic substrate and can guide mapping and ablation. In this review, we focus on best practices for catheter ablation, with emphasis on tailoring ablation strategies, based on the presence or absence of structural heart disease, underlying clinical status, and hemodynamic stability of the ventricular arrhythmia. We discuss steps to make ablation safe and prevent complications, and techniques to improve the efficacy of ablation, including optimal use of electroanatomical mapping algorithms, energy delivery, intracardiac echocardiography, and selective use of mechanical circulatory support.

Ventricular tachycardia (VT) ablation is limited by modest acute and long-term success rates, in part due to the challenges in accurately identifying the arrhythmogenic substrate. The combination of multimodality imaging along with information from electroanatomic mapping allows for a more comprehensive assessment of the arrhythmogenic substrate which facilitates VT ablation, and the use of preprocedural imaging has been shown to improve long-term ablation outcomes. Beyond regional recognition of the arrhythmogenic substrate, advanced imaging techniques can be used to create tailored ablation strategies preprocedurally. This review will focus on how imaging can be used to guide ablation planning and execution with a focus on clinical applications aimed at improving the outcome of VT ablation procedures.

Idiopathic ventricular arrhythmias (VAs) most commonly originate from the ventricular outflow tracts. Because the anatomy of this region is complex and some of those VA origins are intramural and epicardial, it may sometimes be difficult to locate the site of the VA origin. Meticulous mapping in multiple different locations such as the right and left ventricular outflow tracts, endocardial and epicardial sites, and above and below the aortic and pulmonic valves may be required to achieve successful catheter ablation of those VAs. Special ablation techniques may be considered to improve the outcome of catheter ablation of intramural and epicardial VAs.

 Video content accompanies this article at http://www.cardiacep.theclinics.com

The Purkinje system has been found to mediate several monomorphic ventricular tachycardias (VTs). These include fascicular VTs and bundle branch reentrant (BBR) VTs. Previous studies have revealed that VTs involving the His-Purkinje system are composed of multiple discrete subtypes that are best differentiated by their mechanism, drug effect, VT morphology, and successful ablation site. Recognition of the heterogeneity of these VTs and their unique characteristics should facilitate the appropriate diagnosis and therapy and help guide catheter ablation therapy. In this article, we focus on the latest updates of the mechanisms underlying left ventricle fascicular VTs and BBR-VTs as well as the latest catheter ablation techniques.

Percutaneous epicardial ventricular tachycardia ablation can decrease implanted cardioverter defibrillator shocks and hospitalizations; proper patient selection and procedural technique are imperative to maximize the benefit–risk ratio. The best candidates for epicardial ventricular tachycardia will depend on history of prior ablation, type of cardiomyopathy, and specific electrocardiogram and cardiac imaging findings. Complications include hemopericardium, hemoperitoneum, coronary vessel injury, and phrenic nerve injury. Modern epicardial mapping techniques provide new understandings of the 3-dimensional nature of reentrant ventricular tachycardia circuits across cardiomyopathy etiologies. Where epicardial access is not feasible, alternative techniques to reach epicardial ventricular tachycardia sources may be necessary.

Arrhythmogenic right ventricular cardiomyopathy is an inherited desmosomal myopathy characterized by progressive fibrofatty replacement of the myocardium, right ventricular enlargement, and malignant ventricular arrhythmias. Ventricular tachycardias is one of the most common initial presentation of ARVC. This manuscript addresses invasive VT ablation options for the managmnet of VT in patients with ARVC.

 Video content accompanies this article at http://www.cardiacep.theclinics.com

Three decades have passed since the Brugada syndrome (BrS) clinical entity was introduced in the early 1990s. During the first 2 decades, treatment of patients with BrS was challenging because there were limited treatment options, and an implantable cardioverter-defibrillator was the only choice for high-risk patients with BrS, that is, those who had aborted sudden cardiac death or had previous ventricular fibrillation episodes. In this article, the authors focus on these advances and how to treat patients with BrS with catheter ablation.

Implantable cardioverter-defibrillators are the mainstay of therapy for prevention of sudden cardiac death in high-risk patients with hypertrophic cardiomyopathy (HCM). Catheter ablation is a useful option for patients with recurrent, drug refractory monomorphic ventricular tachycardia (VT), and device therapy. Compared with other nonischemic substrates, there are limited data on the role and outcomes of catheter ablation in HCM. The challenges of VT ablation in HCM patients include deep intramural and epicardial substrates, suboptimal power delivery, and higher recurrence due to progression of disease. Patient selection, using cardiac MRI scar localization, and optimizing ablation techniques can improve outcomes in these patients.

Granulomatous myocarditis is an inflammatory disease of the myocardium, characterized by lymphocytic infiltration with characteristic granuloma formation. Although a host of disease processes can elicit myocardial granulomas, two common entities are cardiac sarcoidosis and cardiac tuberculosis. Cardiac arrhythmias in this condition are frequent and management of ventricular arrhythmias can be challenging, especially in those with drug-refractory ventricular tachycardia and electrical storm. In this review, we highlight the role of catheter ablation for ventricular tachycardia and optimal patient selection for catheter ablation, based on cardiac imaging.

has the potential to overcome these limitations. Recent pre-clinical studies suggest that PFA/IRE might be effective and safe for the treatment of cardiac arrhythmias.

The autonomic nervous system plays an integral role in the pathophysiology of ventricular arrhythmias. In the modern era, several therapeutic interventions are available to the clinician for bedside and procedural/surgical management, and there are many ways in which modulation of the autonomic nervous system can provide life-saving benefit. This review discusses some of the current treatment options, the supporting evidence, and also introduce some of the emerging therapies in this expanding field of electrophysiology.

Stereotactic body radiotherapy is a recent promising therapeutic alternative in cases of failed catheter ablation for recurrent ventricular tachycardias (VTs) in patients with structural heart disease. Initial clinical experience with a single radiation dose of 25 Gy shows reasonable efficacy in the reduction of VT recurrences with acceptable acute toxicity. Many unanswered questions remain, including unknown mechanism of action, variable time to effect, optimal method of substrate targeting, long-term safety, and definition of an optimal candidate for this treatment.

Surgery for ventricular tachycardia (VT) is indicated in patients in whom pharmacotherapy or catheter ablation is ineffective or frequent VT attacks are not suppressed or with frequent activation of implantable cardioverter defibrillator. In ischemic VT, resection of fibrous endocardium combined with encircling cryothermia at the border between the infarcted and normal myocardium is performed. In surgery for VT associated with cardiomyopathy, close collaboration between the physician and surgeon is important and intraoperative mapping using electro-anatomic mapping system is helpful. In VT associated with cardiac tumors, cryothermia of the thinned subepicardial myocardium at the edge of the tumor is recommended in addition to resection of tumors.

# CARDIAC ELECTROPHYSIOLOGY CLINICS

---

**SERIES OF RELATED INTEREST**

*Cardiology Clinics*
Available at: https://www.cardiology.theclinics.com/
*Heart Failure Clinics*
Available at: https://www.heartfailure.theclinics.com/
*Interventional Cardiology Clinics*
Available at: https://www.interventional.theclinics.com/

---

**THE CLINICS ARE AVAILABLE ONLINE!**
Access your subscription at:
www.theclinics.com

# Foreword
# Sharing the Journey

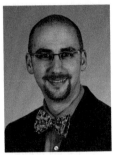  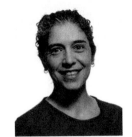

Jordan M. Prutkin, MD, MHS       Emily P. Zeitler, MD, MHS
*Consulting Editors*

We are excited to take the helm as the new editors of *Cardiac Electrophysiology Clinics*. We wish to sincerely thank Drs Ranjan Thakur and Andrea Natale, who edited the journal since its inception in 2009 and have now passed this responsibility to us. Moving forward, we are committed to broadening the reach of the journal by diversifying the topics, guest editors, and authors with special attention to incorporating more international perspectives. We have an exciting lineup of issues and editors already planned into 2024.

This journal has focused on review articles that go in-depth on an important or emerging subject. The first issue in 2009 included an article by Conor Barrett, MBBCH, and coauthors entitled "Ventricular Tachycardia Ablation—For Whom, When, and How?" In the subsequent 13 years, those questions are far from settled, but so much has changed. We now present an entire issue on the topic, "Interventional Management of Ventricular Arrhythmias." Thus, a topic that warranted a single review article in 2009 inspired 18 articles in this issue 13 years later. We have come a long way!

We are thankful to Drs Auras Atreya and Calambur Narasimhan, who edited and guided this issue, and to the numerous authors for their outstanding contributions. This issue takes the readers on a journey through the ablation of ventricular arrhythmias. It includes articles that describe the underlying substrate of ventricular arrhythmias, including mechanisms and imaging. These critical, underlying pathophysiologic discussions, which inform preablation preparation, include a thorough understanding of why the patient is having ventricular arrhythmias to improve the likelihood of success. The issue then explores how to approach ablation for various substrates, including normal hearts, His-Purkinje arrhythmias, epicardial disease, arrhythmogenic right ventricular cardiomyopathy, Brugada syndrome, hypertrophic cardiomyopathy, granulomatous myocarditis, and adult congenital heart disease. Ablation of ventricular fibrillation is discussed as well, with a focus on the elimination of the triggering premature ventricular contractions. Last, there are several articles about ablation using alternative energy sources. Four of these final five articles discuss novel technologies still undergoing testing, and they show us where interventional electrophysiology could be going in the future. This includes the use of alcohol in the arterial or venous systems, pulsed field ablation, neuromodulation, and stereotactic radiotherapy. All of these new technologies have unanswered questions related to safe and effective use, and these articles review the current knowledge and techniques. Surgical ablation is also considered with attention paid to its ongoing use in some specific clinical scenarios.

Card Electrophysiol Clin 14 (2022) xiii–xiv
https://doi.org/10.1016/j.ccep.2022.09.002
1877-9182/22/© 2022 Published by Elsevier Inc.

We look forward to sharing the journey of this journal with you. We hope that you, Reader, will reach out to us if you have ideas for an issue or a specific contribution.

Jordan M. Prutkin, MD, MHS
Division of Cardiology
University of Washington
1959 NE Pacific Street, Box 356422
Seattle, WA 98195, USA

Emily P. Zeitler, MD, MHS
Dartmouth Health and
The Dartmouth Institute
1 Medical Center Drive
Lebanon, NH 03756, USA

E-mail addresses:
jprutkin@uw.edu (J.M. Prutkin)
emily.p.zeitler@hitchcock.org (E.P. Zeitler)

# Preface

# Interventional Management of Ventricular Arrhythmias

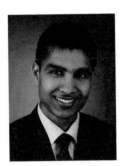
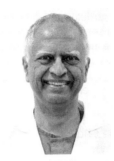

Auras R. Atreya, MD, MPH, FACC, FHRS    Calambur Narasimhan, MD, DM

*Editors*

Ventricular arrhythmias and associated sudden cardiac death remain an important issue in contemporary clinical practice. The foundational principles that guide the complex procedures we perform today are the product of six decades of incremental work in the field. The early days of surgical subendocardial resection, guided by a handheld mapping electrode by Dr Josephson and colleagues, was the precursor of modern catheter-based ablation therapies. The late 1980s and early 1990s saw Drs Stevenson, de Bakker, and Marchlinski elucidate the components of a ventricular tachycardia (VT) circuit—the fundamentals of signal propagation, "zigzag" course of activation in scar-related VT, and the concepts of critical isthmus and bystander circuits were defined. The development of radiofrequency (RF) ablation for supraventricular arrhythmias at the same time allowed for translation of these concepts into catheter-based therapy for ventricular arrhythmias.

Subsequently, great emphasis has been placed on the mechanistic understanding of ventricular arrhythmias in nonischemic cardiomyopathies, and various techniques and strategies have been developed to ablate the intramural and epicardial VT circuits. Over the past three decades, we have witnessed remarkable progress in electroanatomical mapping, epicardial access and ablation, advanced cardiac imaging, high-density mapping catheters, RF energy delivery, and the emergence of alternative energy sources for ablation. This knowledge has allowed us to define the arrhythmogenic substrate better and guide targeted ablation.

While these technological advances have played a key role in arming today's operators with sophisticated mapping and ablation capabilities, it has also added considerable complexity to the management of these patients. In this issue of the *Cardiac Electrophysiology Clinics*, we attempt to deconstruct and crystallize the core concepts of interventional ventricular arrhythmia management. We are truly fortunate to have collaborated with eminent and internationally renowned authors, to aid us in this pursuit.

Broadly, the first section outlines the basics of ventricular arrhythmia pathophysiology and provides an overview of catheter ablation, with an emphasis on pre-procedural imaging and intra-procedural electrogram targets. The next section has articles on catheter ablation of idiopathic ventricular arrhythmias arising from the outflow tracts and left ventricular summit, and VT originating from the conduction system. This is

Card Electrophysiol Clin 14 (2022) xv–xvi
https://doi.org/10.1016/j.ccep.2022.09.001
1877-9182/22/© 2022 Published by Elsevier Inc.

cardiacEP.theclinics.com

followed by a detailed overview of catheter ablation in the epicardial space, and subsequent focused reviews on catheter ablation of ventricular arrhythmias in specific non-ischemic cardiomyopathies (arrhythmogenic right ventricular cardiomyopathy, Brugada syndrome, hypertrophic cardiomyopathy and granulomatous myocarditis). This section ends with articles on ablation of VT in congenital heart disease and ablation of ventricular fibrillation. The final section consists of articles describing the spectrum of non-RF therapies that are used as adjunct to standard catheter ablation (cryothermia, electroporation, alcohol, radiation, autonomic neuromodulation, and surgical ablation).

Our goal, with this issue, is to give the readers of the *Cardiac Electrophysiology Clinics* an in-depth understanding of the entire gamut of interventional management strategies for ventricular arrhythmias. We would like to sincerely thank Drs. Thakur and Natale for inviting us to edit this issue of the Cardiac Electrophysiology Clinics, and we thank all the contributors for helping us synthesize and simplify this rapidly growing field in electrophysiology.

Auras R. Atreya, MD, MPH, FACC, FHRS
AIG Hospitals Institute of Cardiac Sciences and Research
1, Mindspace Road, Gachibowli
Hyderabad, Telangana 500032, India

Division of Cardiovascular Medicine
Electrophysiology Section
University of Arkansas for Medical Sciences
Little Rock, AR, USA

Calambur Narasimhan, MD, DM
AIG Hospitals Institute of Cardiac Sciences and Research
1, Mindspace Road, Gachibowli
Hyderabad, Telangana 500032, India

*E-mail addresses:*
aurasatreya@gmail.com (A.R. Atreya)
calambur1@gmail.com (C. Narasimhan)

# Mechanisms of Ventricular Arrhythmias and Implications for Catheter Ablation

Daniele Muser, MD[a,b], Pasquale Santangeli, MD, PhD[b],
Jackson J. Liang, DO[c],*

## KEYWORDS

- Idiopathic ventricular arrhythmias • Scar related reentry • Catheter ablation
- Structural heart disease • Ventricular tachycardia

## KEY POINTS

- Ventricular arrhythmias are among the most common arrhythmias encountered in everyday clinical practice.
- Catheter ablation can be used to effectively treat ventricular arrhythmias with high efficacy compared with medical therapy with antiarrhythmic drugs.
- Idiopathic ventricular arrhythmias have a focal mechanism and originate from well-defined endocardial and epicardial sites.
- In structural heart disease, myocardial scar plays a central role in the genesis and maintenance of ventricular arrhythmias, with reentry representing the usual underlying mechanism.
- Disruption or isolation of the arrhythmogenic substrate is the main goal of catheter ablation in scar-related ventricular arrhythmias; Accurate characterization is mandatory to achieve effective long-term arrhythmia suppression.

## INTRODUCTION

Ventricular arrhythmias (VA) can be divided into 2 main categories based on their underlying arrhythmogenic mechanism. Those originating in the absence of structural heart disease (SHD) are referred to as idiopathic and are among the most common VA encountered in everyday clinical practice. They can clinically present with frequent monomorphic premature ventricular contractions (PVC), nonsustained ventricular tachycardia (VT) or sustained VT, generally share a benign prognosis and have a focal mechanism originating from specific cardiac sites. Consequently, catheter ablation (CA) mainly relies on activation and pace mapping and may be challenging, especially when it comes to epicardial foci or intracavitary structures such as the papillary muscles and the moderator band. A careful analysis of electrocardiogram (ECG) features of these VAs can help to predict the site of origin (SOO) and plan the procedure. In contrast, VA related to SHD, typically present with sustained VT, are associated with frequent hospitalizations and increased mortality. Scar-related reentry plays a central role in the genesis and maintenance of such VA, and the main

Conflict of interest disclosure: None related to this topic.
[a] Cardiothoracic Department, Udine University Hospital, Udine 33100, Italy; [b] Electrophysiology Section, Division of Cardiology, Hospital of the University of Pennsylvania, 3400 Spruce Street, Philadelphia, PA 19104, USA; [c] Electrophysiology Section, Division of Cardiology, University of Michigan, Frankel Cardiovascular Center, 1425 E. Ann Street, Ann Arbor, MI 48109, USA
* Corresponding author.
E-mail address: liangjac@med.umich.edu

Card Electrophysiol Clin 14 (2022) 547–558
https://doi.org/10.1016/j.ccep.2022.07.006
1877-9182/22/© 2022 Elsevier Inc. All rights reserved.

cardiacEP.theclinics.com

goal of CA is to identify and disrupt critical components of the VT circuits. Ablation can be performed during VT by activation and entrainment mapping or during sinus rhythm by targeting abnormal electrograms (EGM) or sites deemed to be critical for the VT circuit. In this scenario, invasive and noninvasive imaging modalities such as cardiac magnetic resonance (CMR), multidetector computed tomography, and intracardiac echocardiography (ICE) are playing a growing role both in terms of preprocedural planning and intraprocedural guidance by characterizing the arrhythmogenic substrate and allowing the integration of structural and electrophysiological information. In the present review, we provide a comprehensive insight on the main mechanisms of VA and their implication in diagnosis and management with special regard to CA techniques.

## IDIOPATHIC VENTRICULAR ARRHYTHMIAS
### General Concepts

VA arising in the absence of underlying SHD, inherited primary arrhythmia syndromes or metabolic disturbances are referred to as idiopathic. They typically have a focal mechanism and are usually benign. However, in a minority of patients, apparently benign idiopathic VAs can trigger malignant ventricular fibrillation, and in some patients with high arrhythmic burden, frequent VAs can result in reversible left ventricular (LV) dysfunction. Frequent PVCs are the predominant manifestation accounting for approximately 90% of all idiopathic VA but they can be accompanied by nonsustained VT or even sustained VT with the same ECG morphology.[1,2] These idiopathic VAs originate from specific endocardial or epicardial foci, with the most common SOO being the right ventricular outflow tracts (RVOT) and LVOT, accounting for almost 70% of the cases. The remaining 30% of idiopathic VA originate from non-OT structures including the left and right papillary muscles (5%–15%), mitral annulus (5%), tricuspid annulus (8%–10%), left bundle branch fascicles (10%), and moderator band.[3,4] Approximately 4% to 10% of patients with idiopathic VA have an epicardial SOO, with the most common site being the perivalvular epicardium at the LV summit, followed by the cardiac crux region.[4,5] Twelve lead surface ECG characteristics such as frontal plane axis, a bundle branch block pattern, precordial transition, and the QRS width can be used to predict the most likely SOO and guide CA approach. The most frequent SOO of idiopathic VA and their ECG characteristics are schematically represented in **Fig. 1**.

## Mechanisms

Idiopathic VAs are commonly linked with triggered cyclic adenosine monophosphate (cAMP)-mediated afterdepolarizations or increased automaticity.[1] Triggered activity can result from either early or delayed afterdepolarization. Early afterdepolarizations typically are seen with slower heart rates and occur during phase 2 or 3 of the cardiac action potential. Meanwhile, delayed afterdepolarizations occur with faster heart rates and during phase 4 of the action potential. VAs are usually favored by adrenergic tone so that they can be triggered by stress or exertion. The adrenergic stimulus leads to an increased adenylyl cyclase activity with consequent rise of intracellular levels of cAMP, which activates the cAMP-dependent protein kinase (protein kinase A) leading to the phosphorylation of L-type sarcolemmal calcium channels, ryanodine receptor, and phospholamban.[6] All these processes increase intracellular calcium levels by spontaneous diastolic calcium release from the sarcoplasmic reticulum, known as calcium sparks.[7] Eventually, a transient sodium inward current enters the cell and produces delayed afterdepolarizations through the activation of electrogenic sodium–calcium exchanger, generating VA.[8] This mechanism explains some characteristics of idiopathic VA, such as termination by adenosine (by decreasing cAMP in the ventricular myocardium via an inhibitory G-protein cascade) or with vagal maneuvers (by activation of the M2 muscarinic receptor) and response to calcium channel blockers and β-blockers.[9]

Certain cardiac cells, including those in the sinoatrial node, exhibit automaticity at baseline resulting from diastolic depolarization owing to net inward current during phase 4 of the action potential. Under normal conditions, ventricular myocytes do not typically display spontaneous diastolic depolarization. However, in certain scenarios (ie, acute ischemia or myocarditis), abnormal automaticity of ventricular myocytes can occur owing to the release of calcium from the sarcoplasmic reticulum or decrease in $I_{K1}$ resulting in VA.

### Implications for Catheter Ablation

Radiofrequency CA is increasingly being used for the treatment of idiopathic VA.[10] Surface ECG findings, Holter monitoring data, and understanding whether or not a patient has SHD can be helpful to predict the underlying mechanism of VA. For example, OT VAs in patients with structurally normal hearts typically result from triggered activity owing to delayed afterdepolarizations. However, in patients with underlying scar and

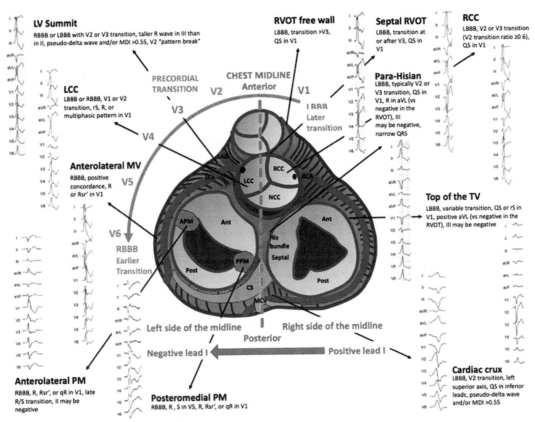

**Fig. 1.** Schematic representation of the main SOO of idiopathic ventricular arrhythmias contractions and their ECG features. (*From* Muser D., Tritto M., Mariani MV., et al. Diagnosis and Treatment of Idiopathic Premature Ventricular Contractions: A Stepwise Approach Based on the Site of Origin. Diagnostics (Basel) 2021;11(10):1840; with permission.)

nonischemic cardiomyopathy (NICM), patients may frequently have multiple VA morphologies and OT VAs in these patients may be more likely to be due to reentry. Examination of the PVC that triggers a VA can be helpful as well. If the triggering PVC has a different morphology than the subsequent VA, the underlying mechanism is more likely to be reentry, whereas with triggered or automatic VAs, the triggering PVC is usually of the same morphology as the subsequent VA. Additionally, gradual increases in the rate at VA onset and deceleration before termination is suggestive of an automatic mechanism.

Procedural planning always starts with the identification of possible SOO by careful evaluation of the surface ECG. In case of OT VA, the RVOT is initially mapped in VA with a left bundle branch block pattern and transition at V3 or higher, whereas the aortic cusps and the LVOTs are mapped first in cases presenting with a right bundle branch block or left bundle branch block with early transition (≤V2).

Activation and pace mapping are the cornerstones to define the SOO and chose the best ablation target. Accurate activation mapping requires a high burden of VA at the time of the procedure. However, when spontaneous VA are infrequent, induction may be attempted with isoproterenol infusion and ventricular or atrial burst pacing. Radiofrequency CA should be performed at the site where earliest activation (≥20 ms before the QRS) is recorded and, ideally, where the pace map is optimal (12/12 leads).[11] When local activation times at multiple adjacent sites such as the great cardiac vein and anterior interventricular vein, left coronary cusp, LV endocardium, and RVOT in cases of OT VA, have similar values and pace maps are suboptimal, an intramural origin should be suspected.[12] For patients with intramural VA, standard unipolar RF ablation may not be successful in eliminating the arrhythmias, even if sequentially delivered from multiple adjacent sites. In these cases, bipolar RF ablation, simultaneous unipolar RF ablation or the use of half-normal saline or nonionic irrigants have been shown to enhance success. Coronary angiography is recommended before ablation from the great cardiac vein, epicardium, and in select cases of ablation at the anterior RVOT, above the pulmonic valve, or within the aortic cusps and radiofrequency energy delivery should be deferred if the site is in proximity (within 5 mm) to major coronary vessels. An adequate distance from the coronary arteries should be confirmed in at least 2 orthogonal fluoroscopic projections and at any moment of the cardiac cycle.[13]

Non-OT VA have several well-defined SOO including papillary muscles, mitral valve annulus and LV summit within the LV and RV papillary muscles, tricuspid annulus, and moderator band within the RV.[14–16] In VA originating from intracavitary structures such as the papillary muscles or a moderator band, the complex anatomy, its variability, and the motion during the cardiac cycle make CA extremely challenging. In these cases, the use of ICE is pivotal to allow real-time visualization and ensure proper catheter contact. Cryoablation may also be an option to improve catheter stability.[15,17,18]

Approximately 4% to 10% of idiopathic VA have an epicardial SOO, represented in most cases by the LV summit and, less frequently, by the cardiac crux. A subxiphoid percutaneous epicardial approach may be pursued when an epicardial origin is suspected on the basis of 12-lead ECG or after failure of an endocardial approach, even if direct epicardial ablation can be challenging owing to the presence of major coronary arterial vessels and epicardial fat.[19] The CA approach must always take into consideration the anatomic structures that are in close proximity and susceptible to injury. In most cases, LV summit arrhythmias can be targeted via the distal coronary venous system (great cardiac vein and anterior interventricular vein), whereas cardiac crux VA can be targeted from the middle cardiac vein.[20,21] When ablation at the earliest epicardial site is not feasible, an anatomic approach targeting adjacent sites or alternative ablation strategies including use of bipolar or simultaneous unipolar ablation or surgical ablation can be considered.[22–29] An anatomic approach has shown to be effective when the distance between the 2 adjacent sites is 12.8 mm or less or when the difference between local activation times is 7 ms or less.[30–32]

## VENTRICULAR ARRHYTHMIAS IN STRUCTURAL HEART DISEASE
### General Concepts

VAs are a major health issue in patients with SHD. Implantable cardioverter defibrillator (ICD) therapy has significantly decreased the risk of SCD in such patients, but has led to frequent ICD shocks as an emerging problem, being associated with a poor quality of life, frequent hospitalizations, and increased mortality.[33] The management of VA in this setting is challenging because of the complexity of the substrate and underlying heart failure (HF). Radiofrequency CA has repeatedly demonstrated its superiority compared with antiarrhythmic drugs in decreasing VT recurrences and ICD shocks, even if a mortality benefit has never been proven convincingly.[34,35] In patients with advanced HF, recurrent VT may simply represent a marker of worsening HF status, with a limited possibility for achieving long-lasting arrhythmia control. However, even if not able to improve survival directly, CA can still result in improved quality of life by decreasing the number of ICD therapies and the need for antiarrhythmic drugs.

Myocardial scar plays a central role in the genesis and maintenance of VA in SHD, and scar-related reentry represents the main underlying mechanism for VT in these patients. In recent years, the evolution of electroanatomic mapping systems together with the integration of noninvasive imaging modalities have significantly improved CA strategies and long-term outcomes. In particular, imaging modalities such as CMR, multidetector computed tomography, and ICE have progressively established their role in characterizing the arrhythmogenic substrate and guiding CA by integrating structural and electrophysiological information, defining anatomy, monitoring catheter location, and recognizing procedural complications.[36,37]

### Mechanisms

The electrophysiological substrate of VA in the setting of SHD is represented by scar-related reentry.[38] In areas of myocardial scar, the presence of surviving myocardial fibers within fibrous tissue leads to the formation of slow conduction pathways as well as to a dispersion of activation and refractoriness that constitute the milieu for reentrant circuits (**Fig. 2**).[39] The elimination or isolation of this arrhythmogenic substrate can potentially prevent VT.[40]

### Implications for Catheter Ablation

The primary goal of CA of scar-related VT is the interruption of critical sites of slow conduction responsible for the development and maintenance of reentrant VT circuits. Traditionally, CA is performed during VT by activation and entrainment mapping to achieve an accurate characterization of the VT circuit, but substrate-based ablation approaches, targeting abnormal EGM or sites deemed to be critical for VT during sinus rhythm,

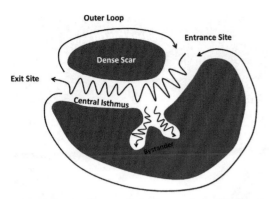

**Fig. 2.** Classic figure-of-eight reentry circuit as described by Stevenson and colleagues in 1993. Blue regions represent areas of dense scar not excitable during tachycardia. The activation wave front propagates around 2 lines of conduction block sharing a central common isthmus. Bystander pathways can be attached to any point in the circuit and represent areas of tissue activated by the wave front but not playing an active role in the reentrant circuit. (*Adapted from* Stevenson WG., Khan H., Sager P., et al. Identification of reentry circuit sites during catheter mapping and radiofrequency ablation of ventricular tachycardia late after myocardial infarction. Circulation 1993;88(4):1647–70. https://doi.org/10.1161/01.CIR.88.4.1647; with permission.)

have progressively emerged as a valuable alternative, especially in patients presenting with unstable or nonsustained arrhythmias precluding activation and entrainment mapping.[41] Some of these strategies target the entire abnormal substrate (ie, late potentials and local abnormal ventricular activity [LAVA] abolition or scar homogenization), whereas others (ie, scar dechanneling, linear ablation, and core isolation) focus on discrete regions within the abnormal substrate that have been proven relevant to the VT. The specific etiology of SHD has a deep impact on the CA strategy, as in ICM the substrate is typically subendocardial following coronary arteries distribution, whereas in NICM, the substrate involves the basal perivalvular region of the LV and the interventricular septum with a high prevalence of midmyocardial or subepicardial substrates.

## Entrainment and Activation Mapping

Entrainment mapping has been the gold standard for the delineation of reentrant circuits. This technique uses overdrive pacing, whereby 2 wavefronts enter the VT circuit to confirm reentry as the underlying mechanism and determine the spatial relationship of the pacing site to the VT circuit.[42,43] Considering the classical figure-of-eight reentry circuit (see **Fig. 2**), a central isthmus, is

bordered between 2 regions of dense scar with an entrance and an exit site, which yields the QRS morphology.[44] This type of circuit manifests a so-called excitable gab determined by the fact that the time it takes the circulating excitation wave to propagate once around the circuit exceeds the refractory period at each point of the circuit. If a pacing stimulus is applied to a site after the site has recovered, but before arrival of the next activation wavefront, the pacing stimulus captures the myocardium, creating 2 wavefronts, with one traveling in the same direction as the tachycardia and resetting the tachycardia itself (orthodromic wavefront), and the other traveling in the opposite direction (antidromic wavefront). During pacing, there is a shortening of the tachycardia cycle length (CL) to the pacing CL with resumption of the intrinsic CL after pacing is terminated. Entrainment does not require the pacing site to be located within the circuit. During pacing there is fixed fusion while pacing at a constant CL and progressive fusion until a fully paced complex is evident while pacing at a faster CL. When pacing terminates, the last paced wavefront goes through the reentrant circuit producing a nonfused QRS complex. The postpacing interval is the interval from the last capturing stimulus to the next activation at the pacing site and a measure of the proximity of the pacing site to the reentry circuit as pacing sites within the circuit will yield a postpacing interval close to the tachycardia CL. When pacing is performed from outside the circuit, the activation at the pacing site will be a composite of the conduction time from the pacing site to the circuit, then through the circuit, and then back to the pacing site resulting in a postpacing interval longer than the tachycardia CL.[39,45] Activation mapping, like entrainment mapping, relies on mapping in VT. It involves the collection of the timing points of most of the VT circuit, which then enables the construction of a color map of activation wavefront. Activation and entrainment mapping allow the identification of the critical components of the VT circuit, which can be targeted with CA (**Fig. 3**). However, accurate entrainment and activation mapping can be challenging, especially in patients with advanced HF or unstable VT.

## Substrate-Based Approaches

The accurate characterization of the arrhythmogenic substrate is critical for any kind of substrate-based CA approach. The current definition of the substrate relies on EGM characteristics (ie, wide, split, and late EGM) together with bipolar and unipolar voltage amplitude thresholds.

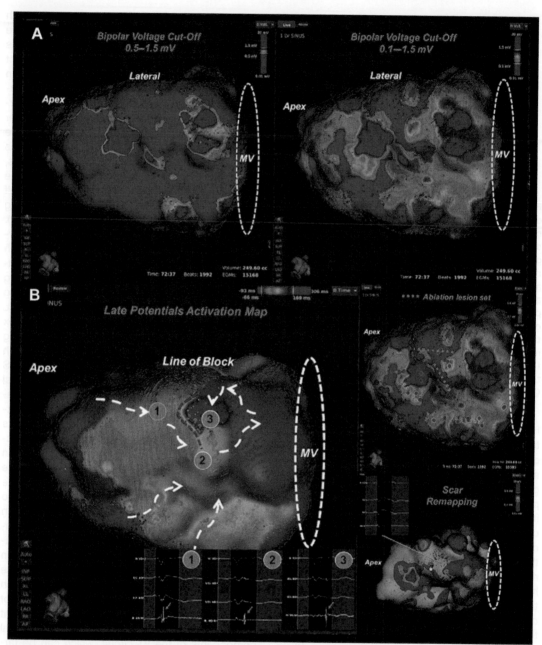

**Fig. 3.** High-density electroanatomic map of a patient showing a large inferior post myocardial infarction scar (*A*), presenting for VT ablation. Activation mapping by manually adjusting the reference activation time to the end of the surface QRS complex (*B*), allowed for identification of conduction channels within the scar (*B–white dotted lines*). In particular, 3 discrete entrance sites (*B–yellow numbers*) were identified at the apical aspect of the scar with a line of block (*B–red dotted line*) at the lateral aspect of the scar. Radiofrequency ablation at the putative entrance sites of the scar, resulted in elimination of late potentials. (*From* Muser D., Kumareswaran R., Santangeli P. Ultrarapid identification of activation channels within the scar using high-density mapping from a basket catheter. HeartRhythm Case Reports 2017;3(1):112–4; with permission.)

Fractionated EGM are the expression of slow heterogeneous conduction (anisotropy) with poor cell-to-cell coupling and are characterized by low amplitude (≤0.5 mV), long duration (≥133 ms), low amplitude to duration ratio (<0.005), and fractionated, split, and late components (**Fig. 4**).[46] Studies in animal models as well as in patients with sustained VT in the setting of coronary artery disease demonstrated that low-voltage regions correlated with infarct regions.[47]

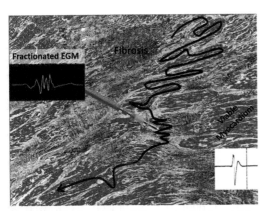

**Fig. 4.** Histologic section of the explanted heart (Masson's trichrome stain) of a patient with post-infarct myocardial scar showing surviving myocardial fibers (*red color*) and fibrotic areas (*blue color*). The "zigzag" course of activation proceeding along slow pathways determined by merging of bundles of surviving myocytes plunged into fibrosis generates fractioned EGM. (*From* Muser D., Liang JJ., Santangeli P. Off-line analysis of electro-anatomical mapping in ventricular arrhythmias. Minerva Cardioangiol 2017;65(4):369–79; with permission.)

In particular, 95% of normal LV endocardial bipolar EGM have been shown to have an amplitude of more than 1.5 mV, leading to the definition of the 1.5 mV as the cut-off for normal voltage.[40] However, the field of view of endocardial bipolar recording is limited and related to electrode size and interelectrode distance and may underestimate or miss deep intramural or epicardial substrates. In this scenario, unipolar endocardial recording, which has a larger field of view, has shown the capability to identify the presence and location of epicardial low bipolar voltage areas.[48] Unipolar voltage evaluates the difference of potential between the endocardial recording site (catheter tip) and a patch applied to the skin of the patient (Wilson's central terminal), including the whole myocardium inside the field of view. In healthy controls, 95% of unipolar EGM exhibit voltages with an amplitude of more than 8.3 mV. Meanwhile, in patients with NICM and VT, the presence of confluent endocardial unipolar low voltage areas identified by the 8.3 mV voltage threshold correlates well with epicardial bipolar low voltage in patients showing normal endocardial bipolar recordings.[48] Recently, advances in imaging techniques have led to a better understanding of arrhythmic substrates, even from a noninvasive point of view. In particular, CMR with late gadolinium enhancement can detect myocardial fibrosis as a potential substrate for reentrant arrhythmias in both ICM and NICM.[49] Late gadolinium enhancement imaging is based on the different wash-in and wash-out kinetics of gadolinium from normal myocardium and tissue with myocardial fibrosis. Gadolinium generally takes a longer time to wash in and out from the regions with replacement fibrosis than normal healthy myocardium; therefore, regions with a greater extracellular volume will have a higher concentration of contrast agent experiencing greater T1 time shortening, which renders the area brighter on T1-weighted images.[50] Critical sites for reentrant VT (ie, VT isthmuses) are frequently located within late gadolinium enhancement regions and such scar information obtained noninvasively from CMR can be imported into electroanatomic mapping systems to facilitate VT mapping and ablation procedures.[51] Based on these findings, several authors have proposed several substrate-based ablation techniques.[52–57]

Extensive substrate ablation approaches involve scar homogenization and ablation of abnormal EGM. In scar homogenization, all abnormal EGMs (any EGM that has >3 deflections, an amplitude of <1.5 mV, and a duration of >70 ms) within the scar defined by bipolar voltage criteria are targeted. The CA end point is either the elimination of the abnormal EGM or the loss of local capture with high-output pacing (20-mA output at a 10-ms pulse width).[53] Ablation of late potentials or LAVAs strictly depends on the definition of abnormal EGMs, which lacks of standardization. Late potentials have been defined variously as any type of EGM with a duration extending beyond the end of the surface QRS, as multiple-component EGMs separated by a more than 50-ms isoelectric signal in sinus rhythm and more than 150 ms during pacing, as distinct EGMs after the QRS separated by 40 ms from an isoelectric interval or a very low amplitude signal of less than 0.1 mV, or as any low-voltage EGM with a single component or multiple continuous delayed electrical components separated from the higher amplitude component of the local ventricular EGM by 20 ms or more and recorded after the end of the surface QRS.[52,55,58,59] The Bordeaux group has recently proposed to include all the different patterns of abnormal EGMs that can be observed within scarred areas as expression of slow conduction pathways under the definition of LAVA.[54] LAVA are defined as sharp high-frequency potentials (not necessarily of low amplitude), distinct from the far-field ventricular EGMs occurring anytime during the local ventricular EGM in sinus rhythm, displaying fractionation or double or multiple components separated by very low amplitude signals or an isoelectric interval. Such EGMs have to be confirmed by pacing maneuvers (ie, pacing from the RV apex introducing short coupled extrastimuli or in sites very proximal to the LAVA recording site with different current outputs) demonstrating a poor coupling with the adjacent myocardium.[60]

More limited substrate-based ablation strategies include all those approaches targeting areas of the substrate deemed to be critical for the development of VT. Linear ablation technique involves the creation of CA lesions from the dense scar area through the border zone and anchoring them to anatomic barriers or normal myocardium. This approach relies on pace mapping techniques to define putative VT exit sites and identify areas within the abnormal substrate where linear lesions should be placed.[40] Scar dechanneling targets channels of viable myocardium within the dense scar who could serve as VT isthmuses. Channels can be delineated by using high-output pacing (10 mA, pulse width 2 ms) to identify electrically unexcitable scar, by adjusting voltage cutoffs on voltage maps or by the high-density reconstruction of channels of activation of late potentials with the end point of eliminating a consecutive series of late potentials by ablation of the earliest late potential.[57,61–63] The core isolation approach has the end point to eliminate all the areas critical for VT within the dense scar and implies initial identification of the area of interest within the scar, including voltage channels, sites with late potentials, sites with good pace maps and long stimulus to QRS intervals, and entrainment-defined isthmus sites. Once identified, the area is targeted with contiguous lesions completely surrounding the region of interest or using anatomic anchors with the end point of inexcitability within the core.[56]

## Specific Etiologies

There are profound differences in the underlying substrate among patients with ICM versus NICM. In ICM, voltage abnormalities are usually confined to the endocardial layer with various degrees of extension through the ventricular wall and are typically restricted to distributions supplied by the affected coronary arteries.[47] Currently, the evolution of reperfusion therapies for acute myocardial infarction has led to early reperfusion, resulting in nontransmural necrosis, with highly heterogeneous infarct cores containing larger bundles of surviving myocytes mixed with fibrotic tissue, surrounded by similarly complex border zones merging into normal myocardium.[64]

In NICM, the substrate typically involves the basal perivalvular region of the LV and the interventricular septum with a high prevalence of midmyocardial or subepicardial substrates with only a modest (<25%) area of endocardial bipolar voltage abnormality.[65,66] The complex 3-dimensional substrate anatomy with variable involvement of the endocardium, epicardium, and presence of intramural circuits in patients with NICM can be a challenge for CA strategies. Therefore, accurate definition of the substrate and determining whether epicardial mapping and ablation may be required is of great importance. Two typical scar patterns (anteroseptal and inferolateral) are found in up to 90% of patients with NICM and VT.[67,68] Two VT morphologies are usually seen in the presence of anteroseptal substrate: a right bundle branch block with an inferior axis and positive concordance throughout the precordial leads or a left bundle branch block with an inferior axis and early (≤V3) precordial transition.[67] A predominant inferolateral substrate can instead be identified in approximately one-half of the patients, and, in the majority of these cases critical components of VT circuits involve the epicardial surface. These patients typically present VT of right bundle branch block morphology with right superior axis and late (≥V5) precordial transition.[67] The distinction between these 2 patterns is of great clinical value in terms of both procedural planning and outcomes. In patients with a predominant anteroseptal substrate, an epicardial approach is largely unnecessary, and the complex local anatomy (ie, proximity to coronary vessels, presence of epicardial fat) usually limits the safety and efficacy of direct epicardial radiofrequency ablation. Conversely, an epicardial approach is often required to achieve VT control in patients with a predominant inferolateral pattern. Even if epicardial coronary vessels and the phrenic nerve may be an obstacle complicating epicardial CA in patients with inferolateral substrate, these patients typically have a more favorable outcome (75% vs 25% VT-free survival at 1.5 years of follow-up) and a lower need for redo procedures (7% vs 59%) compared with patients with an anteroseptal substrate.[69] In patients with septal VT, the intramural location of the substrate can be difficult to address and may require sequential LV and RV CA as well as the use of high radiofrequency energy, potentially leading to collateral injury of the conduction system. Alternative approaches such as bipolar radiofrequency ablation, high-intensity focused ultrasound, retractable needle ablation, and intracoronary ethanol ablation may be necessary to overcome such limitations. A variety of criteria can be used to address the need for epicardial mapping and ablation: (1) a 12-lead ECG of the VT suggesting an epicardial origin (wide QRS complexes [shortest RS complex in precordial leads of $\geq$121 ms], slow initial upstroke of the QRS complex pseudo delta wave of $\geq$34 ms, an intrinsicoid deflection time of $\geq$85 ms, and a maximum deflection Index [shortest QRS onset to maximum precordial deflection/QRS duration] of $\geq$0.55); (2) evidence of epicardial substrate on imaging studies (ie, CMR, ICE), (3) a unipolar voltage abnormality (<8.3 mV) in the presence of no or minimal bipolar (<1.5 mV) abnormality; and (4) failure of endocardial ablation (either early VT recurrence or persistent inducibility of clinical VT). Epicardial ablation approach is usually associated with a higher incidence of complications; moreover, in a substantial proportion of cases (approximately 30%), even if critical VT sites are found on the epicardial surface, CA cannot be safely performed owing to the close proximity of epicardial coronary vessels and the left phrenic nerve or the presence of epicardial fat. Several ECG features have been correlated with epicardial VT origin.70

## SUMMARY

VA are among the most common arrhythmias encountered in everyday clinical practice and can be treated effectively by CA. In this setting, the underlying VA mechanism plays a central role in planning the procedural strategy. Idiopathic VA have a focal mechanism and originate from well-defined SOO that can be predicted based on specific 12-leads ECG characteristics to plan the most effective approach. In contrast, scar-related reentry owing to the coexistence of surviving myocardial fibers within fibrotic tissue is the most common mechanism subtending VT in patients with SHD. The destruction or isolation of the arrhythmic substrate or of its critical components is the main goal of CA of VA in SHD. In this setting, invasive and noninvasive characterization of the arrhythmogenic substrate has progressively led to the development of new ablation strategies and improved outcomes.

## CLINICS CARE POINTS

- Ventricular arrhythmias are among the most common arrhythmias encountered in everyday clinical practice.
- Catheter ablation can be used to effectively treat ventricular arrhythmias with high efficacy compared with medical therapy with antiarrhythmic drugs.

- Idiopathic ventricular arrhythmias have a focal mechanism and originate from well-defined endocardial and epicardial sites.
- Idiopathic ventricular arrhythmias have a focal mechanism and originate from well-defined endocardial and epicardial sites.
- In structural heart disease, myocardial scar plays a central role in the genesis and maintenance of ventricular arrhythmias, with reentry representing the usual underlying mechanism.
- Disruption or isolation of the arrhythmogenic substrate is the main goal of catheter ablation in scar-related ventricular arrhythmias; Accurate characterization is mandatory to achieve effective long-term arrhythmia suppression.

## REFERENCES

1. Lerman BB. Mechanism, diagnosis, and treatment of outflow tract tachycardia. Nat Rev Cardiol 2015; 12(10):597–608.
2. Latif S, Dixit S, Callans DJ. Ventricular arrhythmias in normal hearts. Cardiol Clin 2008;26(3):367–80, vi.
3. Latchamsetty R, Yokokawa M, Morady F, et al. Multicenter outcomes for catheter ablation of idiopathic premature ventricular complexes. JACC Clin Electrophysiol 2015;1(3):116–23.
4. Hayashi T, Liang JJ, Shirai Y, et al. Trends in successful ablation sites and outcomes of ablation for idiopathic outflow tract ventricular arrhythmias. J Am Coll Cardiol EP 2019. https://doi.org/10.1016/j.jacep.2019.10.004.
5. Baman TS, Ilg KJ, Gupta SK, et al. Mapping and ablation of epicardial idiopathic ventricular arrhythmias from within the coronary venous system. Circ Arrhythmia Electrophysiol 2010;3(3):274–9.
6. Schlotthauer K, Bers DM. Sarcoplasmic reticulum Ca(2+) release causes myocyte depolarization. Underlying mechanism and threshold for triggered action potentials. Circ Res 2000;87(9):774–80.
7. Cheng H, Lederer WJ. Calcium sparks. Physiol Rev 2008;88(4):1491–545.
8. Katra RP, Laurita KR. Cellular mechanism of calcium-mediated triggered activity in the heart. Circ Res 2005;96(5):535–42.
9. Lerman BB, Ip JE, Shah BK, et al. Mechanism-specific effects of adenosine on ventricular tachycardia. J Cardiovasc Electrophysiol 2014;25(12):1350–8.
10. Cronin EM, Bogun FM, Maury P, et al. 2019 HRS/EHRA/APHRS/LAHRS expert consensus statement on catheter ablation of ventricular arrhythmias. Heart Rhythm 2019. https://doi.org/10.1016/j.hrthm.2019.03.002.

11. Yamada T, McElderry HT, Doppalapudi H, et al. Idiopathic ventricular arrhythmias originating from the left ventricular summit: anatomic concepts relevant to ablation. Circ Arrhythmia Electrophysiol 2010; 3(6):616–23.

12. Di Biase L, Romero J, Zado ES, et al. Variant of ventricular outflow tract ventricular arrhythmias requiring ablation from multiple sites: intramural origin. Heart Rhythm 2019;16(5):724–32.

13. Stavrakis S, Jackman WM, Nakagawa H, et al. Risk of coronary artery injury with radiofrequency ablation and cryoablation of epicardial posteroseptal accessory pathways within the coronary venous system. Circ Arrhythm Electrophysiol 2014;7(1):113–9.

14. Crawford T, Mueller G, Good E, et al. Ventricular arrhythmias originating from papillary muscles in the right ventricle. Heart Rhythm 2010;7(6):725–30.

15. Enriquez A, Supple GE, Marchlinski FE, et al. How to map and ablate papillary muscle ventricular arrhythmias. Heart Rhythm 2017. https://doi.org/10.1016/j.hrthm.2017.06.036.

16. Yue-Chun L, Wen-Wu Z, Na-Dan Z, et al. Idiopathic premature ventricular contractions and ventricular tachycardias originating from the vicinity of tricuspid annulus: results of radiofrequency catheter ablation in thirty-five patients. BMC Cardiovasc Disord 2012;12:32.

17. Yamada T, McElderry HT, Okada T, et al. Idiopathic focal ventricular arrhythmias originating from the anterior papillary muscle in the left ventricle. J Cardiovasc Electrophysiol 2009;20(8):866–72.

18. Yamada T, Doppalapudi H, McElderry HT, et al. Electrocardiographic and electrophysiological characteristics in idiopathic ventricular arrhythmias originating from the papillary muscles in the left ventricle: relevance for catheter ablation. Circ Arrhythmia Electrophysiol 2010;3(4):324–31.

19. Muser D, Santangeli P. Epicardial ablation of idiopathic ventricular tachycardia. Card Electrophysiol Clin 2020;12(3):295–312.

20. Meininger GR, Berger RD. Idiopathic ventricular tachycardia originating in the great cardiac vein. Heart Rhythm 2006;3(4):464–6.

21. Santangeli P, Marchlinski FE, Zado ES, et al. Percutaneous epicardial ablation of ventricular arrhythmias arising from the left ventricular summit: outcomes and electrocardiogram correlates of success. Circ Arrhythm Electrophysiol 2015;8(2):337–43.

22. Nguyen DT, Tzou WS, Sandhu A, et al. Prospective multicenter experience with cooled radiofrequency ablation using high impedance irrigant to target deep myocardial substrate refractory to standard ablation. JACC Clin Electrophysiol 2018;4(9):1176–85.

23. Futyma P, Sander J, Ciąpała K, et al. Bipolar radiofrequency ablation delivered from coronary veins and adjacent endocardium for treatment of refractory left ventricular summit arrhythmias. J Interv Card Electrophysiol 2019. https://doi.org/10.1007/s10840-019-00609-9.

24. Yamada T, Maddox WR, McElderry HT, et al. Radiofrequency catheter ablation of idiopathic ventricular arrhythmias originating from intramural foci in the left ventricular outflow tract: efficacy of sequential versus simultaneous unipolar catheter ablation. Circ Arrhythm Electrophysiol 2015;8(2):344–52.

25. Yang J, Liang J, Shirai Y, et al. Outcomes of simultaneous unipolar radiofrequency catheter ablation for intramural septal ventricular tachycardia in nonischemic cardiomyopathy. Heart Rhythm 2018. https://doi.org/10.1016/j.hrthm.2018.12.018.

26. Kreidieh B, Rodríguez-Mañero M, Schurmann P, et al. Retrograde coronary venous ethanol infusion for ablation of refractory ventricular tachycardia. Circ Arrhythm Electrophysiol 2016;9(7). https://doi.org/10.1161/CIRCEP.116.004352.

27. Tholakanahalli VN, Bertog S, Roukoz H, et al. Catheter ablation of ventricular tachycardia using intracoronary wire mapping and coil embolization: description of a new technique. Heart Rhythm 2013;10(2):292–6.

28. Choi E-K, Nagashima K, Lin KY, et al. Surgical cryoablation for ventricular tachyarrhythmia arising from the left ventricular outflow tract region. Heart Rhythm 2015;12(6):1128–36.

29. Liang JJ, Betensky BP, Muser D, et al. Long-term outcomes of surgical ablation for refractory ventricular tachycardia in patients with non-ischemic cardiomyopathy. Europace 2016;20(3):e30–41.

30. Jauregui Abularach ME, Campos B, Park K-M, et al. Ablation of ventricular arrhythmias arising near the anterior epicardial veins from the left sinus of Valsalva region: ECG features, anatomic distance, and outcome. Heart Rhythm 2012;9(6):865–73. https://doi.org/10.1016/j.hrthm.2012.01.022.

31. Nagashima K, Choi E-K, Lin KY, et al. Ventricular arrhythmias near the distal great cardiac vein: a challenging arrhythmia for ablation. Circ Arrhythmia Electrophysiol 2014;7(5):906–12. CIRCEP-114.

32. Shirai Y, Santangeli P, Liang JJ, et al. Anatomical proximity dictates successful ablation from adjacent sites for outflow tract ventricular arrhythmias linked to the coronary venous system. Europace 2019; 21(3):484–91.

33. Poole JE, Johnson GW, Hellkamp AS, et al. Prognostic importance of defibrillator shocks in patients with heart failure. N Engl J Med 2008;359(10):1009–17.

34. Santangeli P, Muser D, Maeda S, et al. Comparative effectiveness of antiarrhythmic drugs and catheter ablation for the prevention of recurrent ventricular tachycardia in patients with implantable

cardioverter-defibrillators: a systematic review and meta-analysis of randomized controlled trials. Heart Rhythm 2016;13(7):1552–9.

35. Sapp JL, Wells GA, Parkash R, et al. Ventricular tachycardia ablation versus escalation of antiarrhythmic drugs. N Engl J Med 2016;375(2):111–21.

36. Mahida S, Sacher F, Dubois R, et al. Cardiac imaging in patients with ventricular tachycardia. Circulation 2017;136(25):2491–507.

37. Enriquez A, Saenz LC, Rosso R, et al. Use of intracardiac echocardiography in interventional cardiology: working with the anatomy rather than fighting it. Circulation 2018;137(21):2278–94.

38. Wissner E, Stevenson WG, Kuck K-H. Catheter ablation of ventricular tachycardia in ischaemic and non-ischaemic cardiomyopathy: where are we today? A clinical review. Eur Heart J 2012;33(12):1440–50.

39. Stevenson WG, Khan H, Sager P, et al. Identification of reentry circuit sites during catheter mapping and radiofrequency ablation of ventricular tachycardia late after myocardial infarction. Circulation 1993; 88(4):1647–70.

40. Marchlinski FE, Callans DJ, Gottlieb CD, et al. Linear ablation lesions for control of unmappable ventricular tachycardia in patients with ischemic and nonischemic cardiomyopathy. Circulation 2000;101(11): 1288–96.

41. Di Biase L, Burkhardt JD, Lakkireddy D, et al. Ablation of stable VTs versus substrate ablation in ischemic cardiomyopathy: the VISTA randomized multicenter trial. J Am Coll Cardiol 2015;66(25): 2872–82.

42. Callans DJ, Hook BG, Josephson ME. Comparison of resetting and entrainment of uniform sustained ventricular tachycardia. Further insights into the characteristics of the excitable gap. Circulation 1993;87(4):1229–38.

43. Stevenson WG, Weiss JN, Wiener I, et al. Resetting of ventricular tachycardia: implications for localizing the area of slow conduction. J Am Coll Cardiol 1988; 11(3):522–9.

44. Stevenson WG, Sager PT, Natterson PD, et al. Relation of pace mapping QRS configuration and conduction delay to ventricular tachycardia reentry circuits in human infarct scars. J Am Coll Cardiol 1995;26(2):481–8.

45. Stevenson WG, Friedman PL, Sager PT, et al. Exploring postinfarction reentrant ventricular tachycardia with entrainment mapping. J Am Coll Cardiol 1997;29(6):1180–9.

46. Cassidy DM, Vassallo JA, Marchlinski FE, et al. Endocardial mapping in humans in sinus rhythm with normal left ventricles: activation patterns and characteristics of electrograms. Circulation 1984; 70(1):37–42.

47. Callans DJ, Ren J-F, Michele J, et al. Electroanatomic left ventricular mapping in the porcine model of healed anterior myocardial infarction correlation with intracardiac echocardiography and pathological analysis. Circulation 1999; 100(16):1744–50.

48. Hutchinson MD, Gerstenfeld EP, Desjardins B, et al. Endocardial unipolar voltage mapping to detect epicardial ventricular tachycardia substrate in patients with nonischemic left ventricular cardiomyopathy. Circ Arrhythm Electrophysiol 2011;4(1): 49–55.

49. Simonetti OP, Kim RJ, Fieno DS, et al. An improved MR imaging technique for the visualization of myocardial infarction. Radiology 2001;218(1): 215–23.

50. Mahrholdt H, Wagner A, Judd RM, et al. Assessment of myocardial viability by cardiovascular magnetic resonance imaging. Eur Heart J 2002;23(8):602–19.

51. Desjardins B, Crawford T, Good E, et al. Infarct architecture and characteristics on delayed enhanced magnetic resonance imaging and electroanatomic mapping in patients with post-infarction ventricular arrhythmia. Heart Rhythm 2009;6(5):644–51.

52. Arenal A, Glez-Torrecilla E, Ortiz M, et al. Ablation of electrograms with an isolated, delayed component as treatment of unmappable monomorphic ventricular tachycardias in patients with structural heart disease. J Am Coll Cardiol 2003;41(1):81–92.

53. Di Biase L, Santangeli P, Burkhardt DJ, et al. Endo-epicardial homogenization of the scar versus limited substrate ablation for the treatment of electrical storms in patients with ischemic cardiomyopathy. J Am Coll Cardiol 2012;60(2):132–41.

54. Jais P, Maury P, Khairy P, et al. Elimination of local abnormal ventricular activities: a new end point for substrate modification in patients with scar-related ventricular tachycardia. Circulation 2012;125(18): 2184–96.

55. Vergara P, Trevisi N, Ricco A, et al. Late potentials abolition as an additional technique for reduction of arrhythmia recurrence in scar related ventricular tachycardia ablation. J Cardiovasc Electrophysiol 2012;23(6):621–7.

56. Tzou WS, Frankel DS, Hegeman T, et al. Core isolation of critical arrhythmia elements for treatment of multiple scar-based ventricular tachycardias. Circ Arrhythm Electrophysiol 2015;8(2):353–61.

57. Berruezo A, Fernández-Armenta J, Andreu D, et al. Scar dechanneling: new method for scar-related left ventricular tachycardia substrate ablation. Circ Arrhythm Electrophysiol 2015;8(2):326–36.

58. Cassidy DM, Vassallo JA, Miller JM, et al. Endocardial catheter mapping in patients in sinus rhythm: relationship to underlying heart disease and ventricular arrhythmias. Circulation 1986;73(4):645–52.

59. Nogami A, Sugiyasu A, Tada H, et al. Changes in the isolated delayed component as an endpoint of catheter ablation in arrhythmogenic right ventricular

cardiomyopathy: predictor for long-term success. J Cardiovasc Electrophysiol 2008;19(7):681–8.

60. Sacher F, Lim HS, Derval N, et al. Substrate mapping and ablation for ventricular tachycardia: the LAVA approach: substrate mapping and ablation. J Cardiovasc Electrophysiol 2015;26(4):464–71.

61. Soejima K, Stevenson WG, Maisel WH, et al. Electrically unexcitable scar mapping based on pacing threshold for identification of the reentry circuit isthmus: feasibility for guiding ventricular tachycardia ablation. Circulation 2002;106(13):1678–83.

62. Arenal A, Castillo S del, Gonzalez-Torrecilla E, et al. Tachycardia-related channel in the scar tissue in patients with sustained monomorphic ventricular tachycardias influence of the voltage scar definition. Circulation 2004;110(17):2568–74.

63. Tung R, Mathuria NS, Nagel R, et al. Impact of local ablation on interconnected channels within ventricular scar mechanistic implications for substrate modification. Circ Arrhythm Electrophysiol 2013;6(6):1131–8.

64. Mattfeldt T, Schwarz F, Schuler G, et al. Necropsy evaluation in seven patients with evolving acute myocardial infarction treated with thrombolytic therapy. Am J Cardiol 1984;54(6):530–4.

65. Hsia HH, Callans DJ, Marchlinski FE. Characterization of endocardial electrophysiological substrate in patients with nonischemic cardiomyopathy and monomorphic ventricular tachycardia. Circulation 2003;108(6):704–10.

66. Cano O, Hutchinson M, Lin D, et al. Electroanatomic substrate and ablation outcome for suspected epicardial ventricular tachycardia in left ventricular nonischemic cardiomyopathy. J Am Coll Cardiol 2009;54(9):799–808.

67. Piers SRD, Tao Q, van Huls van Taxis CFB, et al. Contrast-enhanced MRI–derived scar patterns and associated ventricular tachycardias in nonischemic cardiomyopathy implications for the ablation strategy. Circ Arrhythm Electrophysiol 2013;6(5):875–83.

68. Haqqani HM, Tschabrunn CM, Tzou WS, et al. Isolated septal substrate for ventricular tachycardia in nonischemic dilated cardiomyopathy: incidence, characterization, and implications. Heart Rhythm 2011;8(8):1169–76.

69. Oloriz T, Silberbauer J, Maccabelli G, et al. Catheter ablation of ventricular arrhythmia in nonischemic cardiomyopathy: anteroseptal versus inferolateral scar sub-types. Circ Arrhythmia Electrophysiol 2014;7(3):414–23.

70. Berruezo A. Electrocardiographic recognition of the epicardial origin of ventricular tachycardias. Circulation 2004;109(15):1842–7.

# Intracardiac Electrogram Targets for Ventricular Tachycardia Ablation

Sachin Nayyar, MBBS, MD, DM, PhD, FRACP, CCDS, CCEP*

## KEYWORDS

- Ablation • Channel • Electrogram • Fibrosis • Late potential • Pacing • Slow conduction
- Ventricular tachycardia

## KEY POINTS

- Ventricular tachycardia (VT) ablation requires comprehensive knowledge of suitable targets for ablation not only during VT but also in baseline rhythm and during programmed stimulation.
- Differential pacing from multiple ventricular sites can unmask new functional delays in individual electrograms which may improve VT substrate characterization.
- A complete analysis of individual deflections in terms of activation times and voltage sampling within an electrogram at all sites can identify protected segments of surviving myocytes in the scar.

## INTRODUCTION

Ventricular tachycardia (VT) ablation is endorsed by heart rhythm societies across the world as a treatment of choice for recurrent VT not responding to medical treatment.[1] In fact, in case of idiopathic VT, it can be offered as a primary treatment because of remarkable success and low complication rate in those with minimal or no structural heart disease. In contrast, concerns regarding lengthy procedures, hemodynamic instability, multiple VTs, modest success with intramural substrate, need for repeat procedures, and vascular complications diminish the attractiveness of VT ablation as a primary approach in those with cardiomyopathy and ventricular scar. Fundamentally, nonischemic scar-related VTs share common pathophysiology and electrogram targets as ischemic scar VT. However, such targets are patchy and midmyocardial in nonischemic scar, which are less evident, accounting for poorer outcomes.[2,3] Nonetheless, there is enough evidence that VT ablation significantly reduces the burden of ventricular arrhythmias and in fact almost eliminates the risk of recurrent VT storm.[4,5] In this article, we focus on scar-related VTs and discuss specific intracardiac electrogram targets for VT ablation. We will not address idiopathic VT, focal VTs, or VTs with conduction system participation.

## MECHANISM OF VENTRICULAR TACHYCARDIA IN CARDIOMYOPATHY AND VENTRICULAR SCAR

Most VTs in the setting of ventricular scar are due to reentrant mechanism apart from few exceptions.[6] Whenever possible, it is imperative that the mechanism of arrhythmia is defined before ablation. This is important as methods chosen for VT ablation will impact the outcome if critical VT circuit components are missed. Even VTs with apparent outflow tract or papillary muscle exit in diseased ventricles may have an underlying critical zone of slow conduction or conduction system participation, which should always be explored.

Townsville University Hospital, James Cook University, Townsville, Queensland, Australia
* Department of Cardiology, Townsville University Hospital, 100, Angus Smith Drive, Douglas, Queensland 4814, Australia.
E-mail address: sachin.nayyar@health.qld.gov.au

Card Electrophysiol Clin 14 (2022) 559–570
https://doi.org/10.1016/j.ccep.2022.06.001
1877-9182/22/Crown Copyright © 2022 Published by Elsevier Inc. All rights reserved.

## GENERAL CHALLENGES IN VENTRICULAR TACHYCARDIA ABLATION

Ablation of VT requires comprehensive knowledge of suitable targets not only during the arrhythmia but also in baseline rhythm and during programmed stimulation. This approach is necessary as most VTs are poorly tolerated and do not allow time for adequate mapping. Although it gives opportunity to perform an effective ablation in stable baseline rhythm, it is a challenge to identify critical electrogram targets in large ventricular substrate with complex pattern and extensive scarring. The critical components of VT circuit may span variable depth into the myocardium and therefore remain hidden during contemporary mapping. To overcome such difficulties, some groups favor diffuse endo-epicardial ablation to homogenize disease areas in the entire chamber,[7] but benefits of this approach remain controversial.[8] It is worth a mention to the budding electrophysiology readers that historic hallmark targets in substrate-based VT ablation have been frequently rechristened with "new names" in the modern ablation era. This attractiveness in their labeling may have inadvertently introduced some complexities and controversies around VT ablation targets.

### Substrate-Based Mapping: Targets in Sinus (or Paced) Rhythm

1. *Low-voltage electrograms.* Most VT exit sites are in the periphery of scar tissue (ie, borderzone), although the critical isthmus may reside within the dense scar.[9] The reduced availability of membrane $Na^+$ channels and the reduced cell-to-cell electrical coupling due to fibrosis, myofiber malorientation, and connexin redistribution produce slow and discontinuous electrical depolarization that diminish peak electrical voltage. This situation is characteristic of the inhomogeneous substrate associated with myocardial infarction, infiltration, or inflammation, where increased uncoupling between myofiber bundles occurs. Classically, in the ventricular endocardium, bipolar peak-to-peak voltage definitions are used to describe preserved tissue (>1.5 mV), border zone tissue (0.5–1.5 mV), and dense scar (<0.5 mV).[10] In the epicardium, preserved voltage is taken as greater than 1.0 mV to account for voltage attenuation by the overlying epicardial fat.[11] However, peak-to-peak bipolar electrogram voltage depends on several biophysical determinants, especially mapping bipole electrode geometry and orientation, and as such dichotomizing cardiac tissues into scar versus healthy tissues based on single bipolar voltage cutoffs is incorrect[12,13] (**Fig. 1**). Therefore, the practice of anatomic ablation based on low bipolar voltage-based scar or border zone and voltage-based conducting channels is better avoided. In the presence of normal endocardial bipolar voltage, a low tissue unipolar voltage of less than 7.0 mV in the left ventricle (LV) and less than 4.0 mV in the right ventricle (RV) is considered a sensitive marker of diseased

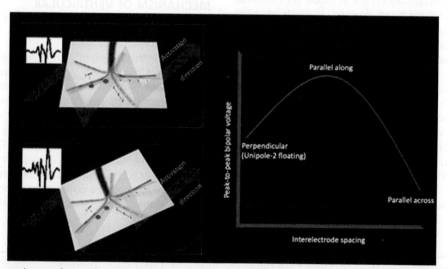

**Fig. 1.** Dependence of a peak-to-peak bipolar electrogram voltage on bipole orientation and interelectrode spacing in relation to the activation direction. A bipole oriented parallel to the tissue along the direction of activation records maximum bipolar voltage and may demonstrate new electrogram components which may not be obvious in other orientations. (Adapted Josephson ME, Anter E: Substrate Mapping for Ventricular Tachycardia Assumptions and Misconceptions. JACC Clin Electrophysiol. 2015; 1:341-52; with permission.)

myocardium under the recording electrode in intramural or epicardial tissues.[14,15] Recent histologic data though suggests that local endocardial bipolar voltage may also decrease due to a remote layer of scar tissue.[3]

2. *Multicomponent or fractionated electrograms.* Fractionated electrograms are considered as indicative of underlying electrically preserved myocardial fibers interspersed within a bed of fibrous scar tissue which may be prone to current or future VTs.[16] The heterogeneities in the cellular electric properties and tissue architecture create regions of discontinuous slow conduction and source-to-sink mismatches, which contribute to the development of unidirectional conduction block and reentrant VT.[17] With reduced intercellular coupling, irregularities seem in local extracellular electrogram as depolarization and propagation of the individual neighboring cells become separated in time to be evident as distinct deflections. The seminal works by Spach and colleagues in 1986 and then Dillon and colleagues in 1988 described the formation of "fractionated" electrograms.[18,19] More recently, in 2014, the term "localized abnormal ventricular activities" (LAVA) were coined by Jais and colleagues to qualify multicomponent electrograms that can be buried within a larger local or far-field electrogram.[20] A normal electrogram has three or fewer sharp intrinsic deflections from baseline, duration less than 70 ms, and/or amplitude: duration greater than 0.046 mV/ms. In contrast, a fractionated electrogram has multiple intrinsic deflections and amplitude: duration ≤0.045 mV/ms (**Fig. 2**).[21]

Current substrate-based ablation strategies emphasize high-density mapping to identify and homogenously target all multicomponent electrograms by catheter ablation.[20,22] However, information pertinent to a VT supporting channel remains obscure in such loose definition of fractionation. Although specific for identifying VT channels, these electrograms have poor sensitivity; not all such electrograms reside in the VT supporting channels, and in fact, many are bystanders (**Fig. 3**).[23,24] Conversely, only 50% of central, proximal or exit sites of reentry circuits have abnormal electrograms.[25] Targeting these electrograms often results in ablation of bystander sites (eg, dead-end pathways) and channels that may not be operative in any clinical VT (non-VT channels).

3. *Late and very late components of fractionated electrograms.* In a multicellular fiber with continuous conduction and normal cellular coupling, the extracellular bipolar electrogram is smooth and activation completes within the duration of the surface QRS complex. The time of local

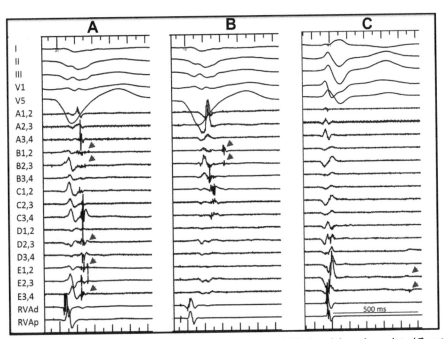

**Fig. 2.** Examples of scar-related abnormal electrograms. Fractionated (*A*), late (*B*), and very late (*C*) potentials are marked with arrows. Channels from top to bottom are surface ECG (I, II, III, V1, and V5), PentaRay mapping catheter in left ventricular scar and right ventricular apical catheter (RVA). d, distal; p, proximal.

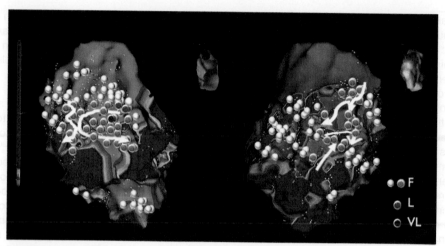

**Fig. 3.** Scar potentials and VT circuits. An endocardial left ventricular bipolar voltage map is shown with abnormal potentials and VT supporting channels. Gray areas represent scar (bipolar voltage <0.5 mV). In a study among patients with ischemic cardiomyopathy and VT,[9] only 25% of abnormal potentials (*yellow* = fractionated, *orange* = late, *blue* = very late) were within the identified VT supporting channels (*white arrows*). The remainders (*white dots*) were distributed elsewhere within the scar.

activation is taken as the moment of steepest negative deflection of the component unipolar electrograms, which coincides with the steepest portion of the upstroke of local action potential (AP) $(dV_m/dt_{max})$ and maximum local depolarizing $Na^+$ current $(I_{Na})$. This relationship does not hold true in tissues with reduced cell-to-cell coupling, and there is no unique local activation time in a multicomponent electrogram.[26,27] Some local tissue depolarization may even be visually split as it is activated late (isolated component ≥20 ms after the end of surface QRS), or very late (isolated component ≥100 ms after the end of surface QRS).[28] Electrograms during sinus rhythm in the delayed isochrones of activation, especially those in regions of steep activation gradient (zone of deceleration with crowding of isochrones), were shown to be in anatomic proximity to critical segments of the VT circuits.[25,29] It is important to realize that ablation target is in the zone of crowded isochrones leading into the latest activated zone, rather than the latest activated zone itself. Recent three-dimensional electroanatomic mapping data have confirmed and relabeled this approach as isochronal late activation mapping, whereby latest activation is annotated at all recorded sites. Ablation is targeted to crowded isochrones defined as color-coded zones encompassing ≥40 ms per 10 cm.[30,31]

Late potential regions in sinus rhythm, however, have a very low sensitivity and moderate specificity for VT channels (see **Fig. 3**).[23,24] This produces frequent "false-negative" and "false-positive" sites of late potentials with

multiple zones of deceleration to identify VT channel regions.[9] Mechanistic studies have also shown that most of the diastolic activation of VT happens in the intra-QRS period during sinus rhythm.[32] Therefore, ablation of late potentials may not only omit key arrhythmogenic regions but also drive excessive ablation of innocuous bystander regions.

## Substrate-Based Mapping: Targets in Differential Pacing and Extrastimulus Pacing

1. *Differential pacing.* Propagating electrical waves in a heterogenous scar interact with anisotropic boundaries which are both physical obstacles such as cell membranes of variably oriented myocytes, connective tissue barriers, and virtual boundaries due to the dispersion of current from a small strand to a large mass of tissue (source-to-sink mismatch).[33] A large mismatch or fibrotic barrier between up and downstream elements produces functional slow conduction or block. Activation recording in multiple wave fronts (sinus rhythm and RV and LV pacing) or by pacing adjacent to the scar can be useful to bring forth such maximal functional slowing in conduction.[34,35] Conduction can instantaneously alter with a different rate or change in the source of activation. In this regard, ventricular as opposed to sinus/atrial pacing disengages myocardial activation of the His–Purkinje conduction and transforms the sequence of ventricular activation into one with pure cell-to-cell conduction.[36] The dynamic responses to

differential pacing can vary among patients depending on their electrophysiological differences in cell-to-cell conduction and unique organization of scar-related fixed conduction abnormalities. For instance, in patients with cardiomyopathy and myocardial scarring, there are fewer entrances to access the protected surviving myocyte network of the heterogeneous scar region.[30,37,38] There is a high probability that a differential activation front will still engage the deep channels through the same entrance in the fibrotic scar, and the deep activation remains relatively unchanged despite altered external activation. Moreover, many long channels or those with long refractory period, when challenged at a rapid activation rate, are prone to complete conduction block or diminution of extracellular electrogram due to their inherent lower safety factor of conduction.[33] The overall reserve for functional conduction variation is therefore paradoxically poorer when there is advanced baseline electrical remodeling. The recently proposed Physio-VT mapping is based on such distinctive responses of individual intracardiac electrograms to RV and LV pacing versus sinus rhythm to improve VT substrate

resolution.[35] Ablation is then restricted to cumulative area of slow activation, defined as the sum of all regions with activation times of $\geq$40 ms per 10 mm ($\geq$4 isochrones within 10 mm).

2. *Extra-stimulus pacing.* Conduction can also instantaneously alter with a different rate of activation. A rate-related decrement in conduction velocity (conduction velocity restitution) is a universal property of the myocardial tissues. The reduced availability of membrane $Na^+$ channels and the reduced cell-to-cell electrical coupling due to altered distribution of gap junction proteins not only contribute to discontinuous slow conduction but also increase susceptibility to further slowing or conduction block at the faster rate.[33,39] This feature is a characteristic of LAVA potentials,[20] also labeled, in principle, as decremental evoked potential (DEEP), the hidden substrate, or the Bart's sense protocol strategy.[40–42] In DEEP mapping, after a 600 ms S1–S1 pulse train, an S2-extrastimulus is delivered from right ventricle at ventricular effective refractory period +20 ms, and a minimum delay of 10 ms is required to be categorized as a DEEP site (**Fig. 4**). The current generation electroanatomic mapping systems have automated some of

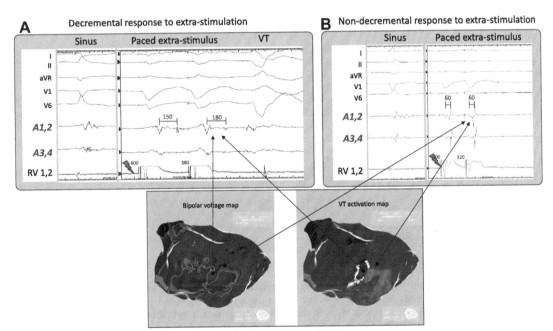

**Fig. 4.** The endocardial left ventricular bipolar voltage and activation map during VT are shown at the bottom. Each of the top panels (A–B) shows the surface ECG channels (I, II, aVR, V1, V6), and Pentaray "A" spline bipoles (A1,2 and A3,4) and right ventricle apex catheter (RV 1,2). The arrows indicate location of the Pentaray A1,2. (*A*) Response of electrograms in sinus rhythm to extra-stimulus pacing from RV. S1-pacing evoked additional conduction delay between electrogram deflections that further pronounced after S2 leading to initiation of VT. (*B*) Adjacent site had multicomponent electrogram in sinus rhythm, but RV-paced extra-stimulation did not induce additional conduction delay.

these tedious pacing and selective latest electrogram annotation approach, improving the efficiency of mapping.

## Substrate-Based Mapping: Targets Using Whole Electrograms

*Electrogram information content-based mapping.* Practically, determination of a unique local activation time or voltage in multiple-deflection bipolar electrograms is difficult. Such electrograms indicate that the electrical activity persists near the bipole in individual local tissue components for the duration of the electrogram. Information content-based strategy considers whole electrogram and assigns individual activation times and sample voltages from all deflections within an electrogram (**Fig. 5**).[29] This approach is based on the original principles of impulse conduction in the branching myofiber networks described by Kucera and is developed partly adapting the method of Ciaccio and others.[29,43,44]

Up to 70% of length of a scar-related VT isthmus may be protected,[6] with few side branch electrical-charge interactions. This is true even when there are multiple VTs from the same region sharing orthogonal multiuse isthmus with different entrance and exits.[45,46] Quantifying information content within an electrogram can predict protected tissue microstructure likely to support VT.[46] Electrograms

from a protected channel can only possess a few states in their voltage (limited to cells of the main strand and its scanty branches if any) and thus low information content. In contrast, load interactions from side branches of an unprotected channel introduce several complex dissimilar voltage deflections and thus high information content. VT isthmus sites can be distinguished based on information content (or entropy) in the voltage domain of sinus or ventricular paced rhythm bipolar electrograms.[46,47] A low-entropy electrogram is practically appreciable as that with relative even amplitude among most of its individual intrinsic deflections. An isolated late potential which is recorded as an upright straight column also has a single even voltage level and can be conceptualized as the most simplistic low-entropy electrogram. A recent small study has also observed that mid-isthmus electrograms may have low voltage and shorter duration (therefore low entropy) in sinus rhythm compared with bystander region.[48] It is, however, important to realize that low-entropy electrogram does not imply low peak-to-peak voltage but is a measure of variation in voltage among individual peaks inscribed within a local electrogram. The congregation of the sites of latest activation and minimum entropy in a region of high dispersion in activation could be predictor of the VT channel location compared with each individual electrogram properties.[47]

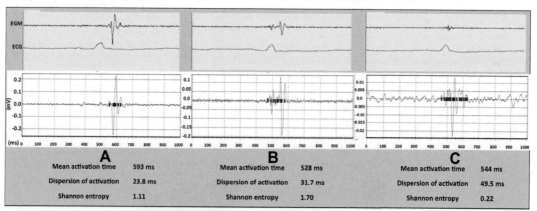

**Fig. 5.** Information content of whole electrogram. The three top panels show electrograms obtained from within the dense scar having low-voltage and multiple intrinsic deflections. The corresponding surface ECG QRS is aligned in the middle of the 1-s recording window. After filtering the electrogram signal at 20 Hz low pass, as in the bottom panels, a local activation point of maximum d$V$/d$t$ is detected (*red marker*) within 300 and 700 ms of the recording window. Annotation is confirmed within each electrogram and slided manually only if there is artifact detection. Every deflection (peak and trough) in a window of 200 ms across maximum d$V$/d$t$, which was ≥1% of the largest peak deflection and had a range ≥5 ms, is assigned an activation time (*green markers*) relative to the start of window (0 ms). The mean and standard deviation of these activation times represent the mean activation time and the dispersion in activation, respectively, at that location. Entropy (Shannon entropy, ShEn) is estimated as the probability distribution in the voltage histogram of each ascribed electrogram. (*A*) Electrogram with the relative late mean activation time, high dispersion, and high ShEn. (*B*) Relative early mean activation time, high dispersion, and high ShEn. (*C*) Relative early mean activation time, high dispersion, and low ShEn.

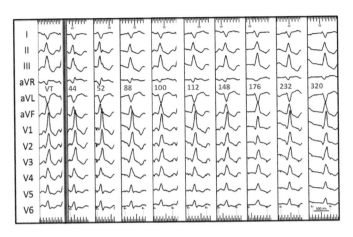

**Fig. 6.** Pace map series for an inducible VT. The left panel shows 12-lead ECG QRS morphology of a VT. The right panel shows the set of pace maps with marked stimulus-QRS intervals of ≥40 ms in an orthodromic sequence and matching QRS morphology (≥11/12 ECG leads) to the VT.

Real-time automated software has been added to the current generation electroanatomic mapping and unmasks electrogram congregation specific for VT ablation (Target-VT study; URL: www. ANZCTR.org.au. Unique identifier: ACTRN12620000049976). When a site with the latest mean activation time (T) is found present adjacent (within 30 mm) to a low-entropy point (S) within a region of high dispersion in activation, a line is drawn along a shortest endocardial path from (T) through (S) to an early activation site near the interface with surrounding low dispersion in activation. The anatomic region in proximity to either side of this line (within a 5-mm rim) is reasoned as the region critical to the maintenance of VT(s).

(**Fig. 6**).[49] VT morphology on the 12-lead electrocardiogram (ECG) and distribution of the underlying abnormal low voltage and multicomponent electrograms and late potentials are relevant in planning selective pace-mapping locations.[51,52] The color-coded sequence (from the best to the poorest matching sites) on the pace maps can identify VT isthmus.[53] Often, however, the 12-lead ECG morphology of the VT itself is not available when treated with a defibrillator or non-inducible at the time of electrophysiologic study. Consequently, pace-mapping becomes of limited additional value finding critical targets in sinus rhythm. Some operators use pace-mapping to differentiate abnormal electrogram sites and recording system noise/artifacts by demonstrating the presence or lack of capture at 10 mA/2 ms, respectively.

## Pace-Mapping

Pacing during sinus rhythm within dense scar can also identify channels.[49,50] Areas of paced latencies ≥40 ms in scar (long stimulus-QRS duration) are observed to collocate with VT isthmus sites

## Ventricular Tachycardia Activation Time Mapping

1. *Mid-isthmus electrogram.* Among those with easily inducible and hemodynamically tolerated

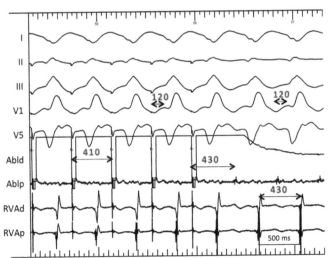

**Fig. 7.** Entrainment pacing (Abld) during VT. Channels from top to bottom are surface ECG (I, II, III, V1, V5), ablation catheter (Abl), and right ventricular apex [RVA, distal (d) and proximal (p)]. Intervals are marked in milliseconds. This pacing site entrained the VT with concealed fusion with post-pacing interval matching tachycardia cycle length. The stimulus-QRS interval (120 ms) matched with the diastolic potential (Ablp) to QRS interval. This site represented mid-diastolic isthmus location for this VT. Abld, Ablation distal; Abl, Ablation; Ablp, Ablation proximal.

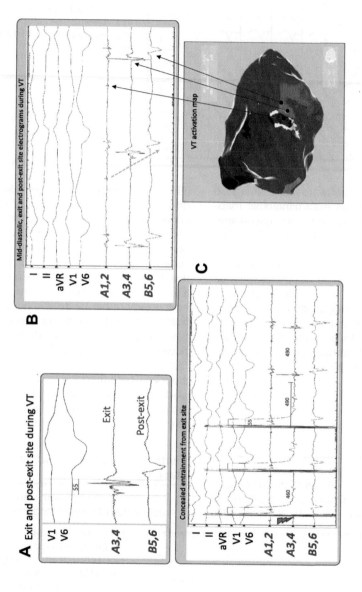

**Fig. 8.** The endocardial left ventricular activation map during VT is shown at the bottom right. Each of the panels A–C shows the surface ECG channels (I, II, aVR, V1, and V6), and Pentaray "A" and "B" spline bipoles (A1,2, A3,4 and B5,6) at the same catheter location. The arrows indicate location of the respective Pentaray bipoles. (A) Electrogram at the VT exit (bipole A3,4) was ahead of surface QRS by 55 ms. It showed multiple initial sharp deflections and a terminal rounded potential, resembling the appearance of a rooster-head. Electrogram at the post-exit site (bipole B5,6) was 5 ms ahead of QRS and had a relatively rounded morphology. (B) Activation during VT marked by pink arrow, demonstrating mid-diastolic (bipole A,1,2), exit (bipole A3,4) and post-exit (bipole B5,6) sites at the same catheter location. (C) Entrainment pacing from the exit site showed concealed response with stimulus-QRS (55 ms) and post-pacing interval matching tachycardia cycle length (490 ms).

VT, point-by-point activation mapping is performed during VT in the wall of interest, focusing on the zone of abnormal sinus rhythm electrograms. If greater than 90% of cycle length is mappable, local electrograms that are activated during mid-diastole with preference toward the middle 25% to 75% of diastole are targeted. Entrainment pacing is recommended to determine proximity and participation of an apparent mid-diastolic signal to the reentrant circuit and determine critical versus bystander segments (**Fig. 7**).[23] A detailed explanation of the entrainment results is beyond the scope of this article. When both sinus rhythm and VT activations are compared in the isthmus region, classic activation direction and polarity reversal of a set of late potentials may be observed.[40] As isthmus may have considerable width (variably reported between 2 and 16 mm depending on the choice of mapping approach),[6,54,55] strategic linear ablation may be required to transect all viable tissue in the isthmus region. The duration of the longest diastolic electrogram has been shown to be inversely correlated with the dimensions of isthmus, whereby a diastolic electrogram duration greater than 26% of tachycardia cycle length is predictive of rapid VT termination by a single radiofrequency application.[56]

2. *Exit site electrogram.* Among those with stable VT, mapping for exit site electrograms with specific temporal component characteristics should be sought when mid-diastolic isthmus cannot be identified or confirmed. Wave front pivoting and deceleration in conduction at the exit site produces typical multicomponent electrograms that have an initial high frequency followed by low-frequency component likely introduced by both low and high current sink conditions, respectively, within the same local region.[31,57,58] A typical VT exit site electrogram is practically appreciable as that with initial multiphasic sharp deflections followed immediately by a biphasic rounded deflection (roosterhead-like appearance) (**Fig. 8**). The median absolute timing of activation in such exit zones is reported to be approximately 60 ms ahead of the surface QRS, which is amid 10% to 29% of the VT cycle length.[6,58] The 60 ms cutoff is in keeping with concealed entrainment response with highest likelihood of termination with ablation, when stimulus-QRS is 15% to 29% of the VT cycle length and post-pacing interval minus VT cycle length of less than 30 ms.[23] The main advantage of awareness about this classical electrogram morphology and timing is to differentiate non-vulnerable post-exit sites from the exit site, without the need of entrainment, thereby providing a practical tool to decide on ablation site among many early electrograms.

3. *Outer loop electrogram.* Activation during outer loop coincides during the QRS interval of VT cycle length. Outer loop activation can change direction and duration with minimal effect on VT-QRS morphology. The VT cycle length, however, can abruptly change with the redirected outer loop. Monomorphic VTs that accelerate or decelerate without change in QRS morphology happen may be due to slow conduction (or block) peripheral to the exit site resulting in a detoured return path.[6,45] Although dense scar location and slow conducted segments with multicomponent electrograms have been reported in the outer loop,[56] ablation targeted to the outer loop is unlikely to be successful.

### Intramural Electrogram Targets

The above-described approaches are of limited value with routine endocardial or epicardial catheter mapping tools if critical segments of the targeted VT are obscured in the mid-myocardium. Low unipolar voltage (<7.0 mV in LV and <4.0 mV in RV) in sinus rhythm, diffuse area of early activation or missing cycle length during VT may be a clue for the presence of diseased myocardium in the intramural tissue. Reconstructed semi-bipolar electrograms using electrodes on either side may give tissue information spanning the width of the intramural wall.[59] Strategic unipolar and semi-bipolar recording with a plunge needle electrode or septal intracoronary wire at selective locations have also been reported.[60]

### CLINICS CARE POINTS

- Careful rapid assessment of electrograms is necessary during ventricular tachycardia (VT) mapping. Targets can be elusive and buried in the intra-QRS electrograms, and whole electrogram analysis and use of pacing maneuvers may be necessary to unmask critical electrograms.

- High-density recordings, preferably with small electrodes and narrow interelectrode spacing, are essential for reliable mapping in either sinus rhythm or VT.

- Pacing maneuvers are time-consuming, difficult to perform, and may invoke unstable

VT. Automatic annotation with electroanatomic mapping can improve performance of pacing maneuvers.

- Consideration should be given to combined endo-epicardial mapping in specific substrates or recurring VT after prior ablation.

## DISCLOSURE

Dr S. Nayyar is examining voltage and time-domain mapping strategy for ventricular tachycardia ablation and is the principal investigator of Target- VT study (URL: www.ANZCTR.org.au. Unique identifier: ACTRN12620000049976). Dr S. Nayyar reports no relationships with industry.

All figures included in this article are from Authors prior published and unpublished works.

## REFERENCES

1. Al-Khatib SM, Stevenson WG, Ackerman MJ, et al. 2017 AHA/ACC/HRS guideline for management of patients with ventricular arrhythmias and the prevention of sudden cardiac death: a report of the American College of Cardiology/American Heart Association Task Force on clinical practice guidelines and the Heart Rhythm Society. Heart Rhythm 2018;15:e73–189.

2. Nakahara S, Tung R, Ramirez RJ, et al. Characterization of the arrhythmogenic substrate in ischemic and nonischemic cardiomyopathy Implications for catheter ablation of hemodynamically unstable ventricular tachycardia. J Am Coll Cardiol 2010;55: 2355–65.

3. Glashan CA, Androulakis AFA, Tao Q, et al. Whole human heart histology to validate electroanatomical voltage mapping in patients with non-ischaemic cardiomyopathy and ventricular tachycardia. Eur Heart J 2018;39:2867–75.

4. Yousuf OK, Zusterzeel R, Sanders W, et al. Trends and outcomes of catheter ablation for ventricular tachycardia in a Community Cohort. JACC Clin Electrophysiol 2018;4:1189–99.

5. Nayyar S, Ganesan AN, Brooks AG, et al. Venturing into ventricular arrhythmia storm: a systematic review and meta-analysis. Eur Heart J 2013;34: 560–71.

6. Martin R, Maury P, Bisceglia C, et al. Characteristics of scar-related ventricular tachycardia circuits using ultra-high-density mapping. Circ Arrhythm Electrophysiol 2018;11:e006569.

7. Di Biase L, Burkhardt JD, Lakkireddy D, et al. Ablation of stable VTs versus substrate ablation in ischemic cardiomyopathy: the VISTA randomized multicenter Trial. J Am Coll Cardiol 2015;66: 2872–82.

8. Nayyar S, Downar E, Bhaskaran AP, et al. Signature signal strategy: electrogram-based ventricular tachycardia mapping. Heart Rhythm 2020;17:2000–9.

9. Nayyar S, Wilson L, Ganesan AN, et al. High-density mapping of ventricular scar: a comparison of ventricular tachycardia (VT) supporting channels with channels that do not support VT. Circ Arrhythm Electrophysiol 2014;7:90–8.

10. Marchlinski FE, Callans DJ, Gottlieb CD, et al. Linear ablation lesions for control of unmappable ventricular tachycardia in patients with ischemic and nonischemic cardiomyopathy. Circulation 2000;101: 1288–96.

11. Tschabrunn CM, Zado ES, Schaller RD, et al. Isolated critical epicardial arrhythmogenic substrate abnormalities in patients with arrhythmogenic right ventricular cardiomyopathy and ventricular tachycardia. Heart Rhythm 2021;19(4):538–45.

12. Josephson ME, Anter E. Substrate mapping for ventricular tachycardia Assumptions and Misconceptions. JACC Clin Electrophysiol 2015;1:341–52.

13. Takigawa M, Relan J, Martin R, et al. Effect of bipolar electrode orientation on local electrogram properties. Heart Rhythm 2018;15:1853–61.

14. Spears DA, Suszko AM, Dalvi R, et al. Relationship of bipolar and unipolar electrogram voltage to scar transmurality and composition derived by magnetic resonance imaging in patients with nonischemic cardiomyopathy undergoing VT ablation. Heart Rhythm 2012;9:1837–46.

15. Venlet J, Piers SRD, Kapel GFL, et al. Unipolar endocardial voltage mapping in the right ventricle: optimal Cutoff values Correcting for Computed Tomography-derived epicardial fat Thickness and their clinical value for substrate delineation. Circ Arrhythm Electrophysiol 2017;10:e005175.

16. Cassidy DM, Vassallo JA, Buxton AE, et al. The value of catheter mapping during sinus rhythm to localize site of origin of ventricular tachycardia. Circulation 1984;69:1103–10.

17. Fast VG, Kleber AG. Role of wavefront curvature in propagation of cardiac impulse. Cardiovasc Res 1997;33:258–71.

18. Dillon SM, Allessie MA, Ursell PC, et al. Influences of anisotropic tissue structure on reentrant circuits in the epicardial border zone of subacute canine infarcts. Circ Res 1988;63:182–206.

19. Spach MS, Dolber PC. Relating extracellular potentials and their derivatives to anisotropic propagation at a microscopic level in human cardiac muscle. Evidence for electrical uncoupling of side-to-side fiber connections with increasing age. Circ Res 1986;58: 356–71.

20. Jais P, Maury P, Khairy P, et al. Elimination of local abnormal ventricular activities: a new end point for

substrate modification in patients with scar-related ventricular tachycardia. Circulation 2012;125: 2184–96.

21. Cassidy DM, Vassallo JA, Marchlinski FE, et al. Endocardial mapping in humans in sinus rhythm with normal left ventricles: activation patterns and characteristics of electrograms. Circulation 1984; 70:37–42.

22. Vergara P, Trevisi N, Ricco A, et al. Late potentials abolition as an additional Technique for reduction of arrhythmia recurrence in scar related ventricular tachycardia ablation. J Cardiovasc Electrophysiol 2012;23:621–7.

23. Harada T, Stevenson WG, Kocovic DZ, et al. Catheter ablation of ventricular tachycardia after myocardial infarction: relation of endocardial sinus rhythm late potentials to the reentry circuit. J Am Coll Cardiol 1997;30:1015–23.

24. Schilling RJ, Davies DW, Peters NS. Characteristics of sinus rhythm electrograms at sites of ablation of ventricular tachycardia relative to all other sites: a noncontact mapping study of the entire left ventricle. J Cardiovasc Electrophysiol 1998;9:921–33.

25. Kocovic D, Harada T, Friedman P, et al. Characteristics of electrograms recorded at reentry circuit sites and bystanders during ventricular tachycardia after myocardial infarction. J Am Coll Cardiol 1999;34: 381–8.

26. Maglaveras N, De Bakker JM, Van Capelle FJ, et al. Activation delay in healed myocardial infarction: a comparison between model and experiment. Am J Physiol 1995;269:H1441–9.

27. Rudy Y, Quan W. Propagation delays across cardiac gap junctions and their reflection in extracellular potentials: a simulation study. J Cardiovasc Electrophysiol 1991;2:299–315.

28. Bogun F, Good E, Reich S, et al. Isolated potentials during sinus rhythm and pace-mapping within scars as guides for ablation of post-infarction ventricular tachycardia. J Am Coll Cardiol 2006;47:2013–9.

29. Ciaccio EJ, Tosti AC, Scheinman MM. Method to predict isthmus location in ventricular tachycardia Caused by reentry with a double-loop pattern. J Cardiovasc Electrophysiol 2005;16:528–36.

30. Irie T, Yu R, Bradfield JS, et al. Relationship between sinus rhythm late activation zones and critical sites for scar-related ventricular tachycardia: systematic analysis of isochronal late activation mapping. Circ Arrhythm Electrophysiol 2015;8:390–9.

31. Anter E, Kleber AG, Rottmann M, et al. Infarct-related ventricular tachycardia: redefining the electrophysiological substrate of the isthmus during sinus rhythm. JACC Clin Electrophysiol 2018;4: 1033–48.

32. Hood MA, Pogwizd SM, Peirick J, et al. Contribution of myocardium responsible for ventricular tachycardia to abnormalities detected by analysis of signal-averaged ECGs. Circulation 1992;86: 1888–901.

33. Kleber A, Rudy Y. Basic mechanisms of cardiac impulse propagation and associated arrhythmias. Physiol Rev 2004;84:431–88.

34. Beheshti M, Nayyar S, Magtibay K, et al. Quantifying the determinants of decremental response in critical ventricular tachycardia substrate. Comput Biol Med 2018;102:260–6.

35. Anter E, Neuzil P, Reddy VY, et al. Ablation of reentry-vulnerable zones determined by left ventricular activation from multiple directions: a novel approach for ventricular tachycardia ablation: a multicenter study (PHYSIO-VT). Circ Arrhythm Electrophysiol 2020;13:e008625.

36. Tung R, Josephson ME, Bradfield JS, et al. Directional influences of ventricular activation on myocardial scar characterization: voltage mapping with multiple wavefronts during ventricular tachycardia ablation. Circ Arrhythm Electrophysiol 2016;9: e004155.

37. Nayyar S, Wilson L, Ganesan A, et al. Electrophysiologic features of protected channels in late postinfarction patients with and without spontaneous ventricular tachycardia. J Interv Card Electrophysiol 2018;51:13–24.

38. Nayyar S, Kuklik P, Tomlinson G, et al. Differential pacing from two sites to diagnose risk of ventricular arrhythmia and death. Pacing Clin Electrophysiol 2019;42:189–200.

39. Kucera JP, Rohr S, Kleber AG. Microstructure, cell-to-cell coupling, and ion currents as determinants of electrical propagation and arrhythmogenesis. Circ Arrhythm Electrophysiol 2017;10.

40. Jackson N, Gizurarson S, Viswanathan K, et al. Decrement evoked potential mapping: basis of a mechanistic strategy for ventricular tachycardia ablation. Circ Arrhythm Electrophysiol 2015;8: 1433–42.

41. Srinivasan NT, Garcia J, Schilling RJ, et al. Multicenter study of dynamic high-density functional substrate mapping improves identification of substrate targets for ischemic ventricular tachycardia ablation. JACC Clin Electrophysiol 2020;6:1783–93.

42. de Riva M, Naruse Y, Ebert M, et al. Targeting the hidden substrate unmasked by right ventricular extrastimulation improves ventricular tachycardia ablation outcome after myocardial infarction. JACC Clin Electrophysiol 2018;4:316–27.

43. Kucera JP, Kléber AG, Rohr S. Slow conduction in cardiac tissue, II: effects of branching tissue geometry. Circ Res 1998;83:795–805.

44. Kucera JP, Rudy Y. Mechanistic insights into very slow conduction in branching cardiac tissue: a model study. Circ Res 2001;89:799–806.

45. Downar E, Saito J, Doig JC, et al. Endocardial mapping of ventricular tachycardia in the intact

human ventricle. III. Evidence of multiuse reentry with spontaneous and induced block in portions of reentrant path complex. J Am Coll Cardiol 1995;25:1591–600.

46. Nayyar S, Downar E, Beheshti M, et al. Information theory to tachycardia Therapy: electrogram entropy predicts diastolic microstructure of reentrant ventricular tachycardia. Am J Physiol Heart Circ Physiol 2018;316:H134–44.

47. Nayyar S, Kuklik P, Ganesan AN, et al. Development of time- and voltage-domain mapping (V-T-Mapping) to localize ventricular tachycardia channels during sinus rhythm. Circ Arrhythm Electrophysiol 2016;9:e004050.

48. Frontera A, Melillo F, Baldetti L, et al. High-density characterization of the ventricular electrical substrate during sinus rhythm in post-myocardial infarction patients. JACC Clin Electrophysiol 2020;6: 799–811.

49. Stevenson WG, Sager PT, Natterson PD, et al. Relation of pace mapping QRS configuration and conduction delay to ventricular tachycardia reentry circuits in human infarct scars. J Am Coll Cardiol 1995;26:481–8.

50. Soejima K, Stevenson W, Maisel W, et al. Electrically unexcitable scar mapping based on pacing threshold for identification of the reentry critical isthmus: Feasibility for guiding ventricular tachycardia ablation. Circulation 2002;106:1678–83.

51. Miller JM, Marchlinski FE, Buxton AE, et al. Relationship between the 12-lead electrocardiogram during ventricular tachycardia and endocardial site of origin in patients with coronary artery disease. Circulation 1988;77:759–66.

52. Brunckhorst CB, Delacretaz E, Soejima K, et al. Identification of the ventricular tachycardia isthmus after infarction by pace mapping. Circulation 2004; 110:652–9.

53. de Chillou C, Groben L, Magnin-Poull I, et al. Localizing the critical isthmus of postinfarct ventricular tachycardia: the value of pace-mapping during sinus rhythm. Heart Rhythm 2014;11:175–81.

54. Pashakhanloo F, Herzka DA, Halperin H, et al. Role of 3-dimensional architecture of scar and surviving tissue in ventricular tachycardia: insights from high-resolution ex vivo porcine models. Circ Arrhythm Electrophysiol 2018;11:e006131.

55. de Chillou C, Lacroix D, Klug D, et al. Isthmus characteristics of reentrant ventricular tachycardia after myocardial infarction. Circulation 2002;105:726–31.

56. Nishimura T, Upadhyay GA, Aziz ZA, et al. Circuit determinants of ventricular tachycardia cycle length: characterization of Fast and unstable human ventricular tachycardia. Circulation 2021;143:212–26.

57. Girouard SD, Pastore JM, Laurita KR, et al. Optical mapping in a new Guinea pig model of ventricular tachycardia reveals mechanisms for multiple wavelengths in a single reentrant circuit. Circulation 1996;93:603–13.

58. Das M, Downar E, Masse S, et al. Temporal-component analysis of diastolic electrograms in ventricular tachycardia differentiates nonvulnerable regions of the circuit. Heart Rhythm 2015;12:1737–44.

59. Bhaskaran A, Niri A, Azam MA, et al. Safety, efficacy, and monitoring of bipolar radiofrequency ablation in beating myopathic human and healthy swine hearts. Heart Rhythm 2021;18:1772–9.

60. Narui R, Tanigawa S, Nakajima I, et al. Irrigated needle ablation compared with other advanced ablation Techniques for Failed endocardial ventricular arrhythmia ablation. Circ Arrhythm Electrophysiol 2021;14:e009817.

# Best Practices for the Catheter Ablation of Ventricular Arrhythmias

Auras R. Atreya, MD, MPH, FACC, FHRS[a,b], Sachin D. Yalagudri, MD, DM[a],
Muthiah Subramanian, MD, DM[a], Vickram Vignesh Rangaswamy, MD, DM[a],
Daljeet Kaur Saggu, MD, DM[a], Calambur Narasimhan, MD, DM[a,*]

## KEYWORDS

- Ventricular arrhythmias • Ventricular tachycardia • Ischemic cardiomyopathy
- Nonischemic cardiomyopathy • Electroanatomical mapping • Catheter ablation
- Substrate ablation • Patient safety

## KEY POINTS

- Ensuring safety and efficacy during catheter ablation requires adequate planning, analysis of VA ECG and stored ICD electrograms, as well as preprocedural imaging (CMRI/CT/PET-CT).
- Defining the underlying arrhythmogenic substrate, disease etiology, and clinical status allows for the development of tailored ablation strategies, particularly for nonischemic cardiomyopathies.
- Patient selection, choice of anesthesia, safe vascular/epicardial access, adequate hemostasis, and postprocedural anticoagulation significantly impact complication prevention.
- Functional substrate mapping techniques in sinus rhythm, including isochronal late activation mapping (ILAM) and decrement evoked potential (DEEP) mapping, are recent refinements that aid in targeted VT ablation.
- VT ablation in the setting of temporary mechanical circulatory devices (Impella, VA-ECMO, TandemHeart) and durable LVADs have expanded the indications for the catheter ablation of VAs in the sicker cohort of patients with advanced heart failure.

## INTRODUCTION

The spectrum of ventricular arrhythmias (VA) seen in clinical practice, ranges from single premature ventricular complexes (PVCs), nonsustained and sustained ventricular tachycardia (VT) and ventricular fibrillation (VF).[1] The initial treatment of these VAs is pharmacologic therapy with antiarrhythmic drugs (AADs) and may include implantable cardioverter defibrillators (ICDs) for those at risk of sudden cardiac death (SCD). Several landmark studies have demonstrated mortality benefit with ICDs for both primary and secondary prevention of SCD, and VT management with antitachycardia pacing and cardioversion.[2–6] As with ICD technology, there has been remarkable progress in the tools and techniques used for the catheter ablation of VAs over the past 3 decades, and catheter ablation is increasingly being used early when AAD therapy fails or as first-line therapy for selected patients.[1,7]

While the core concepts of VA mapping and ablation still hold true, several technical advances, such as high-density electroanatomical (EAM) mapping, intracardiac echocardiography (ICE), open irrigation, contact force sensing ablation catheters, and alternative energy sources have helped improve the outcomes of catheter ablation

[a] Electrophysiology Section, AIG Hospitals Institute of Cardiac Sciences and Research, Hyderabad, India;
[b] Division of Cardiovascular Medicine, Electrophysiology Section, University of Arkansas for Medical Sciences, Little Rock, AR, USA
* Corresponding author. 1, Mindspace Road, Gachibowli, Hyderabad 500032, India.
*E-mail address:* calambur1@gmail.com

Card Electrophysiol Clin 14 (2022) 571–607
https://doi.org/10.1016/j.ccep.2022.08.007

for VAs.[1,7,8] Refinements in advanced cardiac imaging have improved our understanding of the arrhythmogenic substrate and has made imaging an important preprocedural step.[9–12] In this review, we will emphasize best practices for catheter ablation, at every step of the procedure from planning to discharge, that translates to improved clinical outcomes.

## SECTION I: PREPROCEDURAL EVALUATION AND PLANNING

### Preprocedural Clinical, Electrocardiogram, and Device Electrogram Evaluation

Careful clinical evaluation helps to understand triggers and substrate for VA in the individual patient,[7] as some patients with apparently idiopathic VA may have a genetic or inflammatory etiology, and need specific therapeutic approaches for VA management.[13–15] Reversible triggers of VA, such as electrolyte derangement, drug toxicity, ischemia, must be addressed before the consideration of catheter ablation.[7]

Planning for every ablation procedure begins with an analysis of the clinically documented VA; most often this is a 12-lead electrocardiogram (ECG) or an ambulatory ECG tracing. It is important to localize the site of origin (SOO) of the PVC/VT from the 12-lead ECG. This is most accurate for VAs arising in structurally normal hearts whereby the mechanism is focal (triggered activity or abnormal automaticity), and the site of successful ablation tends to be within a 1 to 2 cm radius of the SOO identified on 12-lead ECG.[16,17] In addition to the general rule that VAs arising from the left ventricle (LV) have a right bundle branch block (RBBB) pattern and those arising from the septum or right ventricle (RV) have a left bundle branch block (LBBB) pattern, we find that using a 4-quadrant approach allows for the rapid localization of cardiac structures where the VA may originate.[18] This regionalization can be further refined based on the precordial transition which informs us of basal versus apical SOO. **Fig. 1** shows typical ECG patterns for frequently encountered VA SOOs in structurally normal hearts.[19]

For VTs in patients with structural heart disease arising due to re-entry within scar, related to either ischemic or nonischemic cardiomyopathy, the SOO predicted on the ECG correlates with the exit site rather than the critical isthmus sites or the diastolic corridors of the VT circuit. Depending on the size of the circuit, this exit site may be up to 2 to 5 cm$^2$ away from the critical isthmus.[20,21] Clinical and automated VT-ECG algorithms have been developed with modest ability to predict SOO, but their use remains limited.[20–25]

The 12-lead ECG also offers clues to identify epicardial VT, in which case either epicardial or coronary venous mapping needs to be considered. Several ECG criteria for identifying an epicardial SOO of VAs have been validated over the years, predominantly in patients with structurally normal hearts or those with nonischemic cardiomyopathy (**Table 1**).[26–28] It is important to note that these criteria may not be accurate in the presence of Class I AADs. In clinical practice, it is most useful to use a 4-step algorithm developed by Vallès and colleagues, as it integrates several criteria (each with limited individual predictive value) for predicting epicardial SOO for VT arising in patients with nonischemic cardiomyopathy.[29] **Fig. 2** shows an example of epicardial VT.

In patients with hemodynamically unstable VA that does not allow for 12-lead ECG acquisition, or where ICD therapies terminate the VA before obtaining an ECG, a 12-lead Holter may be used to obtain the VT morphology.[30] Analyzing stored ICD electrograms (near-field and far-field) of VT and comparing them to ICD electrograms during induced VT or by pace mapping (for noninducible VTs) is another strategy for catheter ablation.[31–33]

Finally, a noninvasive mapping strategy that holds promise for VA ablation is the use of electrocardiographic imaging (ECGI), a variant of body surface potential mapping.[34] This method combines a continuous 256-lead ECG recorded by a multi-electrode vest, combined with a noncontrast computed tomography (CT) scan of the chest that provides an anatomic correlate. ECGI has been validated in patients with and without structural heart disease and seems to be accurate for outflow tract VAs and epicardial VAs.[35–38] Commercially available noninvasive multielectrode vest-based mapping systems are now available and are being used to guide stereotactic radioablation, and in the future may be used for selected VA ablations.

### Preprocedural Imaging to Define the Substrate

While analysis of VA ECGs forms the first step of ablation planning, a critically important next step is to obtain imaging data that can guide VA ablation and improve outcomes. Alongside improvements in the resolution of 3D EAM mapping systems, there has been considerable progress in cardiac CT, cardiac magnetic resonance (CMR), and nuclear imaging such as positron-emission tomography (PET) over the past 2 decades.[39] These imaging modalities serve as diagnostic tools and allow for risk stratification before ablation. The most important modality is CMR where late

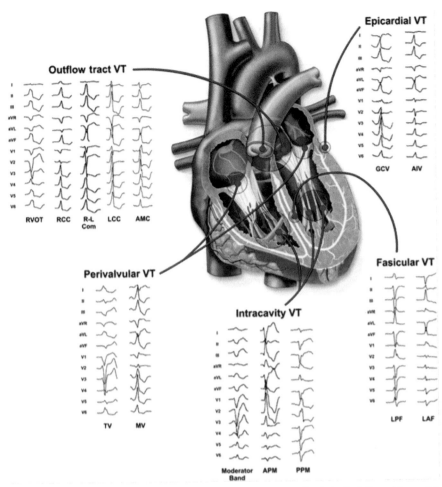

**Fig. 1.** Twelve-lead electrocardiogram morphology of different sites of origin in idiopathic ventricular tachycardia. AIV, anterior interventricular vein; AMC, aortomitral continuity; APM, anterior papillary muscle; GCV, greater cardiac vein; LAF, left anterior fascicle; LCC, left coronary cusp; LPF, left posterior fascicle; MV, mitral annulus; PPM, posterior papillary muscle; RCC, right coronary cusp; R–L com, right–left coronary cusp commissure; RVOT, right ventricular outflow tract; TV, tricuspid annulus. (*From* Tanawuttiwat T., Nazarian S., Calkins H. The role of catheter ablation in the management of ventricular tachycardia. Eur Heart J 2016;37(7):594–609. Doi: 10.1093/eurheartj/ehv421; with permission.)

gadolinium enhancement (LGE) sequences (**Fig. 3**) can define scar burden as well as scar transmurality (which may inform the need to perform epicardial mapping during ablation). Specifically, in nonischemic cardiomyopathy, this information may help distinguish various etiologies (sarcoidosis, myocarditis, amyloidosis) and identify difficult to ablate substrate (intramural scar). Two major limitations for CMR imaging are the limited spatial resolution (restricted to 1- to 2-mm range) in comparison to CT imaging, and imaging artifacts from ICD device generators. Therefore, CMR imaging is best-performed upfront when patients present with VAs, before ICD implantation.[1]

Contrast-enhanced CT imaging is an alternative in patients with ICDs and offers greater spatial

resolution (submillimeter). This allows for the identification of areas of wall thinning (<5 mm), increased fat thickness (>2.8 mm), and calcification, which correlate with arrhythmogenic substrate.[40–43] Studies by Ghannam et al and Takigawa and colleagues identified ridges/channels which denote preserved myocardial tissue surrounded by scar by using CT imaging (with postprocessing using proprietary MUSIC software, IHU LIRYC Bordeaux and Inria Sophia Antipolis, France). These areas were shown to be good target sites for ablation (**Fig. 4**).[44,45] Additionally, CT-detected dense epicardial fat predicts failure of epicardial ablation and can prompt an alternative mapping and ablation strategy (eg, coronary venous system).[41,46–48] CT imaging also identifies epicardial coronary

**Table 1**
**ECG criteria predicting epicardial origin of VT**

| ECG Criteria | Patient Population | Study |
|---|---|---|
| • Pseudodelta wave (earliest ventricular activation to the earliest rapid deflection) in any precordial lead ≥34 ms<br>• Intrinsicoid deflection time (interval measured from the earliest ventricular activation to the peak of the R wave) in lead V2 ≥85 ms<br>• Shortest RS complex duration (earliest ventricular activation to the nadir of the first S wave) in any precordial lead ≥121 ms | Derivation cohort: 6 ICM and 3 NICM with ECG analysis of endocardial and epicardial pacing<br>Validation cohort: 48 ICM and 21 NICM with ECG analysis of RBBB VT | Berruezo et al,[26] 2004 |
| • Maximum Deflection Time (MDI) ≥0.55 in any precordial lead<br>• MDI = time to maximum deflection/QRS duration<br>• Time to maximum deflection = onset of the QRS complex to the maximum deflection in each precordial lead, either above or below the isoelectric line (precordial lead with shortest time is chosen)<br>• QRS duration = interval between the earliest rapid deflection of the ventricular complex in any of the 12 simultaneous leads to the latest offset in any lead | 12 patients with idiopathic VT with the ECG analysis of successful epicardial ablation sites >10 mm from the ASOV | Daniels et al,[27] 2006 |
| • Q waves in lead I predict basal superior and apical superior epicardial VT sites<br>• Q waves in the inferior leads (II, III, aVF) predict basal inferior and apical inferior epicardial VT sites | 15 patients with NICM with ECG analysis of endocardial and epicardial pacing, and epicardial VTs | Bazan et al,[28] 2007 |
| • Algorithm for Basal Superior and Lateral LV Epicardial Origin<br>• Absence of Q waves in inferior leads<br>• Pseudodelta wave ≥75 ms<br>• MDI ≥0.59<br>• Presence of Q waves in lead I | 14 NICM patients with ECG analysis of endocardial and epicardial pacing; and epicardial VT from basal superior and lateral LV sites<br>Validation cohort: 11 NICM patients with epicardial ablation | Vallès et al,[29] 2009 |

*Abbreviations:* ASOV, aortic sinus of Valsalva; ECG, electrocardiogram; ICM, ischemic cardiomyopathy; LV, left ventricle; MDI, maximum deflection index; NICM, nonischemic cardiomyopathy; RBBB, right bundle branch block; VT, ventricular tachycardia.

vessels and the left phrenic nerve, and inadvertent injury can be avoided.[49] Finally, CT imaging may also be used to guide epicardial access and avoid collateral damage to the abdominal viscera and vasculature.[50]

Cardiac anatomy and scar tissue identified by CMR, and CT imaging can be integrated into the EAM systems for guidance during catheter ablation (anatomic landmarks such as the left main coronary artery, aortic root, mitral annulus, LV

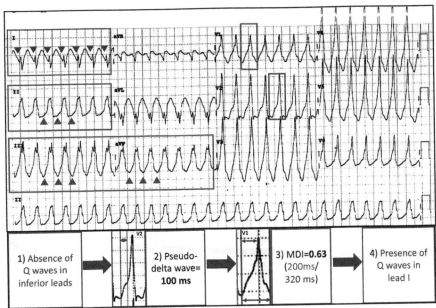

| 1) Absence of Q waves in inferior leads | → | 2) Pseudo-delta wave= **100 ms** | → | 3) MDI=**0.63** (200ms/ 320 ms) | → | 4) Presence of Q waves in lead I |

**Fig. 2.** ECG criteria identifying epicardial tachycardia from the basal superolateral aspect of the LV. 12-lead ECG showing right bundle right inferior axis morphology VT in a patient with nonischemic cardiomyopathy and electrical storm following COVID, that was successfully ablated epicardially in the basal superolateral aspect of the LV. Application of the 4-step algorithm developed by Vallès and colleagues correctly identified the epicardial origin of this VT.[29] (1) Red arrowheads show the absence of Q waves in the inferior leads (2) Pseudo-delta wave measured in lead V2 ≥75 ms (3) MDI measured in lead V1 ≥0.59 (4) Blue arrowheads show the presence of Q waves in lead I. COVID, coronavirus disease; ECG, electrocardiogram; LV, left ventricle; MDI, maximum deflection index; VT, ventricular tachycardia.

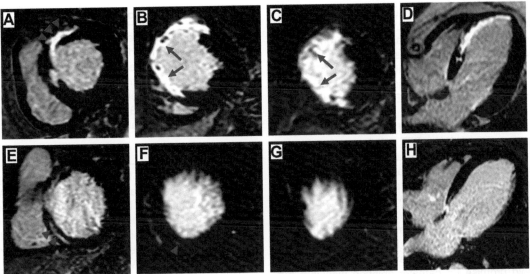

**Fig. 3.** Preprocedural CMR imaging to define the VA substrate and guide ablation planning. LGE-CMR sequences delineate the extent and distribution of arrhythmogenic substrate. Panels A–D show transmural scar location in the anteroseptal left ventricle (red *arrows*) in a patient with ischemic cardiomyopathy. Panels A–C represent short axis cross-sections from base to apex and panel D shows a 4-chamber section. In contrast, nonischemic cardiomyopathy may have midmyocardial or epicardial scar location. Panels E–H are LGE-CMR sequences from a patient with Lamin mutation and midmyocardial inferobasal scar location. CMR, cardiac magnetic resonance imaging; LGE, late gadolinium enhancement; VA, ventricular arrhythmia.

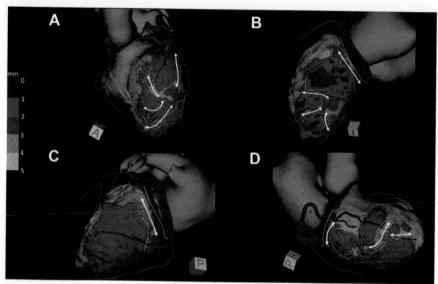

**Fig. 4.** CT-defined wall-thickness identifies channels amid scar tissue. Large area of abnormal myocardial wall thinning (<5 mm) as identified on contrast-enhanced CT scan, with 3-dimensional reconstruction in a patient with postmyocardial infarction VT. This figure highlights ridges or channels [areas of abnormal wall thickness (yellow), with thinner margins on either side (red)]. These CT-channels colocalize with VT isthmus detected by high-density activation mapping. Panels (*A–D*) represent anterior, inferior, lateral and septal aspects of the left ventricle respectively. CT, computed tomography; VT, ventricular tachycardia. (*From* Takigawa M., Duchateau J., Sacher F., et al. Are wall thickness channels defined by computed tomography predictive of isthmuses of postinfarction ventricular tachycardia? Heart Rhythm 2019;16(11):1661–8. Doi: 10.1016/j.hrthm.2019.06.012; with permission.)

apex, or RV ICD lead are used for registration).[51–54] With this technique, areas of scar identified on imaging correlate well with low voltage areas on the EAM system (both unipolar and bipolar voltage maps),[40,55–58] with the caveat that in areas with excessive epicardial fat (>7 mm), falsely low voltages on the EAM system may be seen.[59]

Another imaging modality of value is cardiac PET scanning with [18]F-fluorodeoxyglucose (FDG) and [68]Gallium- DOTATATE, which helps to identify myocardial inflammation and allows distinction between viable tissue and scar.[60] In patients with myocarditis and VAs, PET data become an important decision point, as uptake predicts response to immunosuppressive therapy and may preclude immediate catheter ablation.[61] Indeed, prior studies have shown that in patients with nonischemic cardiomyopathy and VAs, [18]F-FDG-PET imaging identified active inflammation in ~50% of patients.[62,63] Protocols to identify arrhythmogenic substrate and areas with sympathetic denervation hold promise for catheter ablation planning; but are not ready for clinical use as yet.

Our own practice is to obtain CMR imaging in patients being evaluated for elective catheter ablation; and PET imaging if inflammation is suspected. On the other hand, in patients with electrical storm, or pleomorphic VA morphology suggestive of an inflammatory disorder, PET is preferred as the initial imaging modality.

## Developing a Tailored Ablation Strategy

After obtaining all the necessary clinical, ECG, and imaging data, it is important to synthesize a tailored ablation strategy for each patient (**Fig. 5**). Before the procedure, the electrophysiologist must localize the anatomic site where the VA is arising from (based on the VA ECG) and be cognizant of the arrhythmogenic substrate (based on imaging).

## Idiopathic VAs

If all imaging suggests that there is no underlying structural disease, that is, truly idiopathic VA, then the mechanism is likely to be focal (triggered activity, abnormal automaticity) and activation mapping and ablation are highly successful. Invariably, the successful sites of ablation are endocardial structures (LV/RV outflow tracts, aortic/pulmonary cusps, perivalvular, fascicular system, endocavitary structures such as moderator bands or papillary muscles) and epicardial access is rarely required.[64,65] Even when epicardial origin in the LV summit/cardiac crux is suggested by ECG criteria (4%–10% of all idiopathic VAs), mapping in the coronary venous system may provide

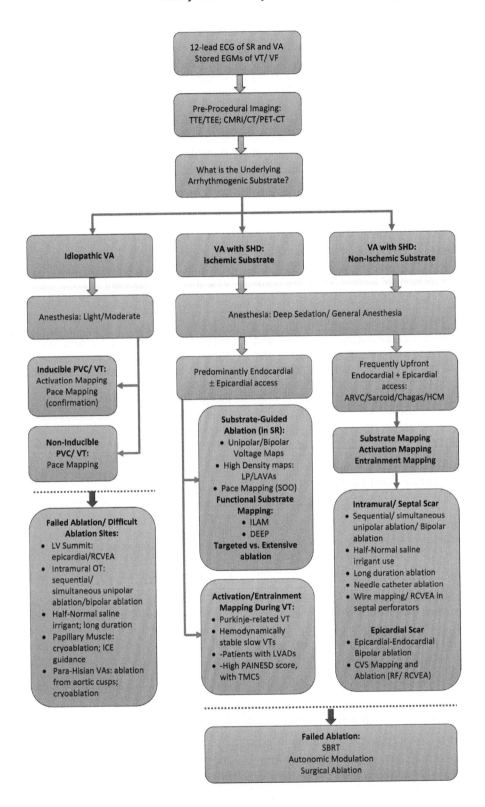

access for mapping and ablation.[66–68] The key issue for idiopathic VAs is inducibility of the clinical arrhythmia. Therefore, withholding antiarrhythmic drugs (if any, for at least 5 half-lives) is important and the use of light to moderate sedation is preferred. If the clinical VA is noninducible, despite extensive programmed stimulation and pharmacologic provocation,[69,70] pace mapping is the next best choice.[71,72] It is important to pace at twice the diastolic threshold and avoid higher output pacing. Comparable outcomes can be achieved with this approach but identifying an optimal endpoint for catheter ablation remains a challenge with pace mapping.

Some possible reasons for the failure of catheter ablation for idiopathic VA include catheter instability on endocavitary structures, para-Hisian VA location, or a difficult LV summit VA where coronary vasculature precludes ablation. Techniques to overcome these challenges have been described[73–76]; Cryoablation, with ICE guidance can be used for endocavitary structures and para-Hisian VAs to achieve catheter stability and avoid collateral damage.[77–81] Ablation strategies for challenging LV summit VAs are discussed in a following chapter by *Yamada*.

### VAs in Structural Heart Disease: Postmyocardial Infarction/Ischemic Substrate

Typically, with ischemic cardiomyopathy, there is an area of dense scar along a coronary artery distribution with a defined border zone that houses several targets for substrate ablation.[82–85] There is increasing interest in modifying the substrate early in the course of VT, including preventive substrate ablation.[86–90] Our approach is to first identify abnormal substrate in sinus rhythm (fractionated electrograms, isolated late potentials, local abnormal ventricular activation [LAVAs]). Pace mapping in areas of abnormal electrograms can identify critical sites close to the re-entrant VT circuit. Pacing close to the exit site produces a good pace match with a short stimulus-to-QRS (S-QRS)

while pacing in the critical isthmus shows a good pace match with long S-QRS. On the other hand, poor pace matching is seen at entrance sites and remote areas.[91–93] Transition from a good pace match to a poor pace match in a small area suggests that the mapping catheter is in the isthmus, and is an excellent site for ablation.[94,95] Functional substrate mapping (discussed in the next section) is helpful in further refining optimal target sites. In some early postmyocardial infarction VT, the Purkinje fibers may serve as a trigger for VT/VF. The ablation of these Purkinje fibers in the infarcted zone helps to eliminate this subset of VT.[96]

If VTs are induced after the initial substrate-guided approach, a combination of further substrate ablation, activation, and entrainment mapping is undertaken to abolish all inducible VTs. It is very important to know if the clinical VT is hemodynamically stable or not; in patients with slow and stable VTs, more time can be spent with activation and entrainment mapping. In sicker patients with reduced LV function, cardiogenic shock, electrical storm, predominantly substrate ablation is a safer approach (70%-75% of VTs are hemodynamically unstable in the electrophysiology laboratory).[97–99] Multidisciplinary management with optimized fluid status before ablation, use of general anesthesia, fluid monitoring and mechanical circulatory support device support are preferred in high-risk patients.

Although transmural substrate is present in ischemic cardiomyopathy, the traditional teaching is that endocardial VT ablation may achieve VA elimination[100]; however, data are emerging in favor of simultaneous endocardial–epicardial mapping and ablation to challenge this paradigm.[101–104]

### VAs in Structural Heart Disease: Nonischemic Substrate

Nonischemic cardiomyopathy is a broad term that comprises several disease entities. Preprocedural imaging with CMR/CT is especially useful as there is wide heterogeneity in scar distribution in

---

**Fig. 5.** Tailored ablation strategy based on the integration of preprocedural electrocardiograms, cardiac imaging, and underlying disease process. ARVC, arrhythmogenic right ventricular cardiomyopathy; CMRI, cardiac magnetic resonance imaging; CT, computed tomography; CVS, coronary venous system; DEEP, decrement evoked potential mapping; ECG, electrocardiogram; EGM, electrogram; HCM, hypertrophic cardiomyopathy; ICE, intracardiac echocardiography; ILAM, isochronal late activation mapping; LAVA, local abnormal ventricular activation; LP, late potential; LV, left ventricle; LVAD, left ventricular assist device; OT, outflow tract; PET-CT, positron emission tomography-computed tomography; PVC, premature ventricular complex; RCVEA, retrograde coronary venous ethanol ablation; RF, radiofrequency; SBRT, stereotactic body radiation therapy; SHD, structural heart disease; SOO, site of origin; SR, sinus rhythm; TMCS, temporary mechanical circulatory support; TEE, transesophageal echocardiogram; TTE, transthoracic echocardiogram; VA, ventricular arrhythmia; VF, ventricular fibrillation; VT, ventricular tachycardia.

nonischemic cardiomyopathies, with a predilection for intramural and epicardial scar location.[105] **Table 2** shows the distribution of scar tissue in commonly encountered nonischemic cardiomyopathies. The approach to VA ablation depends heavily on the substrate one is dealing with. Substrate ablation strategies are preferred in hemodynamically unstable VAs and activation mapping/entrainment mapping is reserved for hemodynamically stable VAs. The key difference between ischemic and nonischemic substrates is the patchiness of scar tissue in the latter. Late potentials and LAVAs are not easily identifiable in nonischemic cardiomyopathy due to discrete low voltage areas. A combination of unipolar/bipolar high-density voltage mapping helps to understand the substrate. Unmasking functional delays, using decrement evoked potential mapping (DeEP) helps to identify targets for ablation. As such, improving techniques for the ablation of VAs in nonischemic substrates represents the true advancing frontier of catheter ablation. A combination of innovative mapping (coronary venous/arterial wire mapping), improved ablation (half-normal saline irrigation, sequential unipolar, simultaneous unipolar, bipolar ablation, ethanol ablation, pulse field ablation, stereotactic radioablation, surgical ablation), and neuromodulation (renal denervation, sympathetic ganglion blockade, cardiac sympathetic denervation) are often needed, in a stepwise fashion.[106] Several of these methods have been described in detail in subsequent articles of this issue.

## SECTION II: PROCEDURAL SAFETY AND EFFICACY
### Anesthesia Choice

The best sedation strategy for an individual patient should be determined by the electrophysiology and anesthesiology teams based on patient age, comorbidities, and the underlying VA.

For idiopathic VA due to triggered activity or automaticity, deep sedation may prevent the induction of VAs, and the use of analgesics (fentanyl) along with short-acting sedatives (midazolam, propofol) are preferred.[107,108] Intravenous anesthetics that reduce sympathetic tone such as dexmedetomidine should also be avoided.[109] Even with the use of midazolam or propofol, VAs can be suppressed, hence minimal sedation is administered and withheld if VA is suppressed.[1,110] It is best practice to obtain templates of the VA in the mapping system before the administration of any sedative, as this allows for pace mapping to target the clinical VA, in case sedation renders the VA noninducible.

For longer procedures, patients with electrical storm, significant LV dysfunction, severe pulmonary hypertension, it is preferable to perform catheter ablation under general anesthesia.[1] However, this may lead to decreased cardiac contractility and hemodynamic compromise, and patients with reduced systolic function often require pharmacologic hemodynamic support.[111] It has also been noted that VAs induced under general anesthesia, may be different from VAs induced under moderate sedation.[111] Therefore, meticulous substrate modification is important as noninducibility of VAs may be misleading. Majority of epicardial ablation procedures are performed under general anesthesia and inspiratory breath holds are helpful in avoiding damage to the diaphragm and abdominal structures.[112,113] For epicardial ablation, short-acting muscle relaxants are preferred to allow phrenic nerve capture and prevent inadvertent injury during epicardial ablation.

### Vascular Access, Epicardial Access, and Approach to Areas of Interest

Most VA ablation procedures will require both arterial and venous access, for hemodynamic monitoring and to map right and left-sided structures. Ultrasound-guided vascular access is the standard of care to minimize the risk of vascular injury and major bleeding during long ablation procedures, on full anticoagulation.[1,114–116]

While transfemoral venous access (occasionally transjugular or transhepatic in patients with vena cava abnormalities) allows for mapping of the entire RV/RVOT,[117,118] there are multiple options to be considered for mapping of the LV (**Fig. 6**). Antegrade transseptal access and retrograde transaortic access both allow adequate LV access. Transseptal access may be preferred in patients with significant aortic atheroma, aorto-iliac tortuosity, and peripheral arterial disease while the retrograde approach is preferred in patients with venous anomalies, mitral valvular pathology/prostheses, and atrial septal closure devices. It should be noted that transseptal access lends itself well to the mapping and ablation of the midinterventricular septum, mid-lateral LV and apical areas, and LV outflow tract (LVOT).[119,120] On the other hand, transaortic access provides easy access to the basal LV segments and the anterior LV.[119] The conduction system (Purkinje-related VAs) can be ablated via either approach. Data suggest that outcomes of catheter ablation are similar between retro-aortic and transseptal approaches,[121,122] but observational data suggest lower cerebral embolic events with transseptal access.[123] To this end, there is an ongoing

**Table 2**
Location of arrhythmogenic substrate in nonischemic cardiomyopathies and ablation strategies

| | Idiopathic NICM | HCM | Sarcoidosis | Chagas | ARVC | Brugada |
|---|---|---|---|---|---|---|
| Substrate Layer | Midmyocardial Epicardial | Midmyocardial | Intramural/ Subepicardial | Epicardial (predominant) | Subepicardial;epicardial | Subepicardial;epicardial |
| Scar Distribution | Patchy | Patchy | Patchy/ Circumferential | Segmental fibrosis | Patchy | Patchy |
| Scar Location | Basal anteroseptal & perivalvular; Inferolateral | Interventricular septum; Apical aneurysm | Basal/mid interventricular septum; Inferolateral | Basal lateral LV | RV/RVOT LV Perivalvular | RV/RVOT Epicardial LV |
| Ablation Strategy | Endo-Epi | Endo > Epi | Endo-Epi | Endo-Epi | Epi > Endo | Predominantly epicardial |
| Adjunct Strategy | Coronary Venous (AIV); Simultaneous Unipolar; Bipolar | Apical aneurysm resection | Simultaneous Unipolar; Bipolar; Needle ablation | Sympathetic denervation | Epicardial DEEP mapping and ablation | Ajmaline or Procainamide administration to unmask RVOT epicardial substrate |

*Abbreviations:* AIV, anterior interventricular vein; ARVC, arrhythmogenic right ventricular cardiomyopathy; DEEP, decrement evoked potential; HCM, hypertrophic cardiomyopathy; ICM, ischemic cardiomyopathy; LV, left ventricle; NICM, nonischemic cardiomyopathy; RV, right ventricle; RVOT, right ventricular outflow tract.

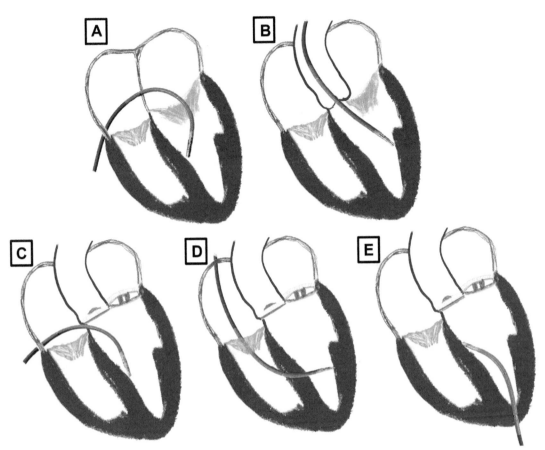

**Fig. 6.** Catheter Access to the Left Ventricle for Mapping and Ablation. (*A*) Antegrade transseptal access via femoral vein-access to the mid interventricular septum, mid lateral LV, apical areas, left posterior fascicular area and LVOT (*B*) Retrograde transaortic access via femoral artery-access to the basal LV segments, conduction system, anterior and lateral LV (*C*) Trans-right atrial to LV access utilizing an RF wire puncture technique into the inferoseptal process of the LV, in the presence of mechanical valves in aortic and mitral position (*D*) Interventricular septal needle puncture and access to the LV, in the presence of mechanical valves in aortic and mitral position. (*E*) Percutaneous or surgical transapical access in the presence of mechanical valves in aortic and mitral position. LV = left ventricle; LVOT = left ventricular outflow tract; RF = radiofrequency.

randomized controlled trial comparing the risk of embolic events with each approach (NCT03946072). Patients with both aortic and mitral mechanical valves present a unique challenge to the electrophysiologist in achieving endocardial LV access. Approaches that have been traditionally used include transapical access (percutaneous or surgical),[124–127] but operators have described interventricular septal access as well as trans-right atrial to LV access.[128–131]

Finally, when epicardial access is required (based on VA ECG, preprocedural imaging, disease etiology, prior failed ablations), it is very important to recognize that this is the most crucial step in the procedure. A subsequent article in this issue, by *Maher and colleagues*, describes safe techniques for epicardial access and ablation.

## Optimal Use of Electroanatomic Mapping Systems to Improve Outcomes

The general concepts of mapping and ablating the endocardial and epicardial spaces have been described in detail by *Muser* et al and *Maher* et al in this issue. A combination of the 4 fundamental mapping techniques is used in every catheter ablation for VA-activation mapping, entrainment mapping, pace mapping, and substrate mapping, depending on the clinical situation and VA being ablated.[132] We will highlight specific advances in EAM-based mapping techniques in this section.

*PVC ablatio*: For the successful ablation of PVCs, activation mapping is preferred (provided the PVCs are frequent during the ablation procedure) and pace mapping is largely confirmatory. All the existing 3D-EAM systems have specific algorithms/modules for activation mapping (LAT, late activation time) and for comparing 12-lead clinical PVC templates with paced QRS complex at each site pace matching (PASO, CARTO 3, Biosense Webster, Diamond Bar, CA; Automap Score Threshold, Abbott EnSite X/Precision, Abbott Laboratories, Abbott Park, IL; Rhythmia, Boston Scientific, Marlborough, MA). One concern during the activation mapping of the PVC is the spatial discordance in catheter position during a PVC and during sinus rhythm. To overcome this, a newer module (LAT hybrid module, CARTO Prime mapping module, Biosense Webster Inc., Diamond Bar, CA) creates an accurate hybrid map integrating the spatial location in sinus rhythm with LAT electrical data from a PVC beat, thereby allowing for RF delivery at the appropriate location. This is particularly helpful in aortic cusp or para-Hisian PVCs, whereby the risk of collateral injury is high (**Fig. 7**).[74,133,134]

Another useful 3D-EAM mapping technique for PVCs arising from endocavitary structures (papillary muscles or moderator band) is point density exclusion (PDX) mapping (Abbott EnSite X/Precision, Abbott Laboratories, Abbott Park, IL). While creating a high-density EAM of the RV or the LV, a volume within these chambers lacking any geometry points (negative space within the chamber EAM) is designated an endocavitary structure (moderator band and papillary muscle, respectively; **Fig. 8**). This technique is simple and in real-time displays the structure of interest which allows for the activation/pace mapping and ablation of PVCs from these areas. Studies have found this technique comparable to ICE-integration with 3D-EAM (CartoSound, Biosense Webster, Diamond Bar, CA).[135,136]

*VT ablation:* Some additional considerations are important for the mapping of VTs. First and foremost, the hemodynamic stability of the VT in the electrophysiology laboratory dictates whether activation mapping and entrainment mapping can be performed. Entrainment mapping is the original technique used to identify critical VT circuits in patients with structural heart disease and is perhaps the one technique that does not rely heavily on 3D-EAM systems.[137-139] Identification of a middiastolic potential or presystolic potential on the EGM recording system during VT is a starting point for entrainment mapping and areas with the entrainment of local EGM, concealed fusion with VT morphology, and a short postpacing interval are identified as critical isthmuses for VT re-entry (**Fig. 9**).

Activation mapping is useful in both re-entrant and focal VTs (identifies the exit site of re-entrant VT circuit and the SOO in focal VTs), with the caveat that the VT should be hemodynamically stable. Newer algorithms that integrate activation mapping data with the vector and velocity of conduction (automated conduction velocity mapping/Coherent Mapping, CARTO 3, Biosense Webster, Diamond Bar, CA) and real-time EGM visualization with amplitude data (Ripple Mapping, CARTO 3, Biosense Webster, Diamond Bar, CA) help delineate VT circuits better. Coherent mapping and low voltage Ripple mapping are 2 modalities that display areas of slow conduction in the ventricular myocardium and identify areas of nonconduction. Initial reports have demonstrated benefits in streamlining the VT mapping workflow, but further validation and more important outcome studies are needed.[133,140-144]

Over the years, substrate mapping has emerged as a critical tool for understanding and ablating hemodynamically unstable VTs and several substrate ablation strategies have been proposed (**Table 3, Fig. 10**).[88,94,102,145-168] The key concept in substrate mapping is to identify the surrogates of the VT isthmus during sinus rhythm, with the isthmus being an area of electrical activation bounded by inexcitable myocardium (anatomic or functional).[169-172] These isthmuses may be identified by different EGM patterns, such as low-voltage or fractionated EGMs, double potentials, isolated late potentials and LAVAs (**Fig. 11**).[173-175] The sensitivity and specificity of identifying critical VT circuits based on EGMs alone is modest at best, and pace mapping in these areas can identify proximity to the VT exit site.[176,177] With current multielectrode high-resolution mapping catheters (Advisor HD-Grid, Abbott, Abbott Park, Illinois; Optrell, Pentaray and Octaray, Biosense Webster, Diamond Bar, California; Orion, Boston Scientific, Marlborough, MA), these regions can be identified readily, and displayed alongside bipolar and unipolar voltage maps, but targeting all these areas for ablation may be impractical and unnecessary.[98,178,179]

Although scar homogenization (extensive ablation to abolish all abnormal EGMs within scar tissue) has been associated with better long-term VA-free survival than clinical VT ablation alone in various subsets,[102,159-161] it is imperative to further define areas that are vital for VT maintenance. We discuss 2 such techniques to identify ablation targets—isochronal late activation mapping (ILAM) and decrement evoked potential mapping (DEEP). ILAM consists of identifying myocardial areas with the steep deceleration of activation during sinus rhythm, and these areas colocalize with VT isthmuses. *Tung and colleagues* described this approach that allows for limited

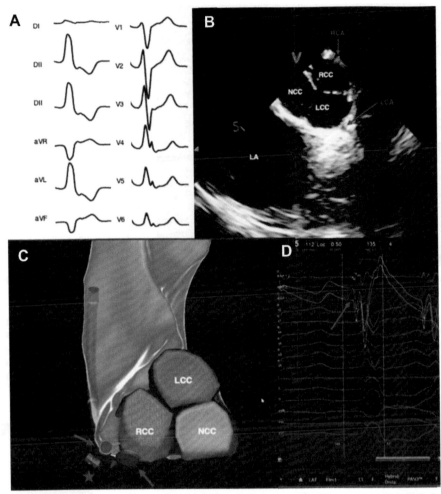

**Fig. 7.** LAT hybrid map showing true location of PVC origin. (*A*) 12-lead surface ECG with LBBB-type PVC with a small R wave in V2 and transition in V3, consistent with an LVOT origin. (*B*) ICE view of the aortic valve, showing the origins and proximal portions of the RCA (green double *line*) and left coronary arteries. (*C*) LAT (local activation time) hybrid activation map of the aortic root (LAO Caudal view) The red pin indicates the point of earliest activation as shown in the LAT hybrid map, and the red tags and red arrow indicate sites of successful ablation. The green point and arrow indicate the earliest activation site on the traditional LAT map, which overlies the RCA ostium (green double *line*). The earliest activation on the LAT hybrid map was relocated 3.3 mm away from the RCA ostium, enabling successful ablation with no damage to the right coronary artery. The red star indicates the intracardiac echocardiography catheter. (*D*) Surface ECG tracings and unipolar signal showing earliest electrogram with a unipolar QS configuration (red *arrow*). ECG, electrocardiogram; ICE, intracardiac echocardiography; LA, left atrium; LAO, left anterior oblique; LAT, late activation time; LBBB, left bundle branch block; LCA, left coronary artery; LCC, left coronary cusp; LVOT, left ventricular outflow tract; NCC, noncoronary cusp; PVC, premature ventricular complex; RCA, right coronary artery; RCC, right coronary cusp. (*From* Compagnucci P., Volpato G., Falanga U., et al. Recent advances in three-dimensional electroanatomical mapping guidance for the ablation of complex atrial and ventricular arrhythmias. J Interv Card Electrophysiol 2021;61(1):37–43. Doi: 10.1007/s10840-020-00781-3; with permission.)

ablation compared with extensive anatomic substrate ablation, with similar ablation outcomes.[180–182] For the visual representation of crowded isochrones or deceleration zones (surrogate for VT isthmus), the activation time in the ventricular myocardium is distributed into 8 equal isochrones of from early to late activation. The procedure of annotating the last local EGM deflection is automated with the Ensite mapping system but needs manual annotation for Carto and Rhythmia systems. Once these zones of isochronal crowding are displayed on the EAM systems, they allow for the targeted ablation of functional re-entrant sites.

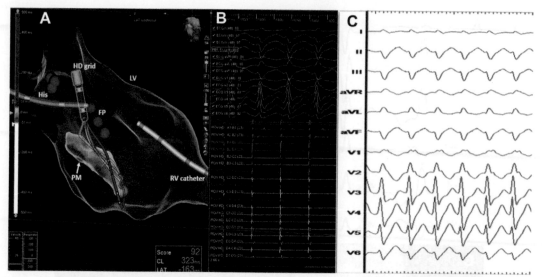

**Fig. 8.** Point density exclusion mapping of endocavitary structures. (*A*) Activation map showing focal VT with earliest activation in the posteromedial papillary muscle. The 3D EAM image shows the posteromedial papillary muscle derived from the usual left ventricular map by applying the PDX mapping technique. The red tags represent the His and the posterior fascicular potentials. (*B*) Pace mapping performed from the A1B1 bipole of the high-density mapping catheter (Advisor HD-Grid, Abbott, Abbott Park, Illinois) in located on the posteromedial papillary muscle revealed a 92% pace match with the clinical VT (*C*) 12-lead ECG showing right bundle left superior axis VT, with V4 transition. EAM, electroanatomic; ECG, electrocardiogram; PDX, point density exclusion; VT, ventricular tachycardia. (*From* Prabhu MA., Saravanan S., Valaparambil AK., et al. Point density exclusion mapping-A useful tool for mapping arrhythmias arising from the endocavitary structures. J Arrhythm 2021;37(5):1371–3. Doi: 10.1002/joa3.12606; with permission.)

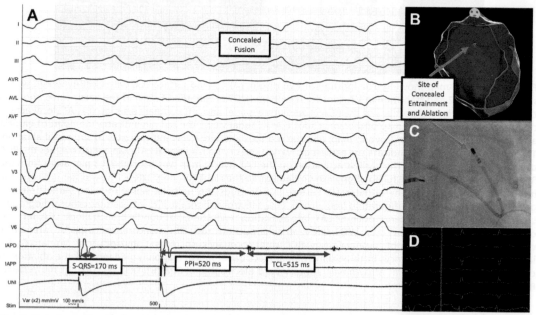

**Fig. 9.** Entrainment mapping in hemodynamically tolerated ventricular tachycardia. Entrainment mapping in a patient with ischemic cardiomyopathy and anterior scar (*A*) Entrainment of a left bundle right inferior axis VT with TCL of 515 ms shows concealed fusion with short PPI-TCL (<10 ms) and S-QRS interval measuring 33% of the TCL, suggestive of a central isthmus site. RF ablation at this anterior LV site (panel B shows an LAO projection of the electroanatomical map and panel C shows the corresponding fluoroscopic position of the ablation catheter via transseptal approach, AP view), terminated the VT (panel D). AP, anteroposterior; LAO, left anterior oblique; LV, left ventricle; PPI, postpacing interval; RF, radiofrequency; S-QRS, stimulus-to-QRS interval; TCL, tachycardia cycle length; VT, ventricular tachycardia.

**Table 3**
Key studies evaluating substrate-guided ablation strategy

| Substrate Ablation Strategy | Study Group | Study Population | Study Endpoint | Outcomes |
|---|---|---|---|---|
| Linear Ablation Strategy | Marchlinski et al,[145] 2000 | 9 ICM and 7 NICM; Linear ablation from dense scar (<0.5 mV) to anatomic boundaries | Noninducibility of VT (~47%) | 75% VA-free survival (median 8 mo) |
| Linear Ablation Strategy | Soejima et al,[146] 2001 | 40 ICM; Linear ablation through critical VT isthmus identified by entrainment or pace mapping | Noninducibility of VT (~58%) | 64% VA-free survival (median 37 mo) |
| Linear Ablation Strategy | Verma et al,[147] 2005 | 22 ARVC; Linear ablation to connect scar/abnormal regions (with good pace map) to a valve continuity or encircle scar/abnormal region | Noninducibility of VT (~82%) | 64% VA-free survival (median 37 mo) |
| Linear Ablation Strategy | Reddy et al,[88] 2007 | 64 ICM; Linear ablation from exit site (good pace map) to center of substrate, and a perpendicular line along the scar border zone | N/A | 88% VA-free survival at 2 y |
| Late Potential Ablation | Arenal et al,[148] 2003 | 21 ICM and 2 NICM; Ablation of all LPs based on EAM | Elimination of LPs and noninducibility (~88%) | 79% VA-free survival (mean 9 mo) |
| Late Potential Ablation | Volkmer et al,[149] 2006 | 25 ICM; Ablation of LPs in scar or border zone (<1.5 mV) | Elimination of LPs and noninducibility (~81%) | 75% VA-free survival (mean 25 mo) |
| Late Potential Ablation | Nogami et al,[150] 2008 | 18 NICM (ARVC); Ablation of endocardial LPs | Elimination or change in LPs and noninducibility (~66%) | 66% VA-free survival (mean 61 mo) |
| Late Potential Ablation | Garcia et al,[151] 2009 | 13 NICM (ARVC); Epicardial ablation of LPs (after failed endocardial ablation) | Elimination of LPs and noninducibility (~85%) | 77% VA-free survival (mean 18 mo) |

(continued on next page)

**Table 3**
*(continued)*

| Substrate Ablation Strategy | Study Group | Study Population | Study Endpoint | Outcomes |
|---|---|---|---|---|
| Late Potential Ablation | Bai et al,[152] 2011 | 26 NICM (ARVC); Endocardial–epicardial ablation of LPs | Elimination of LPs and noninducibility (~100%) | 84% VA-free survival (mean 36 mo) |
| Late Potential Ablation | Vergara et al,[153] 2012 | 36 ICM and 14 NICM; Endocardial–epicardial ablation of LPs | Elimination of LPs (~84%) | 80% VA-free survival at 1 y |
| Late Potential Ablation | Arenal et al,[154] 2013 | 59 ICM; Endocardial ablation of LPs | Elimination of LPs (~97%) | 55% VA-free survival (mean 13 mo) |
| LAVA Ablation | Jaïs et al,[155] 2012 | 56 ICM and 14 NICM; Endocardial and epicardial ablation targeting all LAVAs (identified in ~96% of patients) | Elimination of LAVA and noninducibility (~70%) | 55% VA-free survival (mean 22 mo) |
| LAVA Ablation | Komatsu et al,[156] 2014 | 18 ICM, 13 NICM and 15 ARVC; Endocardial and epicardial ablation targeting all LAVAs (identified in ~96% of patients) | Elimination of LAVA and noninducibility (~70%) | 67% VA-free survival (median 11 mo) |
| LAVA Ablation | Komatsu et al,[157] 2015 | 144 ICM and 51 NICM; Endocardial and epicardial ablation targeting all LAVAs (identified in ~96% of patients) | Elimination of LAVA and noninducibility (~49%) | 59% VA-free survival (median 23 mo) |
| LAVA Ablation | Wolf et al,[158] 2018 | 159 ICM; Endocardial and epicardial ablation targeting all LAVAs (identified in ~92% of patients) | Elimination of LAVA and noninducibility (~64%) | 73% VA-free survival at 1 y 55% VA-free survival (median 47 mo) |
| Scar Homogenization | Di Biase et al,[102] 2012 | 43 ICM with electrical storm; Extensive ablation (endocardial/epicardial) to eliminate all abnormal potentials ± loss of pacing capture within scar tissue | Noninducibility (100%) | 81% VA-free survival (mean 25 mo) |

| | | | |
|---|---|---|---|
| Scar Homogenization | Di Biase et al,[159] 2015 | 58 ICM; Extensive ablation (endocardial/epicardial) to eliminate all abnormal potentials ± loss of pacing capture within scar tissue | Elimination of all abnormal potentials and noninducibility (~84%) | 85% VA-free survival at 1 y |
| Scar Homogenization | Gökoğlan et al,[160] 2016 | 36 NICM; Extensive ablation (endocardial/epicardial) to eliminate all abnormal potentials ± loss of pacing capture within scar tissue | Noninducibility (~69%) | 64% VA-free survival (mean 14 mo) |
| Scar Homogenization | Mohanty et al,[161] 2022 | 70 ICM; Extensive ablation (endocardial/epicardial) to eliminate all abnormal potentials ± loss of pacing capture within scar tissue | Noninducibility (~100%) | 81% VA-free survival at 5 y |
| Scar Dechanneling | Berruezo et al,[162] 2012 | 11 ARVC; Targeted ablation (endocardial/epicardial) of conducting channels within scar tissue | Elimination of all conducting channels and noninducibility (100%) | 91% VA-free survival (median 11 mo) |
| Scar Dechanneling | Tung et al,[163] 2013 | 15 ICM, 4 NICM, 2 ARVC and 1 Chagas; Targeted ablation of earliest late potentials (endocardial ± epicardial) on multipolar catheter, followed by the elimination of entire channels within scar tissue | Noninducibility (~84%) | 86% VA-free survival (median 11 mo) |
| Scar Dechanneling | Berruezo et al,[164] 2015 | 75 ICM and 26 NICM; Targeted ablation (endocardial ± epicardial) of conducting channels within scar tissue | Elimination of all conducting channels and noninducibility (~78%) | 73% VA-free survival (median 21 mo) |

(continued on next page)

**Table 3**
*(continued)*

| Substrate Ablation Strategy | Study Group | Study Population | Study Endpoint | Outcomes |
|---|---|---|---|---|
| Scar Dechanneling | Fernández-Armenta et al,[165] 2016 | 19 ICM and 5 NICM; Upfront targeted ablation (endocardial ± epicardial) of conducting channels within scar tissue | Elimination of all conducting channels and noninducibility (~88%) | 58% VA-free survival (mean 22 mo) |
| Scar Dechanneling | Andreu et al,[166] 2017 | 84 ICM and 21 NICM; Targeted ablation (endocardial ± epicardial) of conducting channels within scar tissue | Elimination of all conducting channels and noninducibility (~50%) | 56% VA-free survival (mean 20 mo) |
| Putative Isthmus Ablation | de Chillou et al,[94] 2014 | 10 ICM; Linear ablation through putative isthmus VT sites identified by abrupt transitions in QRS morphology during pace mapping in sinus rhythm | Noninducibility (~80%) | 50% VA-free survival (mean 65 mo) |
| Core Isolation | Tzou et al,[167] 2015 | 32 ICM and 12 NICM; Circumferentially ablation surrounding putative isthmus or entrance and early exit sites (identified based on pacemapping or entrainment mapping) | Core isolation (~87%) | 86% VA-free survival (mean 18 mo) |
| Imaging-guided Substrate Ablation | Andreu et al,[166] 2017 | 37 ICM and 17 NICM; Elimination of LP channels detected on EAM corroborated by CMRI detected heterogenous tissue channels | Noninducibility (~68%) | 82% VA-free survival (mean 20 mo) |

| Imaging-guided Substrate Ablation | Ghannam et al,[168] 2020 | 29 (predominantly NICM); Extensive ablation targeting all areas of intramural scar identified by DHE-CMRI for scar endocardialization/homogenization | Noninducibility (~42%) | 69% VA-free survival at 1 y |

*Abbreviations:* ARVC, arrhythmogenic right ventricular cardiomyopathy; CMRI, cardiac magnetic resonance imaging; DHE, delayed hyperenhancement; EAM, electroanatomical map; ICM, ischemic cardiomyopathy; LAVA, local abnormal ventricular activation; LP, late potential; NICM, nonischemic cardiomyopathy; VA, ventricular arrhythmia; VT, ventricular tachycardia.

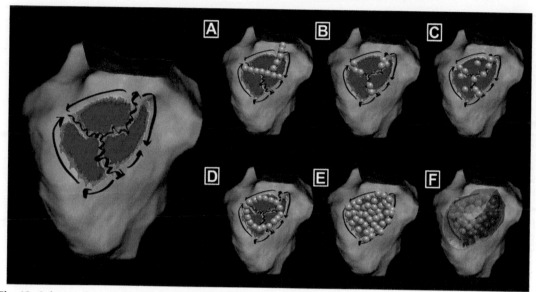

**Fig. 10.** Substrate based ablation strategies. The graphic shows typical substrate that sustains re-entrant VT, with areas of dense scar (red) with border zones (yellow) and channels of conducting tissue in between. This establishes the milieu for multiple macro re-entrant VT circuits (black). Substrate mapping involves the acquisition of imaging, voltage, and EGM information in these areas, with the goal of ablating arrhythmogenic substrate (A) *Linear ablation* consists of lesions placed within dense scar that is responsible for VT, and anchoring these lesions to an anatomic boundary, such as a valvular annulus (B) *Scar dechanneling* is a technique where limited ablation is performed in the entrance sites of conducting channels (delayed EGMs that are consecutively activated), to render the VT circuit inactive (C) *LP/LAVA ablation* targets the ablation of all low voltage abnormal EGMs with single or multiple delayed EGM components. LPs are typically delayed beyond the end of the surface QRS, whereas LAVAs may be noted during or after the QRS complex in sinus rhythm or ventricular pacing. LAVAs also include presystolic abnormal EGMs during VT (D) *Core isolation* is a circumferential lesion set that isolates the arrhythmogenic core (identified by pace mapping and substrate mapping), from the rest of the ventricular myocardium (E) *Scar homogenization* entails the extensive ablation of all abnormal EGMs in the endocardium and epicardium until EGMs fully abate or until loss of capture with high output pacing (F) *Imaging-guided scar homogenization or endothelialization* refers to extensive ablation in areas adjacent to scar tissue as identified by CMR/CT or ICE (yellow overlay), in addition to the ablation of local abnormal EGMs, with the goal of rendering this tissue unexcitable with high output pacing. CMR, cardiac magnetic resonance; CT, computed tomography; EGM, electrogram; ICE, intracardiac echocardiography; LAVA, local abnormal ventricular activity; LP, late potential; VT, ventricular tachycardia.

Another approach to identifying critical functional substrate is DEEP mapping, whereby an extrastimulus (20msec above ventricular effective refractory period) is added to a pacing drivetrain (in areas whereby late potentials have been identified, to unmask or evoke delayed potentials (that correlate with VT substrate, **Fig. 12**).[183,184] It is critical to limit the annotation window to the terminal part of the QRS to detect only the local, delayed EGMs. A practical approach is to perform single extrastimulus pacing (S2) following a continuous drivetrain (S1) and obtain 2 separate EAMs. Potentials that are seen only on the S2 map represent DEEPs and are targets for ablation. This strategy is useful when the targets for ablation are not well defined, such as, nonischemic cardiomyopathies. Multiple studies show that targeted ablation in this fashion can achieve similar results to extensive anatomic substrate ablation.[185,186]

In conclusion, while there have several advancements in 3D-EAM system algorithms and features that enhance the electrophysiologist's ability to successfully ablate VAs, it is important to emphasize that a thorough understanding of EGMs (in sinus rhythm and in VT) is important we should integrate this information with 3D-EAM data, to achieve best results.

## Energy Delivery and Alternative Ablation Strategies

The next major advance after refining our mapping strategies is the improvement in energy delivery during catheter ablation. This is particularly relevant in the dense intramural substrate, whereby deeper lesions are desired. Briefly, the options include (1) making RF ablation more effective (higher power, longer duration, lower ionic irrigant use,

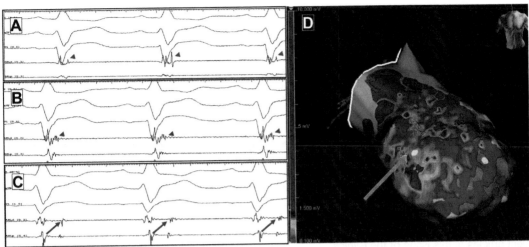

**Fig. 11.** Substrate-guided ablation in hemodynamically unstable ventricular tachycardia. Substrate-guided ablation in a patient with ischemic cardiomyopathy and anterior scar demonstrating several abnormal electrograms. Mapping with an ablation catheter in the area of low voltage shows (*A*) double potentials or split potentials toward the end of the QRS (*B*) highly fractionated, low-amplitude signals denoting local abnormal ventricular activity (LAVA) (*C*) isolated late potentials that are noted well after the end of the QRS. Panel D shows an anteroposterior projection of the bipolar endocardial voltage map (yellow *arrow* shows site with representative abnormal electrograms in the anteroseptal region).

simultaneous unipolar, bipolar ablation, remote magnetic navigation, needle catheter ablation) and (2) using alternative energy sources (cryoablation, alcohol ablation, pulse field electroporation and stereotactic radioablation). Over the past decade, the introduction of contact force sensing and open irrigation RF catheters have greatly optimized energy delivery during ablation.[97,187–191] When greater lesion size is desired, lower ionic irrigant solution (half-normal saline and dextrose) can be utilized with good effect.[192,193] When sequential unipolar ablation is unsuccessful due to intramural

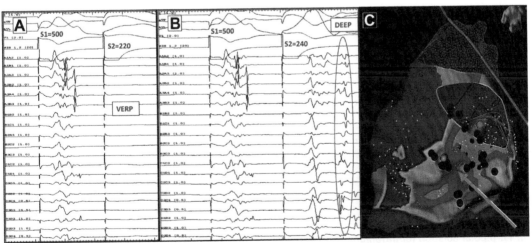

**Fig. 12.** Decrement evoked potential mapping (DEEP) to identify critical functional substrate. DEEP mapping was performed in a patient with ischemic cardiomyopathy and scar in the basal inferior wall of the LV (*A*) Following RV pacing with a drivetrain (S1) of 500 ms, an extrastimulus (S2) at 220 ms demonstrates VERP (*B*) After increasing the S2 coupling interval by 20 ms above VERP, significant decrement in local EGMs is noted (red ellipse) on the multielectrode catheter (Advisor HD-Grid, Abbott, Abbott Park, Illinois) in the inferobasal LV (*C*) PA caudal projection of the electroanatomical map demonstrating the region of the inferobasal LV whereby this DEEP was identified (yellow *arrow*). DEEP, decrement evoked potential; EGM, electrogram; LV, left ventricle; PA, posteroanterior; RV, right ventricle; VERP, ventricular effective refractory period.

substrate (RV/LV ablation for septal VAs and endo-cardial/epicardial ablation for free wall VTs), simultaneous unipolar ablation (2 RF catheters attached to separate RF generators) and bipolar ablation (1 RF catheter attached to output, 1 RF catheter attached to ground) configurations have been used to achieve better results (**Fig. 13**).[194–199] In situations whereby catheter stability is important, remote magnetic navigation (RMN)-guided RF ablation may be helpful. Multiple studies have demonstrated its utility in outflow tract VAs, as well as substrate ablation in the endocardium and epicardium, but randomized trials have been challenging to complete (NCT02637947).[200–204] Use of needle RF catheter ablation and alternative energy sources have been discussed in detail in subsequent articles of this issue of the *Clinics*.

### Adjunctive Use of Intracardiac Echocardiography to Improve Safety and Efficacy

When available, phased array ICE has rapidly become an integral part of VA ablation procedures because of several added benefits. First, it allows for the assessment of anatomic variations at the beginning of the procedure and allows for catheter manipulation in any chamber of the heart while minimizing or eliminating fluoroscopy use.[80] Second, it can be used to safely perform transseptal puncture when antegrade LV access is needed.[205] Third, ICE images can be used to generate a shell

of the RV/LV and can be integrated into the EAM system (CartoSound, Biosense Webster, Diamond Bar, CA).[206,207] Often arrhythmogenic substrate can also be identified on ICE imaging which can aid targeted mapping and ablation.[208] Fourth, ICE is very useful in assessing catheter stability and lesion formation during the ablation of highly mobile, intracavitary structures such as papillary muscles.[209] Finally, ICE imaging offers continuous monitoring for complications (such as pericardial effusion, thrombus, char formation) and in avoiding injury to cardiac structures (valves and coronary arteries). Previous articles in the *Clinics* have addressed these points in detail and are a useful reference for practicing interventional electrophysiologists.[79,210–213] Several observational studies have been published showing better outcomes in patients with ICE-guided VT ablation, but randomized studies are lacking.[214–216]

### Managing Procedural Complications

Patients being brought to the EP laboratory for VA ablation represent a high-risk population in whom a range of procedural complications has been described. While the complication rates vary widely among studies (largely due to differences in patient characteristics and disease acuity), vascular complications seem to be the most common complication in most studies (2%–7%).[217–219] Potential complications range from vascular site complications to intraprocedural mortality

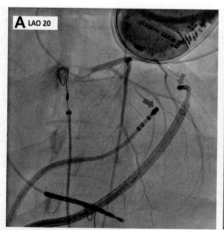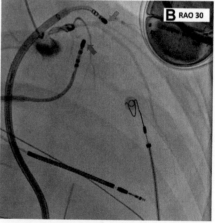

**Fig. 13.** Bipolar ablation for intramural VT substrate. VT originating from intramural scar in the basal anterolateral region of the LV in a patient with late-stage cardiac sarcoidosis. Sequential endocardial and epicardial ablation failed to abolish the VT; therefore, bipolar ablation was performed with one ablation catheter in the LV endocardium (red *arrow*) serving as the active electrode, and one ablation catheter in the epicardium (yellow *arrow*) serving as the ground electrode. VT terminated within seconds after bipolar ablation was initiated. Panels (*A*) and (*B*) show LAO and RAO fluoroscopic projections of catheter positions during simultaneous left coronary angiography. The LV endocardial catheter is positioned via a transseptal approach and the epicardial catheter is positioned via a posterior subxiphoid puncture. LAO, left anterior oblique; LV, left ventricle; RAO, right anterior oblique; VT, ventricular tachycardia.

(**Table 4**). Although procedural death may be related to cardiac perforation and tamponade, coronary injury, and/or major bleeding, the most likely cause is recurrent VT with resultant cardiogenic shock and hemodynamic collapse. Therefore, strategies that focus on the refinement of ablation technique (integrating preprocedural imaging data, intracardiac EGMs, anatomic and functional substrate data) are likely to minimize time spent in VT and the risk of HF decompensation and/or cardiogenic shock.[217,219–221]

## SECTION III: POSTABLATION CARE

There are 3 key areas to consider following the catheter ablation of VAs (1) vascular site and pericardial space management, (2) postprocedural anticoagulation, and (3) duration of AADs. Since the most common complication is a vascular site complication, ensuring adequate hemostasis is crucial after the completion of the ablation. Manual hemostasis of arterial and venous sites has been the standard of care, but several operators are now using vascular closure devices for arteriotomy sites and purse-string sutures/figure of 8 sutures for venous sites. A recent randomized controlled study of a dedicated venous vascular closure device versus manual hemostasis showed the improved time to hemostasis and ambulation.[222] Protamine administration has also been shown to reduce time to hemostasis and ambulation, without increasing thrombotic complications.[223] Similarly, the pericardial access site needs great care if epicardial ablation has been performed. The majority of operators instill steroids in the pericardium to prevent pericarditis and adhesions (which may impact a redo epicardial procedure).[224] Most often, a pericardial drain/pigtail catheter is left in place and monitored for the accumulation of pericardial fluid/blood and removed a day later once the output is minimal.

Once access sites are free of complications, it is important to address postprocedural anticoagulation. In patients with extensive endocardial ablation, who are at risk for thromboembolic complications, it is advisable to bridge with low dose unfractionated heparin (600–900 units/h, 6–8 hours after hemostasis) and then transition to oral anticoagulants for at least 3 months (either warfarin or direct agents).[1,225,226] In patients with less extensive ablation, an antiplatelet agent alone is usually sufficient for short-term use.[1,97]

Finally, AAD prescription after ablation is not well studied; most studies have left it to the operator's discretion, while some have advocated for 3 months of use post-ablation. In our experience, if the burden of VA was significant before ablation,

structural heart disease is present and extensive ablation is needed, we continue AADs for up to 3 months, and reassess clinical and ICD data before discontinuing AADs. In cases where minimal ablation is required, the heart is structurally normal, AADs are discontinued after the ablation. Noninvasive programmed ventricular stimulation (NIPS) performed via ICD 2 to 4 days after ablation may identify patients who would benefit from the continuation of AAD and a select few may need repeat catheter ablation.[227]

## SECTION IV: SPECIAL CONSIDERATIONS
### Ventricular Tachycardia Ablation in Patients with Temporary Mechanical Circulatory Devices

Increasingly, patients with advanced structural heart disease are presenting with VT/electrical storm and concomitant cardiogenic shock. Patients with this clinical overlap of electrical storm and cardiogenic shock who are brought to the electrophysiology laboratory for catheter ablation are the sickest cohort electrophysiologists must care for, and the procedural mortality alone may be well more than 5%.[220] To manage cardiogenic shock, a host of temporary mechanical circulatory devices (TMCS) are available—intra-aortic balloon pump (IABP), Veno-arterial Extracorporeal membrane oxygenation, (VA-ECMO), Tandem Heart (LivaNova, UK) and Impella (Abiomed, Danvers, MA).[228] While an IABP provides minimal support (∼1 L/min), the remaining TMCS devices all provide 3.5–4 L/min of circulatory support and can prevent hemodynamic decompensation during VT. It is important to consider LV access in the presence of TMCS. As the Impella is placed in the LV across the aortic valve, VT ablation must be performed via antegrade transseptal access. With a Tandem-Heart, there is a large bore cannula (21F) across the interatrial septum, and it is best to use a retroaortic access for VT ablation. This is perhaps one reason why peripheral VA-ECMO is the most widely used TMCS for VT ablation, as either antegrade or retrograde LV access remains feasible.[229] There are several observational studies evaluating outcomes in patients undergoing catheter ablation in the presence of TMCS,[98,230–236] and nearly all observational comparative studies have consistently demonstrated higher mortality in the group using TMCS, attributable to selection bias. In one study comparing pre-emptive TMCS before ablation versus rescue TMCS after hemodynamic decompensation, 30-day mortality was very high in the rescue group (58%), while 30-day mortality in the pre-emptive TMCS group was similar to those not needing any TMCS (4% vs 3%).[234]

**Table 4**
Complications of ventricular arrhythmia ablation

| Complication | Incidence | Mechanism | Management | Prevention | References |
|---|---|---|---|---|---|
| Procedural Mortality | 0%–0.6% | Pericardial effusion/ tamponade; intracranial bleeding; retroperitoneal bleeding; stroke, pulmonary embolism; refractory VT and cardiogenic shock | Cause-specific intervention (eg, surgical pericardial repair or vascular bleed repair); followed by the multi-disciplinary management of sick patients | Following procedural best practices; patient clinical status optimization before ablation | 217,220,243 |
| In-Hospital/Early Mortality | 1.5%–5% | Refractory VT and cardiogenic shock | Management of ES; ganglion blockade, and/or sympathectomy; Bailout TMCS; Multidisciplinary HF management | Risk stratification of patients at risk of hemodynamic decompensation (PAINESD/ RIVA score): prophylactic TMCS | 218,220,221 |
| Pericardial Effusion/ Cardiac Tamponade | 0.4%–3% | Cardiac perforation during transseptal puncture, catheter manipulation; epicardial injury | Urgent pericardiocentesis; heparin reversal; cardiac surgical repair in few cases; | Imaging-guided transseptal puncture; contact force sensing catheter use | 217–219,221 |
| Stroke, TIA, Cerebral Bleeding* | 0.4%–6.5% | Emboli from left ventricle; aortic valve/aorta (retrograde approach) | Thrombolytic therapy; mechanical thrombectomy | Anticoagulation throughout left-sided ablation (ACT > 300sec); cerebral protection device in high-risk cases | 217–219,226 |
| Heart Failure Decompensation or Cardiogenic Shock | 0.4%–11% | ES/CS prior to ablation; prolonged procedure; LV dysfunction; prolonged time in VT; anesthetic agents | Pharmacologic and/or mechanical circulatory support | Preoptimization; risk assessment (PAINESD/RIVA score) with prophylactic TMCS; substrate ablation-based strategy; hemodynamic monitoring | 219,238 |
| Vascular Complications | 2.5%–6.9% | High or low arterial puncture; pseudoaneurysm/laceration/ perforation due to catheter manipulation/sheath removal | Ultrasound-guided compression, thrombin injection, and surgical closure | Ultrasound-guided vascular access; vascular closure devices; protamine administration | 217–219 |

| Coronary Artery Injury | 0.1%–1.9% | Proximity to coronary artery with unipolar/bipolar ablation; mechanical injury during epicardial ablation or catheter manipulation in the aortic root | Coronary angiography and/or stenting | Coronary angiography before ablation in high-risk sites; ablation to be avoided within 5 mm of coronary arteries | 218,244,245 |
|---|---|---|---|---|---|
| Valvular Injury | <1% | Catheter manipulation through the aortic and mitral valve; papillary muscle dysfunction after ablation | Transthoracic/transesophageal echocardiography to determine the severity; May need surgical intervention for hemodynamically significant severe valvular regurgitation | ICE and/or fluoroscopic guidance during catheter manipulation across valves | 97,246 |
| Conduction System Injury | ≤1.5% | Ablation near conduction system (para-Hisian or distal conduction system/left bundle branch block) | Temporary and/or permanent pacing | Use of adjacent sites for ablation (aortic cusps, right atrium, right/left ventricular septum); Pacing maneuvers to distinguish near-field and far-field His signals; ICE guidance Cryoablation | 74,217 |
| Phrenic Nerve Injury | ≤0.5% | Epicardial ablation along the lateral wall leading to left phrenic injury | Immediate cessation of ablation; Supportive care | High output pacing before ablation in the epicardial lateral wall; CT-guided detection of phrenic nerve location; Air Insufflation or saline Instillation in pericardium; Balloon-guided mechanical separation of visceral and parietal pericardium | 219,247,248 |

*Abbreviations:* ACT, activated clotting time; CS, cardiogenic shock; CT, computed tomography; ES, electrical storm; HF, heart failure; ICE, intracardiac echocardiography; LV, left ventricle; TMCS, temporary mechanical circulatory support; VT, ventricular tachycardia.

Therefore, there has been considerable interest in estimating the risk of hemodynamic decompensation during VT ablation; the PAINESD score and the RIVA score are useful clinical scores derived from such studies.[220,221,235,237,238] Using the PAINESD score, it has been demonstrated that prophylactic TMCS may significantly improve outcomes in high-risk VT ablation.[237] Further refinements are needed in our risk stratification. Until then it is prudent to choose substrate-based strategies for ablation, to minimize the risk of hemodynamic collapse in these high-risk patients and prophylactic TMCS may be considered in patients with high PAINESD scores.

### Ventricular Tachycardia Ablation in Patients with Durable Mechanical Circulatory Devices

As the burden of advanced heart failure increases, there is a sharp increase in patients with durable left ventricular assist device (LVAD) implants, either as a bridge-to-transplant or destination therapy.[239] While these patients are at increased risk for VT and mortality (particularly if they had VT before LVAD implant), they often tolerate VT without any hemodynamic compromise or symptoms.[240] When the VT is drug refractory and persistent, catheter ablation may be considered to prevent RV dysfunction, LVAD malfunction and long-term mortality.[1] The mechanism of VT is predominantly scar-related

re-entry (~90%). Bundle-branch re-entrant VT and focal/micro-re-entrant VT are responsible for a minority of VTs.[241] It is important to note that up to 20% of VT critical sites may be close to the LVAD inflow cannula (**Fig. 14**).[241] This area needs careful mapping and ablation, with the knowledge that contact with the inflow cannula may produce artifact with impedance drops.[242] Contrary to common perception, catheter entrapment is rare.[241,242] As the EAM systems may not accurately demonstrate catheter position due to electromagnetic interference, it is important to use fluoroscopy, transesophageal echocardiography (TEE) or ICE to visualize the catheter position when close to the inflow cannula.[241] It is important to know that the 12-lead ECG does not accurately predict the VT SOO, as the anatomy of the heart and chest is altered following an LVAD implant. Both ECGs and intracardiac EGMs should have low-pass filters set to 40 Hz to reduce noise. While retro-aortic access has been described in the literature, it is prudent to choose antegrade transseptal access to avoid damage to the aortic valve (aortic insufficiency would adversely affect LVAD functioning).[241,242] If ICE or TEE imaging suggests a small left atrium, it may be necessary to increase preload temporarily for transseptal access to distend the left atrium and minimize complications. One of the major advantages of VT ablation in patients with LVAD is hemodynamic stability. This

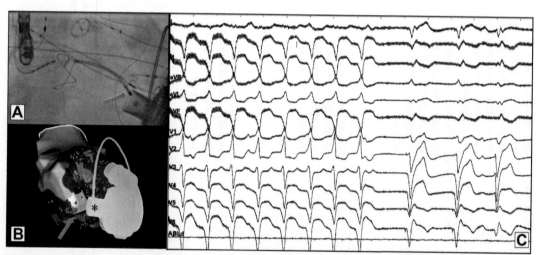

**Fig. 14.** VT ablation in the presence of an LVAD. Catheter ablation for incessant VT in a patient with nonischemic cardiomyopathy, mechanical AVR and Heart Mate 3 LVAD (Abbott, Abbott Park, Illinois) (*A*) Fluoroscopic RAO projection showing the ablation catheter position (yellow *arrow*) close to the LVAD inflow cannula (red star). Continuous TEE monitoring was performed to prevent catheter entrapment (*B*) AP projection of the electroanatomical map, with superimposed image of the LVAD from a chest X-ray, showing the ablation catheter position (yellow *arrow*) close to the LVAD inflow cannula (red star). Activation mapping showed early ventricular activation in this region during VT (white) (*C*) The right bundle left superior axis VT, with V3 transition, terminated during RF ablation at this site. Note the electromagnetic interference on ECG leads despite low-pass filter set to 40 Hz. AP, anteroposterior; AVR, aortic valve; LVAD, left ventricular assist device; RAO, right anterior oblique; RF, radiofrequency; TEE, transesophageal echocardiogram; VT, ventricular tachycardia.

allows activation mapping with confirmation using entrainment mapping. Once the clinical VT is terminated, the adjacent abnormal substrate can be targeted for ablation using previously described techniques. It is important to note that pace mapping may be severely hampered by high-frequency noise from the LVAD. Unlike routine VA ablations, these patients should receive prophylactic antibiotics and as far as possible ablation should be performed with uninterrupted anticoagulation to prevent LVAD pump thrombosis. Finally, it is important to understand and set expectations around outcomes. Although VT storm can be addressed successfully with catheter ablation, VT recurrence (>40%), mortality (~35%, albeit not due to recurrent VT) and need for heart transplantation (~25%) remain high in these patients.[241,242]

## SUMMARY

We are in an exciting era of catheter ablation with an array of advances in mapping and ablation technology. As a result, our ability to characterize the underlying arrhythmogenic substrate has improved, translating into greater efficacy of catheter ablation for VAs. It is crucial to couple these accomplishments with high levels of peri-procedural safety, by using best practices to achieve optimal long-term outcomes. Enhanced safety and efficacy in clinical trials and practice, will help identify the cohort of patients in whom catheter ablation for VAs can be the initial approach. In this review, we discuss preprocedure planning strategies, appropriate use of mapping technologies, and best practices for VA ablation. Additionally, we highlight the role of VT ablation in the presence of mechanical circulatory devices as the next step in the evolution of catheter ablation for VAs.

## CLINICS CARE POINTS

- Catheter ablation for VAs has improved in efficacy and is increasingly being offered as first-line therapy.
- Fundamental mapping techniques for VA ablation include activation, entrainment, pace mapping, substrate mapping.
- Appropriate patient selection, pre-procedural preparation, and peri-procedural protocol-based care are important to avoid complications.
- Choosing substrate based ablation strategies may improve safety during VT ablation.

## ACKNOWLEDGEMENT

The authors would like to acknowledge Drs. Preetam Krishnamurthy, Malav Jhala, and Basavaraj Sutar for their assistance with figures.

## CONFLICT OF INTEREST DISCLOSURE

Dr A.R. Atreya receives honoraria or consultancy fees from Abbott, Connected Care, and Abiomed. Dr S.D. Yalagudri receives honoraria or consultancy fees from Boston Scientific, Medtronic, and Johnson & Johnson. Dr C. Narasimhan and Dr D.K Saggu receive support for the fellowship program from Medtronic. Dr D.K. Saggu receives honoraria from Boston Scientific. All other authors have no conflicts of interest to disclose relevant to the content of this article.

## REFERENCES

1. Cronin EM, Bogun FM, Maury P, et al. 2019 HRS/EHRA/APHRS/LAHRS expert consensus statement on catheter ablation of ventricular arrhythmias: Executive summary. Heart Rhythm 2020;17(1):e155–205.
2. Moss AJ, Hall WJ, Cannom DS, et al. Improved survival with an implanted defibrillator in patients with coronary disease at high risk for ventricular arrhythmia. Multicenter Automatic Defibrillator Implantation Trial Investigators. N Engl J Med 1996;335(26):1933–40.
3. Antiarrhythmics versus Implantable Defibrillators (AVID) Investigators A comparison of antiarrhythmic-drug therapy with implantable defibrillators in patients resuscitated from near-fatal ventricular arrhythmias. N Engl J Med 1997;337(22):1576–83.
4. Buxton AE, Lee KL, Fisher JD, et al. A randomized study of the prevention of sudden death in patients with coronary artery disease. Multicenter Unsustained Tachycardia Trial Investigators. N Engl J Med 1999;341(25):1882–90.
5. Greenberg H, Case RB, Moss AJ, et al. Analysis of mortality events in the multicenter automatic defibrillator implantation trial (MADIT-II). J Am Coll Cardiol 2004;43(8):1459–65.
6. Bardy GH, Lee KL, Mark DB, et al. Amiodarone or an implantable cardioverter-defibrillator for congestive heart failure. N Engl J Med 2005;352(3):225–37.
7. Al-Khatib SM, Stevenson WG, Ackerman MJ, et al. 2017 AHA/ACC/HRS guideline for management of patients with ventricular arrhythmias and the prevention of sudden cardiac death: a report of the American College of Cardiology/American heart association Task force on clinical practice

Guidelines and the heart rhythm Society. Heart Rhythm 2018;15(10):e73–189.

8. Vaseghi M, Hu TY, Tung R, et al. Outcomes of catheter ablation of ventricular tachycardia based on etiology in nonischemic heart disease: an International ventricular tachycardia ablation center Collaborative study. JACC Clin Electrophysiol 2018;4(9):1141–50.

9. Mukherjee RK, Whitaker J, Williams SE, et al. Magnetic resonance imaging guidance for the optimization of ventricular tachycardia ablation. Europace 2018;20(11):1721–32.

10. Ghannam M, Liang JJ, Attili A, et al. Cardiac magnetic resonance imaging and ventricular tachycardias involving the Sinuses of Valsalva in patients with nonischemic cardiomyopathy. JACC Clin Electrophysiol 2021;7(10):1243–53.

11. Muser D, Nucifora G, Castro SA, et al. Myocardial substrate characterization by CMR T1 mapping in patients with NICM and No LGE undergoing catheter ablation of VT. JACC Clin Electrophysiol 2021;7(7):831–40.

12. Maccabelli G, Tsiachris D, Silberbauer J, et al. Imaging and epicardial substrate ablation of ventricular tachycardia in patients late after myocarditis. Europace 2014;16(9):1363–72.

13. Lukas Laws J, Lancaster MC, Ben Shoemaker M, et al. Arrhythmias as Presentation of genetic cardiomyopathy. Circ Res 2022;130(11):1698–722.

14. Thachil A, Christopher J, Sastry BKS, et al. Monomorphic ventricular tachycardia and mediastinal adenopathy due to granulomatous infiltration in patients with preserved ventricular function. J Am Coll Cardiol 2011;58(1):48–55.

15. Muser D, Santangeli P, Castro SA, et al. Risk stratification of patients with apparently idiopathic premature ventricular contractions: a multicenter International CMR Registry. JACC Clin Electrophysiol 2020;6(6):722–35.

16. Park K-M, Kim Y-H, Marchlinski FE. Using the surface electrocardiogram to localize the origin of idiopathic ventricular tachycardia. Pacing Clin Electrophysiol 2012;35(12):1516–27.

17. de Riva M, Watanabe M, Zeppenfeld K. Twelve-lead ECG of ventricular tachycardia in structural heart disease. Circ Arrhythm Electrophysiol 2015; 8(4):951–62.

18. Enriquez A, Baranchuk A, Briceno D, et al. How to use the 12-lead ECG to predict the site of origin of idiopathic ventricular arrhythmias. Heart Rhythm 2019;16(10):1538–44.

19. Tanawuttiwat T, Nazarian S, Calkins H. The role of catheter ablation in the management of ventricular tachycardia. Eur Heart J 2016;37(7):594–609.

20. Miller JM, Marchlinski FE, Buxton AE, et al. Relationship between the 12-lead electrocardiogram during ventricular tachycardia and endocardial site of origin in patients with coronary artery disease. Circulation 1988;77(4):759–66.

21. Kuchar DL, Ruskin JN, Garan H. Electrocardiographic localization of the site of origin of ventricular tachycardia in patients with prior myocardial infarction. J Am Coll Cardiol 1989;13(4):893–903.

22. Segal OR, Chow AWC, Wong T, et al. A novel algorithm for determining endocardial VT exit site from 12-lead surface ECG characteristics in human, infarct-related ventricular tachycardia. J Cardiovasc Electrophysiol 2007;18(2):161–8.

23. Yokokawa M, Liu T-Y, Yoshida K, et al. Automated analysis of the 12-lead electrocardiogram to identify the exit site of postinfarction ventricular tachycardia. Heart Rhythm 2012;9(3):330–4.

24. Sapp JL, Bar-Tal M, Howes AJ, et al. Real-time localization of ventricular tachycardia origin from the 12-lead electrocardiogram. JACC Clin Electrophysiol 2017;3(7):687–99.

25. Zhou S, AbdelWahab A, Horáček BM, et al. Prospective assessment of an automated intraprocedural 12-lead ECG-based system for localization of early left ventricular activation. Circ Arrhythm Electrophysiol 2020;13(7):e008262.

26. Berruezo A, Mont L, Nava S, et al. Electrocardiographic recognition of the epicardial origin of ventricular tachycardias. Circulation 2004;109(15): 1842–7.

27. Daniels DV, Lu Y-Y, Morton JB, et al. Idiopathic epicardial left ventricular tachycardia originating remote from the sinus of Valsalva: electrophysiological characteristics, catheter ablation, and identification from the 12-lead electrocardiogram. Circulation 2006;113(13):1659–66.

28. Bazan V, Gerstenfeld EP, Garcia FC, et al. Site-specific twelve-lead ECG features to identify an epicardial origin for left ventricular tachycardia in the absence of myocardial infarction. Heart Rhythm 2007;4(11):1403–10.

29. Vallès E, Bazan V, Marchlinski FE. ECG criteria to identify epicardial ventricular tachycardia in nonischemic cardiomyopathy. Circ Arrhythm Electrophysiol 2010;3(1):63–71.

30. Steinberg JS, Varma N, Cygankiewicz I, et al. 2017 ISHNE-HRS expert consensus statement on ambulatory ECG and external cardiac monitoring/telemetry. Heart Rhythm 2017;14(7):e55–96.

31. Yoshida K, Liu T-Y, Scott C, et al. The value of defibrillator electrograms for recognition of clinical ventricular tachycardias and for pace mapping of post-infarction ventricular tachycardia. J Am Coll Cardiol 2010;56(12):969–79.

32. Tschabrunn CM, Anter E, Marchlinski FE. Identifying non-inducible ventricular tachycardia origin utilizing defibrillator electrograms. J Interv Card Electrophysiol 2013;36(3):243–6.

33. Yokokawa M, Kim HM, Sharaf Dabbagh G, et al. Targeting Noninducible clinical ventricular tachycardias in patients with prior myocardial infarctions based on stored electrograms. Circ Arrhythm Electrophysiol 2019;12(7):e006978.

34. J Shah A, Hocini M, Pascale P, et al. Body surface electrocardiographic mapping for non-invasive identification of arrhythmic sources. Arrhythm Electrophysiol Rev 2013;2(1):16–22.

35. Wang Y, Cuculich PS, Zhang J, et al. Noninvasive electroanatomic mapping of human ventricular arrhythmias with electrocardiographic imaging. Sci Transl Med 2011;3(98). 98ra84.

36. Rudy Y. Noninvasive electrocardiographic imaging of arrhythmogenic substrates in humans. Circ Res 2013;112(5):863–74.

37. Varma N, Strom M, Chung MK. Noninvasive voltage and activation mapping of ARVD/C using ECG imaging. JACC Cardiovasc Imaging 2013; 6(12):1346–7.

38. Zhang J, Cooper DH, Desouza KA, et al. Electrophysiologic scar substrate in relation to VT: Noninvasive high-resolution mapping and risk assessment with ECGI. Pacing Clin Electrophysiol 2016;39(8):781–91.

39. Njeim M, Desjardins B, Bogun F. Multimodality imaging for guiding EP ablation procedures. JACC Cardiovasc Imaging 2016;9(7):873–86.

40. Esposito A, Palmisano A, Antunes S, et al. Cardiac CT with delayed enhancement in the characterization of ventricular tachycardia structural substrate: relationship between CT-Segmented scar and electro-anatomic mapping. JACC Cardiovasc Imaging 2016;9(7):822–32.

41. Desjardins B, Morady F, Bogun F. Effect of epicardial fat on electroanatomical mapping and epicardial catheter ablation. J Am Coll Cardiol 2010; 56(16):1320–7.

42. Cheniti G, Sridi S, Sacher F, et al. Post-myocardial infarction scar with fat Deposition shows specific electrophysiological Properties and Worse outcome after ventricular tachycardia ablation. J Am Heart Assoc 2019;8(15):e012482.

43. Alyesh DM, Siontis KC, Sharaf Dabbagh G, et al. Postinfarction myocardial calcifications on cardiac computed tomography: implications for mapping and ablation in patients with Nontolerated ventricular tachycardias. Circ Arrhythm Electrophysiol 2019;12(5):e007023.

44. Ghannam M, Cochet H, Jais P, et al. Correlation between computer tomography-derived scar topography and critical ablation sites in postinfarction ventricular tachycardia. J Cardiovasc Electrophysiol 2018;29(3):438–45.

45. Takigawa M, Duchateau J, Sacher F, et al. Are wall thickness channels defined by computed tomography predictive of isthmuses of postinfarction

ventricular tachycardia? Heart Rhythm 2019; 16(11):1661–8.

46. Piers SRD, van Huls van Taxis CFB, Tao Q, et al. Epicardial substrate mapping for ventricular tachycardia ablation in patients with non-ischaemic cardiomyopathy: a new algorithm to differentiate between scar and viable myocardium developed by simultaneous integration of computed tomography and contrast-enhanced magnetic resonance imaging. Eur Heart J 2013;34(8):586–96.

47. Baman TS, Ilg KJ, Gupta SK, et al. Mapping and ablation of epicardial idiopathic ventricular arrhythmias from within the coronary venous system. Circ Arrhythm Electrophysiol 2010;3(3):274–9.

48. Carrigan TP, Patel S, Yokokawa M, et al. Anatomic relationships between the coronary venous system, surrounding structures, and the site of origin of epicardial ventricular arrhythmias. J Cardiovasc Electrophysiol 2014;25(12):1336–42.

49. Yamashita S, Sacher F, Mahida S, et al. Role of high-resolution image integration to visualize left phrenic nerve and coronary arteries during epicardial ventricular tachycardia ablation. Circ Arrhythm Electrophysiol 2015;8(2):371–80.

50. Subramanian M, Ravilla VV, Yalagudri S, et al. CT-guided percutaneous epicardial access for ventricular tachycardia ablation: a proof-of-concept study. J Cardiovasc Electrophysiol 2021;32(10):2665–72.

51. Bogun FM, Desjardins B, Good E, et al. Delayed-enhanced magnetic resonance imaging in nonischemic cardiomyopathy: utility for identifying the ventricular arrhythmia substrate. J Am Coll Cardiol 2009;53(13):1138–45.

52. Desjardins B, Yokokawa M, Good E, et al. Characteristics of intramural scar in patients with nonischemic cardiomyopathy and relation to intramural ventricular arrhythmias. Circ Arrhythm Electrophysiol 2013;6(5):891–7.

53. Yamashita S, Sacher F, Mahida S, et al. Image integration to guide catheter ablation in scar-related ventricular tachycardia. J Cardiovasc Electrophysiol 2016;27(6):699–708.

54. Piers SRD, Tao Q, de Riva Silva M, et al. CMR-based identification of critical isthmus sites of ischemic and nonischemic ventricular tachycardia. JACC Cardiovasc Imaging 2014;7(8):774–84.

55. Perin EC, Silva GV, Sarmento-Leite R, et al. Assessing myocardial viability and infarct transmurality with left ventricular electromechanical mapping in patients with stable coronary artery disease: validation by delayed-enhancement magnetic resonance imaging. Circulation 2002; 106(8):957–61.

56. Desjardins B, Crawford T, Good E, et al. Infarct architecture and characteristics on delayed enhanced magnetic resonance imaging and electroanatomic mapping in patients with postinfarction

ventricular arrhythmia. Heart Rhythm 2009;6(5):644–51.

57. Codreanu A, Odille F, Aliot E, et al. Electroanatomic characterization of post-infarct scars comparison with 3-dimensional myocardial scar reconstruction based on magnetic resonance imaging. J Am Coll Cardiol 2008;52(10):839–42.

58. Cochet H, Komatsu Y, Sacher F, et al. Integration of merged delayed-enhanced magnetic resonance imaging and multidetector computed tomography for the guidance of ventricular tachycardia ablation: a pilot study. J Cardiovasc Electrophysiol 2013;24(4):419–26.

59. van Huls van Taxis CF, Wijnmaalen AP, Piers SR, et al. Real-time integration of MDCT-derived coronary anatomy and epicardial fat: impact on epicardial electroanatomic mapping and ablation for ventricular arrhythmias. JACC Cardiovasc Imaging 2013;6(1):42–52.

60. Gormsen LC, Haraldsen A, Kramer S, et al. A dual tracer (68)Ga-DOTANOC PET/CT and (18)F-FDG PET/CT pilot study for detection of cardiac sarcoidosis. EJNMMI Res 2016;6(1):52.

61. Subramanian M, Swapna N, Ali AZ, et al. Pre-treatment myocardial 18FDG uptake predicts response to immunosuppression in patients with cardiac sarcoidosis. JACC Cardiovasc Imaging 2021;14(10):2008–16.

62. Tung R, Bauer B, Schelbert H, et al. Incidence of abnormal positron emission tomography in patients with unexplained cardiomyopathy and ventricular arrhythmias: the potential role of occult inflammation in arrhythmogenesis. Heart Rhythm 2015;12(12):2488–98.

63. Lakkireddy D, Turagam MK, Yarlagadda B, et al. Myocarditis causing premature ventricular contractions: Insights from the MAVERIC Registry. Circ Arrhythm Electrophysiol 2019;12(12):e007520.

64. Muser D, Tritto M, Mariani MV, et al. Diagnosis and treatment of idiopathic premature ventricular contractions: a stepwise approach based on the site of origin. Diagnostics (Basel) 2021;11(10):1840.

65. Sabzwari SRA, Rosenberg MA, Mann J, et al. Limitations of unipolar signals in guiding successful outflow tract premature ventricular contraction ablation. JACC Clin Electrophysiol 2022;8(7):843–53.

66. Yamada T, McElderry HT, Doppalapudi H, et al. Idiopathic ventricular arrhythmias originating from the left ventricular summit: anatomic concepts relevant to ablation. Circ Arrhythm Electrophysiol 2010;3(6):616–23.

67. Kawamura M, Gerstenfeld EP, Vedantham V, et al. Idiopathic ventricular arrhythmia originating from the cardiac crux or inferior septum: epicardial idiopathic ventricular arrhythmia. Circ Arrhythm Electrophysiol 2014;7(6):1152–8.

68. Muser D, Santangeli P. Epicardial ablation of idiopathic ventricular tachycardia. Card Electrophysiol Clin 2020;12(3):295–312.

69. Shinoda Y, Komatsu Y, Nogami A, et al. Stepwise approach to induce infrequent premature ventricular complex using bolus isoproterenol and epinephrine infusion. Pacing Clin Electrophysiol 2020;43(5):437–43.

70. Gopi A, Nair SG, Shelke A, et al. A stepwise approach to the induction of idiopathic fascicular ventricular tachycardia. J Interv Card Electrophysiol 2015;44(1):17–22.

71. Azegami K, Wilber DJ, Arruda M, et al. Spatial resolution of pacemapping and activation mapping in patients with idiopathic right ventricular outflow tract tachycardia. J Cardiovasc Electrophysiol 2005;16(8):823–9.

72. Bennett R, Campbell T, Kotake Y, et al. Catheter ablation of idiopathic outflow tract ventricular arrhythmias with low intraprocedural burden guided by pace mapping. Heart Rhythm 2021;2(4):355–64.

73. Briceño DF, Liang JJ, Shirai Y, et al. Clinical and electrophysiological characteristics of idiopathic ventricular arrhythmias originating from the slow pathway region. Heart Rhythm 2019;16(9):1421–8.

74. Enriquez A, Tapias C, Rodriguez D, et al. How to map and ablate parahisian ventricular arrhythmias. Heart Rhythm 2018;15(8):1268–74.

75. Mariani MV, Piro A, Magnocavallo M, et al. Catheter ablation for papillary muscle arrhythmias: a systematic review. Pacing Clin Electrophysiol 2022;45(4):519–31.

76. Tschabrunn CM, Santangeli P. Maximizing papillary muscle radiofrequency ablation size: Importance of catheter orientation. J Cardiovasc Electrophysiol 2022;33(4):696–7.

77. Gordon JP, Liang JJ, Pathak RK, et al. Percutaneous cryoablation for papillary muscle ventricular arrhythmias after failed radiofrequency catheter ablation. J Cardiovasc Electrophysiol 2018;29(12):1654–63.

78. Di Biase L, Al-Ahmad A, Santangeli P, et al. Safety and outcomes of cryoablation for ventricular tachyarrhythmias: results from a multicenter experience. Heart Rhythm 2011;8(7):968–74.

79. Campbell T, Bennett RG, Kumar S. Intracardiac echocardiography to guide the ablation of parahisian arrhythmias. Card Electrophysiol Clin 2021;13(2S):e1–16.

80. Enriquez A, Saenz LC, Rosso R, et al. Use of intracardiac echocardiography in interventional Cardiology: Working with the anatomy rather than Fighting it. Circulation 2018;137(21):2278–94.

81. Whitaker J, Batnyam U, Kapur S, et al. Safety and efficacy of cryoablation for right ventricular moderator band-papillary muscle complex ventricular

arrhythmias. JACC Clin Electrophysiol 2022;8(7): 857–68.

82. Hsia HH, Lin D, Sauer WH, et al. Anatomic characterization of endocardial substrate for hemodynamically stable reentrant ventricular tachycardia: identification of endocardial conducting channels. Heart Rhythm 2006;3(5):503–12.

83. Frontera A, Pagani S, Limite LR, et al. Outer loop and isthmus in ventricular tachycardia circuits: characteristics and implications. Heart Rhythm 2020;17(10):1719–28.

84. Martin R, Hocini M, Haïsaguerre M, et al. Ventricular tachycardia isthmus characteristics: Insights from high-density mapping. Arrhythm Electrophysiol Rev 2019;8(1):54–9.

85. Ciaccio EJ, Anter E, Coromilas J, et al. Structure and function of the ventricular tachycardia isthmus. Heart Rhythm 2022;19(1):137–53.

86. Sapp JL, Wells GA, Parkash R, et al. Ventricular tachycardia ablation versus Escalation of antiarrhythmic drugs. N Engl J Med 2016;375(2):111–21.

87. Arenal Á, Ávila P, Jiménez-Candil J, et al. Substrate ablation vs antiarrhythmic drug therapy for Symptomatic ventricular tachycardia. J Am Coll Cardiol 2022;79(15):1441–53.

88. Reddy VY, Reynolds MR, Neuzil P, et al. Prophylactic catheter ablation for the prevention of defibrillator therapy. N Engl J Med 2007;357(26):2657–65.

89. Willems S, Tilz RR, Steven D, et al. Preventive or Deferred ablation of ventricular tachycardia in patients with ischemic cardiomyopathy and implantable defibrillator (BERLIN VT): a multicenter randomized trial. Circulation 2020;141(13): 1057–67.

90. Atti V, Vuddanda V, Turagam MK, et al. Prophylactic catheter ablation of ventricular tachycardia in ischemic cardiomyopathy: a systematic review and meta-analysis of randomized controlled trials. J Interv Card Electrophysiol 2018;53(2):207–15.

91. Stevenson WG, Sager PT, Natterson PD, et al. Relation of pace mapping QRS configuration and conduction delay to ventricular tachycardia reentry circuits in human infarct scars. J Am Coll Cardiol 1995;26(2):481–8.

92. Sadek MM, Schaller RD, Supple GE, et al. Ventricular tachycardia ablation - the right approach for the right patient. Arrhythm Electrophysiol Rev 2014;3(3):161–7.

93. Nayyar S, Wilson L, Ganesan AN, et al. High-density mapping of ventricular scar: a comparison of ventricular tachycardia (VT) supporting channels with channels that do not support VT. Circ Arrhythm Electrophysiol 2014;7(1):90–8.

94. de Chillou C, Groben L, Magnin-Poull I, et al. Localizing the critical isthmus of postinfarct ventricular tachycardia: the value of pace-mapping during sinus rhythm. Heart Rhythm 2014;11(2):175–81.

95. de Chillou C, Sellal J-M, Magnin-Poull I. Pace mapping to localize the critical isthmus of ventricular tachycardia. Card Electrophysiol Clin 2017;9(1): 71–80.

96. Bogun F, Good E, Reich S, et al. Role of Purkinje fibers in post-infarction ventricular tachycardia. J Am Coll Cardiol 2006;48(12):2500–7.

97. Stevenson WG, Wilber DJ, Natale A, et al. Irrigated radiofrequency catheter ablation guided by electroanatomic mapping for recurrent ventricular tachycardia after myocardial infarction: the multicenter thermocool ventricular tachycardia ablation trial. Circulation 2008;118(25):2773–82.

98. Dukkipati SR, Koruth JS, Choudry S, et al. Catheter ablation of ventricular tachycardia in structural heart disease: indications, strategies, and outcomes-Part II. J Am Coll Cardiol 2017;70(23): 2924–41.

99. Shirai Y, Liang JJ, Santangeli P, et al. Comparison of the ventricular tachycardia circuit between patients with ischemic and nonischemic cardiomyopathies: Detailed characterization by entrainment. Circ Arrhythm Electrophysiol 2019;12(7):e007249.

100. Richardson TD, Kanagasundram AN, Stevenson WG. Epicardial ablation of ventricular tachycardia in ischemic cardiomyopathy. Card Electrophysiol Clin 2020;12(3):313–9.

101. Acosta J, Fernández-Armenta J, Penela D, et al. Infarct transmurality as a criterion for first-line endo-epicardial substrate-guided ventricular tachycardia ablation in ischemic cardiomyopathy. Heart Rhythm 2016;13(1):85–95.

102. Di Biase L, Santangeli P, Burkhardt DJ, et al. Endo-epicardial homogenization of the scar versus limited substrate ablation for the treatment of electrical storms in patients with ischemic cardiomyopathy. J Am Coll Cardiol 2012;60(2):132–41.

103. Tung R, Michowitz Y, Yu R, et al. Epicardial ablation of ventricular tachycardia: an institutional experience of safety and efficacy. Heart Rhythm 2013; 10(4):490–8.

104. Romero J, Cerrud-Rodriguez RC, Di Biase L, et al. Combined endocardial-epicardial versus endocardial catheter ablation alone for ventricular tachycardia in structural heart disease: a systematic review and meta-analysis. JACC Clin Electrophysiol 2019;5(1):13–24.

105. Kuo L, Liang JJ, Nazarian S, et al. Multimodality imaging to guide ventricular tachycardia ablation in patients with non-ischaemic cardiomyopathy. Arrhythm Electrophysiol Rev 2020;8(4):255–64.

106. Bhaskaran A, Tung R, Stevenson WG, et al. Catheter ablation of VT in non-ischaemic cardiomyopathies: endocardial, epicardial and intramural approaches. Heart Lung Circ 2019;28(1):84–101.

107. Servatius H, Höfeler T, Hoffmann BA, et al. Propofol sedation administered by cardiologists for patients

undergoing catheter ablation for ventricular tachycardia. Europace 2016;18(8):1245–51.

108. Wutzler A, Mueller A, Loehr L, et al. Minimal and deep sedation during ablation of ventricular tachycardia. Int J Cardiol 2014;172(1):161–4.

109. Lü F, Lin J, Benditt DG. Conscious sedation and anesthesia in the cardiac electrophysiology laboratory. J Cardiovasc Electrophysiol 2013;24(2): 237–45.

110. Mulpuru SK, Patel DV, Wilbur SL, et al. Electrical storm and termination with propofol therapy: a case report. Int J Cardiol 2008;128(1):e6–8.

111. Nof E, Reichlin T, Enriquez AD, et al. Impact of general anesthesia on initiation and stability of VT during catheter ablation. Heart Rhythm 2015;12(11): 2213–20.

112. Mandel JE, Hutchinson MD, Marchlinski FE. Remifentanil-midazolam sedation provides hemodynamic stability and comfort during epicardial ablation of ventricular tachycardia. J Cardiovasc Electrophysiol 2011;22(4):464–6.

113. Nazer B, Woods C, Dewland T, et al. Importance of ventricular tachycardia induction and mapping for patients Referred for epicardial ablation. Pacing Clin Electrophysiol 2015;38(11):1333–42.

114. Sharma PS, Padala SK, Gunda S, et al. Vascular complications during catheter ablation of cardiac arrhythmias: a comparison between vascular ultrasound guided access and Conventional vascular access. J Cardiovasc Electrophysiol 2016;27(10): 1160–6.

115. Sobolev M, Shiloh AL, Di Biase L, et al. Ultrasound-guided cannulation of the femoral vein in electrophysiological procedures: a systematic review and meta-analysis. Europace 2017;19(5):850–5.

116. Bohnen M, Stevenson WG, Tedrow UB, et al. Incidence and predictors of major complications from contemporary catheter ablation to treat cardiac arrhythmias. Heart Rhythm 2011;8(11):1661–6.

117. Han S, Park H-W, Lee YS, et al. Catheter ablation of left ventricular tachycardia through internal jugular vein: refining the continuous line. J Cardiovasc Electrophysiol 2013;24(5):596–9.

118. Singh SM, Neuzil P, Skoka J, et al. Percutaneous transhepatic venous access for catheter ablation procedures in patients with interruption of the inferior vena cava. Circ Arrhythm Electrophysiol 2011; 4(2):235–41.

119. Tilz RR, Makimoto H, Lin T, et al. In vivo left-ventricular contact force analysis: comparison of antegrade transseptal with retrograde transaortic mapping strategies and correlation of impedance and electrical amplitude with contact force. Europace 2014;16(9):1387–95.

120. Ouyang F, Mathew S, Wu S, et al. Ventricular arrhythmias arising from the left ventricular outflow tract below the aortic sinus cusps: mapping and

catheter ablation via transseptal approach and electrocardiographic characteristics. Circ Arrhythm Electrophysiol 2014;7(3):445–55.

121. Pluta S, Lenarczyk R, Pruszkowska-Skrzep P, et al. Transseptal versus transaortic approach for radiofrequency ablation in patients with cardioverter-defibrillator and electrical storm. J Interv Card Electrophysiol 2010;28(1):45–50.

122. Pratola C, Baldo E, Notarstefano P, et al. Feasibility of the transseptal approach for fast and unstable left ventricular tachycardia mapping and ablation with a non-contact mapping system. J Interv Card Electrophysiol 2006;16(2):111–6.

123. Whitman IR, Gladstone RA, Badhwar N, et al. Brain Emboli after left ventricular endocardial ablation. Circulation 2017;135(9):867–77.

124. Hsieh CHC, Thomas SP, Ross DL. Direct transthoracic access to the left ventricle for catheter ablation of ventricular tachycardia. Circ Arrhythm Electrophysiol 2010;3(2):178–85.

125. Li A, Hayase J, Do D, et al. Hybrid surgical vs percutaneous access epicardial ventricular tachycardia ablation. Heart Rhythm 2018;15(4):512–9.

126. Koya T, Watanabe M, Kamada R, et al. Hybrid epicardial ventricular tachycardia ablation with lateral thoracotomy in a patient with a history of left ventricular reconstruction surgery. J Cardiol Cases 2022;25(1):37–41.

127. Soejima K, Nogami A, Sekiguchi Y, et al. Epicardial catheter ablation of ventricular tachycardia in no entry left ventricle: mechanical aortic and mitral valves. Circ Arrhythm Electrophysiol 2015;8(2): 381–9.

128. Vaseghi M, Macias C, Tung R, et al. Percutaneous interventricular septal access in a patient with aortic and mitral mechanical valves: a novel technique for catheter ablation of ventricular tachycardia. Heart Rhythm 2013;10(7):1069–73.

129. Santangeli P, Shaw GC, Marchlinski FE. Radiofrequency wire Facilitated interventricular septal access for catheter ablation of ventricular tachycardia in a patient with aortic and mitral mechanical valves. Circ Arrhythm Electrophysiol 2017;10(1):e004771.

130. Santangeli P, Hyman MC, Muser D, et al. Outcomes of percutaneous trans-right atrial access to the left ventricle for catheter ablation of ventricular tachycardia in patients with mechanical aortic and mitral valves. JAMA Cardiol 2020. https://doi.org/10. 1001/jamacardio.2020.4414.

131. Santangeli P. Right atrium to left ventricle puncture for VT ablation in patients with mechanical aortic and mitral valves: a step-by-step approach. J Cardiovasc Electrophysiol 2022. https://doi.org/ 10.1111/jce.15467.

132. Guandalini GS, Liang JJ, Marchlinski FE. Ventricular tachycardia ablation: past, present, and future

perspectives. JACC Clin Electrophysiol 2019; 5(12):1363–83.

133. Compagnucci P, Volpato G, Falanga U, et al. Recent advances in three-dimensional electroanatomical mapping guidance for the ablation of complex atrial and ventricular arrhythmias. J Interv Card Electrophysiol 2021;61(1):37–43.

134. De Potter T, Iliodromitis K, Bar-On T, et al. Premature ventricular contractions cause a position shift in 3D mapping systems: analysis, quantification, and correction by hybrid activation mapping. Europace 2020;22(4):607–12.

135. Miller JD, Dewland TA, Henrikson CA, et al. Point density exclusion electroanatomic mapping for ventricular arrhythmias arising from endocavitary structures. Heart Rhythm 2020;1(5):394–8.

136. Prabhu MA, Saravanan S, Valaparambil AK, et al. Point density exclusion mapping-A useful tool for mapping arrhythmias arising from the endocavitary structures. J Arrhythm 2021;37(5):1371–3.

137. Stevenson WG, Khan H, Sager P, et al. Identification of reentry circuit sites during catheter mapping and radiofrequency ablation of ventricular tachycardia late after myocardial infarction. Circulation 1993;88(4 Pt 1):1647–70.

138. Stevenson WG, Friedman PL, Sager PT, et al. Exploring postinfarction reentrant ventricular tachycardia with entrainment mapping. J Am Coll Cardiol 1997;29(6):1180–9.

139. Bogun F, Bahu M, Knight BP, et al. Comparison of effective and ineffective target sites that demonstrate concealed entrainment in patients with coronary artery disease undergoing radiofrequency ablation of ventricular tachycardia. Circulation 1997;95(1):183–90.

140. Xie S, Kubala M, Liang JJ, et al. Utility of ripple mapping for identification of slow conduction channels during ventricular tachycardia ablation in the setting of arrhythmogenic right ventricular cardiomyopathy. J Cardiovasc Electrophysiol 2019; 30(3):366–73.

141. Katritsis G, Luther V, Kanagaratnam P, et al. Arrhythmia mechanisms revealed by ripple mapping. Arrhythm Electrophysiol Rev 2018;7(4):261–4.

142. Hoshiyama T, Nagakura T, Kanazawa H, et al. Coherent mapping helps identify abnormal potentials and improves the treatment of multiple ventricular tachycardia: a case report. Heartrhythm Case Rep 2021;7(6):408–12.

143. Sciacca V, Fink T, Bergau L, et al. Combination of high-density and Coherent mapping for ablation of ventricular arrhythmia in patients with structural heart disease. J Clin Med 2022;11(9):2418.

144. Hawson J, Anderson RD, Al-Kaisey A, et al. Functional assessment of ventricular tachycardia circuits and Their underlying substrate using automated conduction velocity mapping. JACC Clin Electrophysiol 2022;8(4):480–94.

145. Marchlinski FE, Callans DJ, Gottlieb CD, et al. Linear ablation lesions for control of unmappable ventricular tachycardia in patients with ischemic and nonischemic cardiomyopathy. Circulation 2000;101(11):1288–96.

146. Soejima K, Suzuki M, Maisel WH, et al. Catheter ablation in patients with multiple and unstable ventricular tachycardias after myocardial infarction: short ablation lines guided by reentry circuit isthmuses and sinus rhythm mapping. Circulation 2001;104(6):664–9.

147. Verma A, Kilicaslan F, Schweikert RA, et al. Short- and long-term success of substrate-based mapping and ablation of ventricular tachycardia in arrhythmogenic right ventricular dysplasia. Circulation 2005;111(24):3209–16.

148. Arenal A, Glez-Torrecilla E, Ortiz M, et al. Ablation of electrograms with an isolated, delayed component as treatment of unmappable monomorphic ventricular tachycardias in patients with structural heart disease. J Am Coll Cardiol 2003;41(1):81–92.

149. Volkmer M, Ouyang F, Deger F, et al. Substrate mapping vs. tachycardia mapping using CARTO in patients with coronary artery disease and ventricular tachycardia: impact on outcome of catheter ablation. Europace 2006;8(11):968–76.

150. Nogami A, Sugiyasu A, Tada H, et al. Changes in the isolated delayed component as an endpoint of catheter ablation in arrhythmogenic right ventricular cardiomyopathy: predictor for long-term success. J Cardiovasc Electrophysiol 2008;19(7):681–8.

151. Garcia FC, Bazan V, Zado ES, et al. Epicardial substrate and outcome with epicardial ablation of ventricular tachycardia in arrhythmogenic right ventricular cardiomyopathy/dysplasia. Circulation 2009;120(5):366–75.

152. Bai R, Di Biase L, Shivkumar K, et al. Ablation of ventricular arrhythmias in arrhythmogenic right ventricular dysplasia/cardiomyopathy: arrhythmia-free survival after endo-epicardial substrate based mapping and ablation. Circ Arrhythm Electrophysiol 2011;4(4):478–85.

153. Vergara P, Trevisi N, Ricco A, et al. Late potentials abolition as an additional technique for reduction of arrhythmia recurrence in scar related ventricular tachycardia ablation. J Cardiovasc Electrophysiol 2012;23(6):621–7.

154. Arenal Á, Hernández J, Calvo D, et al. Safety, long-term results, and predictors of recurrence after complete endocardial ventricular tachycardia substrate ablation in patients with previous myocardial infarction. Am J Cardiol 2013;111(4):499–505.

155. Jaïs P, Maury P, Khairy P, et al. Elimination of local abnormal ventricular activities: a new end point for

substrate modification in patients with scar-related ventricular tachycardia. Circulation 2012;125(18): 2184–96.

156. Komatsu Y, Daly M, Sacher F, et al. Endocardial ablation to eliminate epicardial arrhythmia substrate in scar-related ventricular tachycardia. J Am Coll Cardiol 2014;63(14):1416–26.

157. Komatsu Y, Maury P, Sacher F, et al. Impact of substrate-based ablation of ventricular tachycardia on cardiac mortality in patients with implantable cardioverter-defibrillators. J Cardiovasc Electrophysiol 2015;26(11):1230–8.

158. Wolf M, Sacher F, Cochet H, et al. Long-term outcome of substrate modification in ablation of post-myocardial infarction ventricular tachycardia. Circ Arrhythm Electrophysiol 2018;11(2):e005635.

159. Di Biase L, Burkhardt JD, Lakkireddy D, et al. Ablation of stable VTs versus substrate ablation in ischemic cardiomyopathy: the VISTA randomized multicenter trial. J Am Coll Cardiol 2015;66(25): 2872–82.

160. Gökoğlan Y, Mohanty S, Gianni C, et al. Scar homogenization versus limited-substrate ablation in patients with nonischemic cardiomyopathy and ventricular tachycardia. J Am Coll Cardiol 2016; 68(18):1990–8.

161. Mohanty S, Trivedi C, Di Biase L, et al. Endocardial scar-homogenization with vs without epicardial ablation in VT patients with ischemic cardiomyopathy. JACC Clin Electrophysiol 2022;8(4):453–61.

162. Berruezo A, Fernández-Armenta J, Mont L, et al. Combined endocardial and epicardial catheter ablation in arrhythmogenic right ventricular dysplasia incorporating scar dechanneling technique. Circ Arrhythm Electrophysiol 2012;5(1):111–21.

163. Tung R, Mathuria NS, Nagel R, et al. Impact of local ablation on interconnected channels within ventricular scar: mechanistic implications for substrate modification. Circ Arrhythm Electrophysiol 2013; 6(6):1131–8.

164. Berruezo A, Fernández-Armenta J, Andreu D, et al. Scar dechanneling: new method for scar-related left ventricular tachycardia substrate ablation. Circ Arrhythm Electrophysiol 2015;8(2):326–36.

165. Fernández-Armenta J, Penela D, Acosta J, et al. Substrate modification or ventricular tachycardia induction, mapping, and ablation as the first step? A randomized study. Heart Rhythm 2016; 13(8):1589–95.

166. Andreu D, Penela D, Acosta J, et al. Cardiac magnetic resonance-aided scar dechanneling: Influence on acute and long-term outcomes. Heart Rhythm 2017;14(8):1121–8.

167. Tzou WS, Frankel DS, Hegeman T, et al. Core isolation of critical arrhythmia elements for treatment of multiple scar-based ventricular tachycardias. Circ Arrhythm Electrophysiol 2015;8(2):353–61.

168. Ghannam M, Siontis KC, Kim HM, et al. Stepwise approach for ventricular tachycardia ablation in patients with predominantly intramural scar. JACC Clin Electrophysiol 2020;6(4):448–60.

169. Kitamura T, Martin CA, Vlachos K, et al. Substrate mapping and ablation for ventricular tachycardia in patients with structural heart disease: How to identify ventricular tachycardia substrate. J Innov Card Rhythm Manag 2019;10(3):3565–80.

170. Josephson ME, Anter E. Substrate mapping for ventricular tachycardia: assumptions and misconceptions. JACC Clin Electrophysiol 2015;1(5):341–52.

171. Anter E. Limitations and Pitfalls of substrate mapping for ventricular tachycardia. JACC Clin Electrophysiol 2021;7(4):542–60.

172. Sacher F, Lim HS, Derval N, et al. Substrate mapping and ablation for ventricular tachycardia: the LAVA approach. J Cardiovasc Electrophysiol 2015;26(4):464–71.

173. Santangeli P, Marchlinski FE. Substrate mapping for unstable ventricular tachycardia. Heart Rhythm 2016;13(2):569–83.

174. Cassidy DM, Vassallo JA, Miller JM, et al. Endocardial catheter mapping in patients in sinus rhythm: relationship to underlying heart disease and ventricular arrhythmias. Circulation 1986;73(4):645–52.

175. Frontera A, Melillo F, Baldetti L, et al. High-density characterization of the ventricular electrical substrate during sinus rhythm in post-myocardial infarction patients. JACC Clin Electrophysiol 2020;6(7):799–811.

176. Anter E, Kleber AG, Rottmann M, et al. Infarct-related ventricular tachycardia: Redefining the electrophysiological substrate of the isthmus during sinus rhythm. JACC Clin Electrophysiol 2018; 4(8):1033–48.

177. Tung R. Substrate mapping in ventricular arrhythmias. Card Electrophysiol Clin 2019;11(4):657–63.

178. Jiang R, Beaser AD, Aziz Z, et al. High-density Grid catheter for detailed mapping of sinus rhythm and scar-related ventricular tachycardia: comparison with a linear Duodecapolar catheter. JACC Clin Electrophysiol 2020;6(3):311–23.

179. Cheung JW. Targeting abnormal electrograms for substrate-based ablation of ventricular tachycardia: can We ablate Smarter? JACC Clin Electrophysiol 2020;6(7):812–4.

180. Irie T, Yu R, Bradfield JS, et al. Relationship between sinus rhythm late activation zones and critical sites for scar-related ventricular tachycardia: systematic analysis of isochronal late activation mapping. Circ Arrhythm Electrophysiol 2015;8(2):390–9.

181. Aziz Z, Tung R. Novel mapping strategies for ventricular tachycardia ablation. Curr Treat Options Cardiovasc Med 2018;20(4):34.

182. Aziz Z, Shatz D, Raiman M, et al. Targeted ablation of ventricular tachycardia guided by Wavefront

Discontinuities during sinus rhythm: a new functional substrate mapping strategy. Circulation 2019;140(17):1383–97.

183. Jackson N, Gizurarson S, Viswanathan K, et al. Decrement evoked potential mapping: Basis of a mechanistic strategy for ventricular tachycardia ablation. Circ Arrhythm Electrophysiol 2015;8(6):1433–42.

184. Bhaskaran A, Fitzgerald J, Jackson N, et al. Decrement evoked potential mapping to guide ventricular tachycardia ablation: Elucidating the functional substrate. Arrhythm Electrophysiol Rev 2020;9(4):211–8.

185. Porta-Sánchez A, Jackson N, Lukac P, et al. Multicenter study of ischemic ventricular tachycardia ablation with decrement-evoked potential (DEEP) mapping with Extra stimulus. JACC Clin Electrophysiol 2018;4(3):307–15.

186. Srinivasan NT, Garcia J, Schilling RJ, et al. Multicenter study of Dynamic high-density functional substrate mapping improves identification of substrate targets for ischemic ventricular tachycardia ablation. JACC Clin Electrophysiol 2020;6(14):1783–93.

187. Aryana A, d'Avila A. Contact force during VT ablation: vector orientation is key. Circ Arrhythm Electrophysiol 2014;7(6):1009–10.

188. Jesel L, Sacher F, Komatsu Y, et al. Characterization of contact force during endocardial and epicardial ventricular mapping. Circ Arrhythm Electrophysiol 2014;7(6):1168–73.

189. Ariyarathna N, Kumar S, Thomas SP, et al. Role of contact force sensing in catheter ablation of cardiac arrhythmias: evolution or history repeating itself? JACC Clin Electrophysiol 2018;4(6):707–23.

190. Elbatran AI, Li A, Gallagher MM, et al. Contact force sensing in ablation of ventricular arrhythmias using a 56-hole open-irrigation catheter: a propensity-matched analysis. J Interv Card Electrophysiol 2021;60(3):543–53.

191. Leshem E, Zilberman I, Barkagan M, et al. Temperature-controlled radiofrequency ablation using irrigated catheters: maximizing ventricular lesion Dimensions while reducing Steam-Pop formation. JACC Clin Electrophysiol 2020;6(1):83–93.

192. Nguyen DT, Olson M, Zheng L, et al. Effect of irrigant characteristics on lesion formation after radiofrequency energy delivery using ablation catheters with actively Cooled Tips. J Cardiovasc Electrophysiol 2015;26(7):792–8.

193. Nguyen DT, Tzou WS, Sandhu A, et al. Prospective multicenter experience with Cooled radiofrequency ablation using high impedance irrigant to target deep myocardial substrate refractory to standard ablation. JACC Clin Electrophysiol 2018;4(9):1176–85.

194. Yamada T, Maddox WR, McElderry HT, et al. Radiofrequency catheter ablation of idiopathic ventricular arrhythmias originating from intramural foci in the left ventricular outflow tract: efficacy of sequential versus simultaneous unipolar catheter ablation. Circ Arrhythm Electrophysiol 2015;8(2):344–52.

195. Yang J, Liang J, Shirai Y, et al. Outcomes of simultaneous unipolar radiofrequency catheter ablation for intramural septal ventricular tachycardia in non-ischemic cardiomyopathy. Heart Rhythm 2019;16(6):863–70.

196. Chang RJ, Stevenson WG, Saxon LA, et al. Increasing catheter ablation lesion size by simultaneous application of radiofrequency current to two adjacent sites. Am Heart J 1993;125(5 Pt 1):1276–84.

197. Sivagangabalan G, Barry MA, Huang K, et al. Bipolar ablation of the interventricular septum is more efficient at creating a transmural line than sequential unipolar ablation. Pacing Clin Electrophysiol 2010;33(1):16–26.

198. Koruth JS, Dukkipati S, Miller MA, et al. Bipolar irrigated radiofrequency ablation: a therapeutic option for refractory intramural atrial and ventricular tachycardia circuits. Heart Rhythm 2012;9(12):1932–41.

199. Neira V, Santangeli P, Futyma P, et al. Ablation strategies for intramural ventricular arrhythmias. Heart Rhythm 2020;17(7):1176–84.

200. Aryana A, d'Avila A, Heist EK, et al. Remote magnetic navigation to guide endocardial and epicardial catheter mapping of scar-related ventricular tachycardia. Circulation 2007;115(10):1191–200.

201. Bauernfeind T, Akca F, Schwagten B, et al. The magnetic navigation system allows safety and high efficacy for ablation of arrhythmias. Europace 2011;13(7):1015–21.

202. Aagaard P, Natale A, Briceno D, et al. Remote magnetic navigation: a focus on catheter ablation of ventricular arrhythmias. J Cardiovasc Electrophysiol 2016;27(Suppl 1):S38–44.

203. Xie Y, Liu A, Jin Q, et al. Novel strategy of remote magnetic navigation-guided ablation for ventricular arrhythmias from right ventricle outflow tract. Sci Rep 2020;10(1):17839.

204. Bennett RG, Campbell T, Sood A, et al. Remote magnetic navigation compared to contemporary manual techniques for the catheter ablation of ventricular arrhythmias in structural heart disease. Heliyon 2021;7(12):e08538.

205. Žižek D, Antolič B, Prolič Kalinšek T, et al. Intracardiac echocardiography-guided transseptal puncture for fluoroless catheter ablation of left-sided tachycardias. J Interv Card Electrophysiol 2021;61(3):595–602.

206. Packer DL, Johnson SB, Kolasa MW, et al. New generation of electro-anatomic mapping: full intracardiac ultrasound image integration. Europace 2008;10(Suppl 3):iii35–41.

207. Rossillo A, Indiani S, Bonso A, et al. Novel ICE-guided registration strategy for integration of electroanatomical mapping with three-dimensional CT/MR images to guide catheter ablation of atrial fibrillation. J Cardiovasc Electrophysiol 2009;20(4):374–8.

208. Bunch TJ, Weiss JP, Crandall BG, et al. Image integration using intracardiac ultrasound and 3D reconstruction for scar mapping and ablation of ventricular tachycardia. J Cardiovasc Electrophysiol 2010;21(6):678–84.

209. Hijazi ZM, Shivkumar K, Sahn DJ. Intracardiac echocardiography during interventional and electrophysiological cardiac catheterization. Circulation 2009;119(4):587–96.

210. Qian PC, Tedrow UB. Intracardiac echocardiography to guide catheter ablation of ventricular arrhythmias in ischemic cardiomyopathy. Card Electrophysiol Clin 2021;13(2):285–92.

211. Hanson M, Enriquez A. Intracardiac echocardiography to guide catheter ablation of idiopathic ventricular arrythmias. Card Electrophysiol Clin 2021; 13(2):325–35.

212. Barrett C, Tzou WS. Utility of intracardiac echocardiography for guiding ablation of ventricular tachycardia in nonischemic cardiomyopathy. Card Electrophysiol Clin 2021;13(2):337–43.

213. Campbell T, Haqqani H, Kumar S. Intracardiac echocardiography to guide mapping and ablation of arrhythmias in patients with Congenital heart disease. Card Electrophysiol Clin 2021;13(2):345–56.

214. Field ME, Gold MR, Reynolds MR, et al. Real-world outcomes of ventricular tachycardia catheter ablation with versus without intracardiac echocardiography. J Cardiovasc Electrophysiol 2020;31(2):417–22.

215. Field ME, Goldstein L, Yu Lee SH, et al. Intracardiac echocardiography use and outcomes after catheter ablation of ventricular tachycardia. J Comp Eff Res 2020;9(5):375–85.

216. Kitamura T, Nakajima M, Kawamura I, et al. Safety and effectiveness of intracardiac echocardiography in ventricular tachycardia ablation: a nationwide observational study. Heart Vessels 2021; 36(7):1009–15.

217. Peichl P, Wichterle D, Pavlu L, et al. Complications of catheter ablation of ventricular tachycardia: a single-center experience. Circ Arrhythm Electrophysiol 2014;7(4):684–90.

218. Palaniswamy C, Kolte D, Harikrishnan P, et al. Catheter ablation of postinfarction ventricular tachycardia: ten-year trends in utilization, in-hospital complications, and in-hospital mortality in the United States. Heart Rhythm 2014;11(11):2056–63.

219. Ding WY, Pearman CM, Bonnett L, et al. Complication rates following ventricular tachycardia ablation in ischaemic and non-ischaemic cardiomyopathies: a systematic review. J Interv Card Electrophysiol 2022;63(1):59–67.

220. Santangeli P, Frankel DS, Tung R, et al. Early mortality after catheter ablation of ventricular tachycardia in patients with structural heart disease. J Am Coll Cardiol 2017;69(17):2105–15.

221. Mathew S, Fink T, Feickert S, et al. Complications and mortality after catheter ablation of ventricular arrhythmias: risk in VT ablation (RIVA) score. Clin Res Cardiol 2022;111(5):530–40.

222. Natale A, Mohanty S, Liu PY, et al. Venous vascular closure system versus manual Compression following multiple access electrophysiology procedures: the AMBULATE trial. JACC Clin Electrophysiol 2020;6(1):111–24.

223. Ghannam M, Chugh A, Dillon P, et al. Protamine to expedite vascular hemostasis after catheter ablation of atrial fibrillation: a randomized controlled trial. Heart Rhythm 2018;15(11):1642–7.

224. Aryana A, Tung R, d'Avila A. Percutaneous epicardial approach to catheter ablation of cardiac arrhythmias. JACC Clin Electrophysiol 2020;6(1): 1–20.

225. Siontis KC, Jamé S, Sharaf Dabbagh G, et al. Thromboembolic prophylaxis protocol with warfarin after radiofrequency catheter ablation of infarct-related ventricular tachycardia. J Cardiovasc Electrophysiol 2018;29(4):584–90.

226. Lakkireddy D, Shenthar J, Garg J, et al. Safety/efficacy of DOAC versus aspirin for reduction of risk of Cerebrovascular events following VT ablation. JACC Clin Electrophysiol 2021;7(12):1493–501.

227. Muser D, Hayashi T, Castro SA, et al. Noninvasive programmed ventricular stimulation-guided management following ventricular tachycardia ablation. JACC Clin Electrophysiol 2019;5(6):719–27.

228. Arora S, Atreya AR, Birati EY, et al. Temporary mechanical circulatory support as a bridge to heart transplant or durable left ventricular assist device. Interv Cardiol Clin 2021;10(2):235–49.

229. Vallabhajosyula S, Vallabhajosyula S, Vaidya VR, et al. Venoarterial Extracorporeal membrane oxygenation support for ventricular tachycardia ablation: a systematic review. ASAIO J 2020; 66(9):980–5.

230. Miller MA, Dukkipati SR, Chinitz JS, et al. Percutaneous hemodynamic support with Impella 2.5 during scar-related ventricular tachycardia ablation (PERMIT 1). Circ Arrhythm Electrophysiol 2013;6(1):151–9.

231. Aryana A, Gearoid O'Neill P, Gregory D, et al. Procedural and clinical outcomes after catheter ablation of unstable ventricular tachycardia supported by a percutaneous left ventricular assist device. Heart Rhythm 2014;11(7):1122–30.

232. Turagam MK, Vuddanda V, Atkins D, et al. Hemodynamic support in ventricular tachycardia ablation: an International VT ablation center Collaborative group study. JACC Clin Electrophysiol 2017;3(13):1534–43.

233. Aryana A, d'Avila A, Cool CL, et al. Outcomes of catheter ablation of ventricular tachycardia with mechanical hemodynamic support: an analysis of the Medicare database. J Cardiovasc Electrophysiol 2017;28(11):1295–302.

234. Mathuria N, Wu G, Rojas-Delgado F, et al. Outcomes of pre-emptive and rescue use of percutaneous left ventricular assist device in patients with structural heart disease undergoing catheter ablation of ventricular tachycardia. J Interv Card Electrophysiol 2017;48(1):27–34.

235. Muser D, Castro SA, Liang JJ, et al. Identifying risk and management of acute Haemodynamic decompensation during catheter ablation of ventricular tachycardia. Arrhythm Electrophysiol Rev 2018; 7(4):282–7.

236. Grimaldi M, Marino MM, Vitulano N, et al. Cardiopulmonary support during catheter ablation of ventricular arrhythmias with hemodynamic instability: the role of inducibility. Front Cardiovasc Med 2021;8:747858.

237. Muser D, Liang JJ, Castro SA, et al. Outcomes with prophylactic use of percutaneous left ventricular assist devices in high-risk patients undergoing catheter ablation of scar-related ventricular tachycardia: a propensity-score matched analysis. Heart Rhythm 2018;15(10):1500–6.

238. Santangeli P, Muser D, Zado ES, et al. Acute hemodynamic decompensation during catheter ablation of scar-related ventricular tachycardia: incidence, predictors, and impact on mortality. Circ Arrhythm Electrophysiol 2015;8(1):68–75.

239. Miller L, Birks E, Guglin M, et al. Use of ventricular assist devices and heart transplantation for advanced heart failure. Circ Res 2019;124(11): 1658–78.

240. Galand V, Flécher E, Auffret V, et al. Early ventricular arrhythmias after LVAD implantation is the Strongest predictor of 30-day post-Operative mortality. JACC Clin Electrophysiol 2019;5(8):944–54.

241. Anderson RD, Lee G, Virk S, et al. Catheter ablation of ventricular tachycardia in patients with a ventricular assist device: a systematic review of procedural characteristics and outcomes. JACC Clin Electrophysiol 2019;5(1):39–51.

242. Sacher F, Reichlin T, Zado ES, et al. Characteristics of ventricular tachycardia ablation in patients with continuous flow left ventricular assist devices. Circ Arrhythm Electrophysiol 2015;8(3):592–7.

243. Tilz RR, Lin T, Eckardt L, et al. Ablation outcomes and predictors of mortality following catheter ablation for ventricular tachycardia: data from the German multicenter ablation Registry. J Am Heart Assoc 2018;7(6):e007045.

244. Pothineni NV, Kancharla K, Katoor AJ, et al. Coronary artery injury related to catheter ablation of cardiac arrhythmias: a systematic review. J Cardiovasc Electrophysiol 2019;30(1):92–101.

245. Castaño A, Crawford T, Yamazaki M, et al. Coronary artery pathophysiology after radiofrequency catheter ablation: review and perspectives. Heart Rhythm 2011;8(12):1975–80.

246. Kuck K-H, Schaumann A, Eckardt L, et al. Catheter ablation of stable ventricular tachycardia before defibrillator implantation in patients with coronary heart disease (VTACH): a multicentre randomised controlled trial. Lancet 2010;375(9708):31–40.

247. Buch E, Vaseghi M, Cesario DA, et al. A novel method for preventing phrenic nerve injury during catheter ablation. Heart Rhythm 2007;4(1):95–8.

248. Muser D, Santangeli P, Castro SA, et al. Long-term outcome after catheter ablation of ventricular tachycardia in patients with nonischemic Dilated cardiomyopathy. Circ Arrhythm Electrophysiol 2016;9(10):e004328.

# Improving Outcomes in Ventricular Tachycardia Ablation Using Imaging to Identify Arrhythmic Substrates

Michael Ghannam, MD*, Frank Bogun, MD

## KEYWORDS

- Ventricular tachycardia • Radiofrequency ablation • Computed tomography
- Cardiac magnetic resonance imaging • Nuclear cardiac imaging • Intracardiac echocardiography

## KEY POINTS

- Ventricular tachycardia (VT) ablations have modest acute- and long-term success rates, in part due to the challenges in accurately identifying the arrhythmogenic substrate.
- Multimodality imaging can be integrated with electroanatomic mapping to aid in the planning and execution of ablation procedures and has been shown to improve long-term outcomes.
- Further work is needed to assess the widespread applicability of imaging techniques and to reduce the time and expertise demands these approaches require.

## INTRODUCTION

Ventricular tachycardia (VT) is a complex arrhythmia that may occur in patients with structural heart disease. Catheter ablation is an effective therapy that can reduce the burden of VT and, in patients with incessant arrhythmias, can be a lifesaving therapy. Despite advances in mapping and ablation technology, the procedure is limited by modest success and high recurrence rates[1,2] A major barrier to success is the complex and heterogeneous nature of arrhythmogenic substrate capable of supporting VT circuits. Traditional approaches relying upon electroanatomic mapping alone have limitations in their ability to identify these critical substrates. This is particularly true in patients with apparently normal hearts or minimal structural heart disease, as well as those with non-ischemic cardiomyopathy (NICM). Various imaging modalities including nuclear imaging, computed tomography (CT), and cardiac magnetic resonance (CMR) imaging not only define cardiac anatomy but can characterize the composition of cardiac tissue itself (such as the identification of fibrosis or scar), surrounding structures (epicardial coronary arteries, coronary venous system, phrenic nerves), and tissue innervation properties. The combination of multimodality imaging along with information from electroanatomic mapping allows for a more comprehensive assessment of the arrhythmogenic substrate which facilitates VT ablation. Advanced imaging integration techniques can be used to plan specific ablation lesion sets independently of an electrogram (EGM)-guided approach.

This review will focus on how imaging can be used to guide ablation planning and execution with a focus on clinical applications aimed at improving the outcome of VT ablation procedures.

## VENTRICULAR TACHYCARDIA PATHOPHYSIOLOGY AND CARDIAC SUBSTRATE

Ventricular tachycardia may be due to localized regions of abnormal cardiac tissue (such as in the case of abnormal automaticity or triggered activity)

Division of Cardiovascular Medicine, University of Michigan, 1500 E. Medical Center Dr., SPC5853, Ann Arbor, Michigan 48109-5853, USA
* Corresponding author.
*E-mail address:* mousajab@med.umich.edu

Card Electrophysiol Clin 14 (2022) 609–620
https://doi.org/10.1016/j.ccep.2022.06.009
1877-9182/22/© 2022 Elsevier Inc. All rights reserved.

or abnormal conductive tissue; however, it is more commonly encountered in the setting of structural heart disease which supports reentrant tachycardias.[3] Myocardial fibrosis and scar can create anatomically distinct pathways with different conductive properties. VT circuits can be created through blocked conduction in one pathway and slow propagation through another, which allows recovery of the initially blocked pathway, such that the propagation can occur and enter the other pathway in a retrograde manner. These observations have been supported through histological studies as well as with high-density electroanatomic mapping during VT. Complex VT circuits involve both fixed and functional components. Critical elements of this reentrant circuit may involve endocardial, epicardial, and intramural layers of the myocardium. A substrate modification approach, where all areas with abnormal electrical properties are targeted for ablation, is an effective ablation strategy[3]; however, a more ideal strategy would focus on areas critical to arrhythmogenesis to avoid unnecessary mapping and ablation. The goal of preprocedural imaging is to define the ventricular scar substrate in 3-D to guide the operator toward sites critical for arrhythmogenesis.

## ECHOCARDIOGRAPHY

Real-time intracardiac echocardiography (ICE) can provide detailed information on cardiac anatomy and can be integrated into electroanatomic mapping data. This can be used to facilitate navigation within the heart and to identify intracardiac thrombus that may be overlooked with transthoracic echocardiography.[4] The high-spatial resolution of ICE catheters can identify areas of wall thinning, aneurysmal segments, and areas of dyskinesia/hypokinesia suggestive of underlying

scar and arrhythmic substrate. Myocardial fibrosis leads to an increased reflection of ultrasound, resulting in the bright, hyperechoic images indicative of scar.[5] These feature has been validated in patients with both ischemic cardiomyopathy and NICM[6,7] (Fig. 1).

In a correlative study, Bunch and colleagues were able to demonstrate that both transthoracic and ICE information can identify myocardial segments concordant with EGM-defined scar with high accuracy.[8] ICE has particular utility in accurately classifying basal segments which may not be well visualized with transthoracic imaging. Quantitative assessment of tissue echogenicity on ICE imaging correlates with local bipolar EGMs, allowing for the identification of normal tissue, dense scar, and border zone scar[7] on ICE imaging alone. A retrospective analysis of health billing data suggests that the use of ICE results in reduced rates of VT-related readmission and lower rates of repeat VT ablation procedures among patients undergoing VT ablation.[9] Prospective studies are needed to better understand how ICE can be fully leveraged to improve VT ablation outcomes.

## NUCLEAR CARDIAC IMAGING

Nuclear perfusion imaging can be integrated into electroanatomic mapping to aid in the identification of cardiac scar. Hybrid positron emission tomography (PET)/CT imaging with 18-fluorodeoxyglucose imaging ($^{18}$F-FDG) imaging is highly accurate for discerning viable from scarred myocardium but is limited by relatively poor spatial resolution[10] compared to other modalities. Reports on the correlation between metabolic activity maps and EGM-defined scar have been variable[11]; however, the identification of metabolically active channels has been shown to correlate with VT isthmus sites not identified by voltage

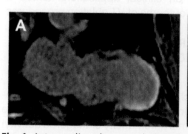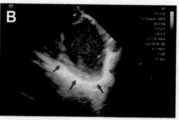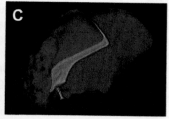

**Fig. 1.** Intracardiac ultrasound identification of ischemic substrate. Cardiac fibrosis and scar lead to an increase in ultrasound reflection compared to healthy myocardium, resulting in bright hyperechoic findings on ICE which can be used to identify the arrhythmogenic substrate. (*A*) Delayed enhancement magnetic resonance (DE-CMR) imaging in a patient with a large left anterior descending artery infarction, demonstrated wall thinning and transmural infarction pattern through the anterior wall, apex, and distal inferior wall. (*B*) An abrupt transition from healthy tissue to scar tissue is seen on ICE imaging, corresponding to DE-CMR findings. (*C*) Electroanatomic mapping during the ablation procedure confirms an aneurysmal apex with low voltage (red indicates local bipolar voltage <0.5mv, purple indicates >1.5 mV).

mapping.[12] Ghzally and colleagues reported on 56 patients with ischemic cardiomyopathy who had [18]F-FDG PET imaging maps overlayed with electroanatomic maps during VT ablation procedures.[13] Metabolic activity maps over-estimated both dense and border zone scar areas defined by electroanatomic mapping, consistent with prior reports. Thirty-one percent of metabolically identified channels were found to harbor clinical VT target sites, and overall, 90% of VT target sites were located at or adjacent to areas of abnormal metabolic activity. Nuclear perfusion imaging with [23]I-meta-iodobenzylguanidine examining cardiac denervation (indicative of ischemic scar) similarly has been shown to over-estimate EGM-defined scar areas,[14] yet has utility in localizing regions where VT target sites may be found. Taken together, nuclear imaging can be used to provide useful information on ischemic VT substrate, albeit with limited anatomic detail and specificity compared to other modalities.

## Cardiac Computed Tomography

Cardiac CT provides a comprehensive anatomic evaluation of cardiac and extra-cardiac structures relevant to VT ablations. Multidetector CT scans (MDCT) provide submillimeter voxel spatial resolution allowing for detailed anatomic reconstructions of ventricular chamber size and morphology. In patients with postinfarction-related VT, MDCT-derived areas of wall thinning correlated with areas of low endocardial voltage as well as the presence of local abnormal ventricular activity (LAVA).[15] A segmental assessment of wall thinning can help rapidly narrow down the area of interest; however, more detailed 3D reconstructions can identify conducting channels present on ridges of preserved tissue thickness within these larger areas[16] (Fig. 2). In a study by Takigawa and colleagues among patients with postinfarction VT, over half of all MDCT-defined channels were found to harbor VT isthmus sites.[17] CT also has excellent utility in identifying myocardial calcifications, which may be present in patients with well-healed myocardial infarctions. Alyesh and colleagues examined 56 patients undergoing ablations for postinfarction-related VT who underwent preprocedure CT scans.[18] Myocardial calcifications were present in 70% of patients and corresponded to areas of unexcitability when overlayed onto electroanatomic maps. Myocardial calcifications represented only a small fraction of the total scar area defined by EGM analysis (0.5 cm2 vs 88 cm2), yet over 35% of mapped VTs were located near areas of myocardial calcifications, often between 2 areas of calcification or another fixed anatomical barrier. Identification of myocardial calcification and ridges with more preserved wall thickness embedded in areas of thinning is beneficial in

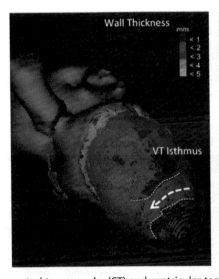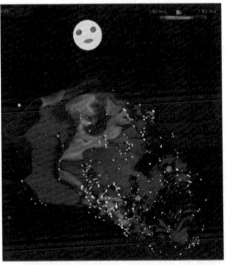

**Fig. 2.** Computed tomography (CT) and ventricular tachycardia (VT) target sites. Computed tomography can provide a detailed topography based on wall-thickness in patients with postinfarction ventricular tachycardia. Left panel demonstrates a color-coded scheme of wall thickness, showing a ridge of tissue with relatively preserved wall thickness in the anterior apical left ventricle. Right panel shows registration with electroanatomic mapping; 2 sites (*yellow tags*) were identified as isthmus target sites through entrainment mapping, VT terminated with ablation along this ridge of tissue. (*From* Ghannam M, Cochet H, Jais P, et al. Correlation between computer tomography-derived scar topography and critical ablation sites in postinfarction ventricular tachycardia. J Cardiovasc Electrophysiol 2018;29:438–45. doi:10.1111/jce.13441; with permission.)

identifying conduction channels within large post-infarction scars and focusing on areas most likely to harbor VT target sites.

Similar to gadolinium-based contrast agents used in delayed enhancement (DE)-CMR, iodinated-based contrast agents display altered diffusion kinetics in the presence of cardiac scar.[19] Accordingly, DE-CT can be used to define anatomic (wall-thinning) and tissue properties consistent with myocardial scar and fibrosis.[20,21] Esposito and colleagues were able to show good agreement between DE-CT derived scars and areas of low-amplitude voltages during VT ablation among patients with both ischemic cardiomyopathy and NICM.[22] DE-CT has also shown to be effective in delineating between endocardial, intramural, and epicardial scar,[22,23] with comparable agreement with delayed enhancement-cardiac magnetic resonance (DE-CMR)[24] (see **Fig. 4**).

During epicardial ablation procedures, cardiac CT can identify the course of structures such as the epicardial coronary arteries and phrenic nerves which may help minimize the risk of injury to these structures.[25] Zeppenfeld and colleagues demonstrated that the epicardial fat pads can also be identified and merged onto electroanatomic maps.[26] The presence of the epicardial fat pads impacts local bipolar EGMs with greater fat thickness leading to more attenuation of EGM amplitude voltage. Identification of the epicardial fat can be critical to avoid the misclassification of the epicardial voltage-defined substrate.[27]

### Delayed Enhancement-Cardiac Magnetic Resonance Imaging

Delayed enhancement-cardiac magnetic resonance (DE-CMR) imaging provides a comprehensive evaluation of cardiac substrate and has important roles in both the diagnostic evaluation of patients with VT.[3] Even among patients with apparently normal hearts and ventricular arrhythmia, DE-CMR can detect intracardiac scar in 25% of cases.[28] DE-CMR has the advantage of not utilizing ionizing radiation which can be an important consideration in patients who will be undergoing lengthy ablation procedures associated with long duration of fluoroscopy. Unlike iodinated contrast agents, gadolinium-based contrast agents are not associated with acute kidney injury[29] and are safer for patients with renal insufficiency. Gadolinium-based agents have been associated with nephrogenic systemic fibrosis (NSF), a debilitating condition that is reported to occur in patients with severe kidney function. New evidence has shown that with the selection of the appropriate type of gadolinium-based agent, the risk of developing NSF in patients with even advanced kidney disease (eGFR<30 mL/min per 1.73 m$^2$) is thought to be very low (<0.07%).[30] Recent consensus statements recommend that the harm of withholding these agents should be balanced against the very low risk of NSF.[31] While DE-CMR does not provide the temporal or spatial resolution of CT or echocardiography, modern imaging protocols can provide an excellent definition (voxel size 1.25 × 1.25 × 2.5 mm).[32]

Delayed enhancement-cardiac magnetic resonance can be performed safely for the vast majority of patients with implantable cardiac defibrillators.[33] With proper protocols, DE-CMR has been shown to be safe in patients with devices and factors traditionally deemed to be contraindications to imaging, such as abandoned leads, battery depletion, or recently implanted devices.[34] Despite this excellent safety profile, metal artifacts from defibrillators remain an issue particularly in the anterior and apical wall segments which are in closer proximity to the pulse generators.[35] With optimized imaging sequencing, metal artifacts from cardiac implantable electronic devices (CIEDs) can be minimized.[36] The use of modified wideband inversion recovery technique was found to eliminate all mild-to-moderate instances of metal artifact and substantially reduced the volume of severe artifact compared to traditional sequencing in patients with CIEDs undergoing preablation VT planning.[37]

### Delayed Enhancement-Cardiac Magnetic Resonance Scar Localization

DE-CMR is the gold standard for noninvasive identification of cardiac scar and can accurately detail the location, transmurality, and the extent of scar in ischemic cardiomyopathy and nonischemic cardiomyopathies.[38–40] Scar identification relies on the altered uptake and washout properties of gadolinium-based contrast agents in regions of myocardial fibrosis, allowing for enhancement in areas of scaring with a "nulling" or blackening out of normal myocardium.[41] DE-CMR is more sensitive than DE-CT for scar detection[42] and has superior contrast resolution compared to DE-CT.[19] Multiple studies have demonstrated that VT isthmus sites in both ischemic cardiomyopathy and nonischemic cardiomyopathies colocalize to regions of gadolinium uptake.[11] Additionally, the volume of abnormal tissue can be quantified with DE-CMR based on the voxel signal-intensity of contrast uptake, allowing for the identification of dense scar and border zone scar intermixed with healthy and fibrotic tissue.[43] Larger border zone scar sizes have been associated with higher rates of ventricular arrhythmias in patients with ischemic cardiomyopathy and NICM[44] and are more likely to contain VT target sites during ablation procedures.[45]

The localization of cardiac scar has major implications for patients with NICM undergoing ablation procedures. The presence of epicardial scar is a major contribution to the failure of endocardial ablation procedures. Routine use of an endocardial and epicardial approach may not improve ablation outcomes in mixed populations of patients with NICM undergoing ablation[46]; however, the use of a combined approach in patients with epicardial scar identified on DE-CMR may improve ablation outcomes.[47] Percutaneous epicardial ablation is associated with increased procedural risks compared to an endocardial only approach[46] but should be considered if imaging findings demonstrate an epicardial substrate. Alternatively, DE-CMR may identify patients whose epicardial substrate is accessible from the coronary venous system (CVS) and who may not require percutaneous epicardial approaches. Patients with NICM often have a basal-predominant scar pattern accessible through the CVS. In a series of 41 patients with NICM undergoing VT ablation with preprocedure DE-CMR, patients with and without VT ablation targets in the CVS were examined.[48] No patient characteristics, including overall scar size, were associated with the presence of CVS VT targets;

however, the proximity of the scar to the CVS and its tributaries was strongly associated with the presence of such targets. A minimum distance of 9 mm from the CVS to the border zone regions of scar best predicted the presence of CVS VT (**Fig. 3**).

Identification of intramural scar on DE-CMR can aid in procedural planning. Intramural scar is often encountered in patients with NICM but is present among patients with postinfarction VT as well.[49] Identification of intramural scar based on EGMs alone has limitations; traditional bipolar cut-off valves (1.5 mV) will not reliably identify intramural scar.[50] Unipolar EGM analysis may improve detection, but the optimal cut-off values are not well defined and there is a large overlap of unipolar low voltage areas with DE-CMR-defined scar vs areas without DE-CMR-defined scar.[51,52] In these patients, a DE-CMR-based approach to ablation may improve outcomes over ablation based solely upon electroanatomic mapping data (**Fig. 4**). Our study examining this approach included 42 patients with intramural scar on preprocedural imaging who underwent a stepwise ablation approach with ablation targeted initially through conventional mapping criteria. Among patients who remained inducible for VT after this approach, additional ablation was performed in regions with intramural scar identified on overlayed DE-CMR images. Patients with this image-guided approach had improved arrhythmia-free survival compared

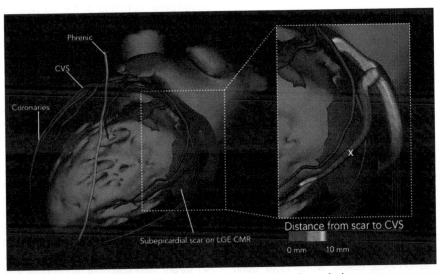

**Fig. 3.** Identification of ventricular tachycardia ablation sites accessible through the coronary venous system. Delayed enhancement CMR imaging is shown in a patient with subepicardial scar (*light blue*) along with reconstructions of the endocardium (*gray*) and the coronary venous system (CVS) (*dark blue*). A color-coded map is shown in the insert panel, displaying the proximity between a lateral branch of the CVS and the arrhythmogenic substrate. In this patient, ventricular tachycardia target sites were accessible through the CVS without the need for subxiphoid epicardial access. (*From* Ghannam M, Siontis KC, Cochet H, et al. Value of mapping and ablation of ventricular tachycardia targets within the coronary venous system in patients with nonischemic cardiomyopathy. Heart Rhythm 2020;17:520–6. doi:10.1016/j.hrthm.2020.01.010; with permission.)

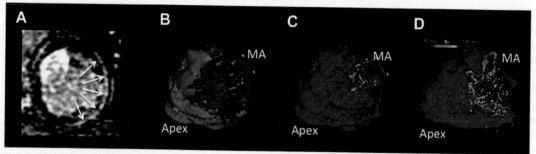

**Fig. 4.** Intramural scar and ventricular tachycardia (VT) ablation. (*A*): Delayed enhancement cardiac magnetic resonance imaging (DE-CMR) identified intramural scar prior to ventricular tachycardia ablation (*white arrows*). (*B*): The scar was then registered to the electroanatomic map during the ablation procedure. (*C*): Bipolar mapping was performed demonstrating preserved voltage overlaying the scar area at a cut-off of 1.5 mV. After an ablation targeting conventional electrogram-based targets, the patient remained inducible for VT. (*D*): an extensive ablation was performed targeting scar based on DE-CMR registration in areas of preserved bipolar voltage. After this approach, the patient was no longer inducible for VT. (*From* Ghannam M, Siontis KC, Kim HM, et al. Stepwise Approach for Ventricular Tachycardia Ablation in Patients With Predominantly Intramural Scar. JACC Clin Electrophysiol 2020;6:448–60. doi:10.1016/j.jacep.2019.11.020; with permission.)

to a historic cohort without image guidance.[45] Additionally, patients with larger volumes of deeper-seated scar, particularly scar deeper than 5 mm from the endocardial surface, had worse arrhythmia-free survival as this substrate was difficult to target even with combined endo and epicardial approaches. DE-CMR may, therefore, be helpful in identifying patients who require adjunctive ablation measures, such as bipolar ablation, simultaneous unipolar ablation, or alcohol-based ablation.[53]

## RIGHT VENTRICULAR SCAR LOCALIZATION

Delayed enhancement-cardiac magnetic resonance has allowed for the characterization of the right ventricular (RV) substrate which has implications for VT originating in this chamber. Patients with arrhythmogenic right ventricular cardiomyopathy (ARVC) display fibrofatty infiltration primarily affected by the epicardial layers[54] which creates anisotropic conduction and the substate for VT.[55] DE-CMR plays a critical role in the diagnosis of this condition but can also yield information useful during ablation procedures. In a series of 10 patients with ARVC undergoing epicardial ablation for VT, the location of DE-CMR-defined scar closely correlated with regions of low EGM voltage. Regions of DE-CMR were also highly specific for areas containing late-potentials on local EGMs, which have been shown to be highly important targets for patients with VT related to ARVC.[56] Imaging the thin walled and mobile RV with DE-CMR remains challenging, with some investigators reporting that nearly half of electrically defined endocardial scar is not confirmed by DE-CMR in patients with ARVC who undergo ablation procedures.[57] Incorporation of

RV strain imaging to identify contractile abnormalities associated with RV scar along with DE-CMR imaging has been shown to further increase the ability to identify VT target sites.[58]

## ASSESSING POSTABLATION LESION FORMATION

VT recurrence or arrhythmia exacerbation after an ablation procedure is associated with poor long-term outcomes.[59] Poor lesion formation and incomplete targeting of the arrhythmic substrate can result in recurrence of a previously seen VT; however, new scar formed through successful ablation lesions may also contribute to new VT circuits.[60] Successful ablation lesions result in changes in the myocardium that evolve from acute inflammation and edema to a chronic phase consistent with microvascular obstruction and scar deposition.[61–63] When imaged in the chronic postablation phase, DE-CMR can identify areas of successful ablation lesions which can help guide repeat ablation procedures (see **Fig. 4**). In patients with postinfarction-related VT undergoing repeat ablation procedures, prior ablation sites may manifest as a dark confluent structure located upon areas of contrast enhancement representing native scar.[62] These sites correlate with areas of noninducibility and are often in close proximity to VT target sites and may function as a fixed border for new or modified reentry circuits.[64,65] In contrast, Ilg and colleagues demonstrated that ablation lesions in patients without structural heart disease manifest hyper-enhancement consistent with scar deposition.[66] Other studies have shown that a transition from a dark-core (microvascular obstruction) to a hyper-enhanced region (scar deposition) can occur with serial DE-CMR imaging.[63] More work is needed to define the optimal timing and imaging protocols to identify postablation lesions (**Fig. 5**).[67]

## T1-WEIGHTED IMAGING

DE-CMR relies upon regional differences in tissue gadolinium contrast uptake to identify cardiac scarring. In patients with NICM and diffuse fibrotic disease, the relative differences in uptake may not reach a critical threshold for detection and will appear as "normal" nonenhanced regions, despite the presence of fibrotic tissue with arrhythmogenic potential.[68–70] T1 mapping allows for the identification of myocardial extracellular collagen and fibrosis in a quantitative manner[71] and identification of fibrosis has implications for VT ablation procedures. Muser and colleagues examined 51 patients with NICM and no evidence of DE-CMR-defined scar who underwent ablation procedures for VT.[72] Patients in this series had a septal predominant scar pattern, and the average midseptal T1 measurements were correlated with the extent of EGM-defined scar as well as long-term ablation outcomes. Patients with more extensive fibrosis on T1 mapping were found to have larger abnormal electrical substrates and worse long-term arrhythmia outcomes. While this technique lacks precise anatomic correlation, T1 mapping may provide further procedural and prognostic

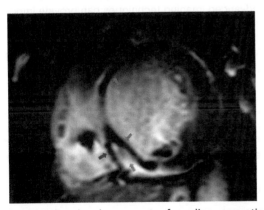

**Fig. 5.** Delayed enhancement of cardiac magnetic resonance and postablation lesions. Ablation lesions may be identified on delayed enhancement cardiac magnetic resonance (DE-CMR). DE-CMR imaging is shown three weeks postablation. The intrinsic intramural scar appears as bright, contrast-enhanced segments seen throughout the septum (*green arrow*). A dark confluent core consistent with ablation lesions is seen throughout the left ventricle endocardium (*blue arrows*). Ablation was also performed from the right ventricle (RV) to target the deep-seated intramural scar and appears as a dark confluent core along the RV septum (*red arrow*).

information among this challenging population undergoing VT ablation.

## T2-WEIGHTED IMAGING

Acute myocardial inflammation can be assessed with T2-weighted images[73] which also has applications for planning VT ablations. Ventricular arrhythmias can complicate the acute and chronic phases of myocarditis. Patients in the chronic phase of myocarditis present with scar-related VT similar to other forms of structural heart disease. Maccabelli and colleagues examined 26 patients with VT and a remote history of myocarditis who underwent preprocedure DE-CMR.[74] Nearly all patients displayed basal-mid inferolateral scarring in an epicardial and intramural distribution pattern, correlating with findings on endocardial and epicardial mapping. No patients in this series had inflammatory findings on T2-weighted imaging, and 77% of patients remained arrhythmia free after a median of 23 months follow-up. In contrast, Pretto and colleagues enrolled 125 patients with myocarditis undergoing ablation including patients in the acute phase (n = 47) and chronic phase (n = 78) of myocarditis, assessed through multimodality imaging and myocardial biopsy. T2-weighted sequencing on CMR demonstrated myocardial inflammation in all patients with acute-phase myocarditis and in no patients in the chronic phase.[75] Ablation during the acute phase was associated with a greater recurrence than during ablation in the chronic phase (HR 9.5, 95%CI 2.6–35.3, P < 0.001). Similarly, T2-weighted sequences can be used to identify patients with active versus chronic cardiac sarcoidosis.[76] A recent multicenter study demonstrated that patients with active inflammation related to cardiac sarcoidosis have higher rates of postablation VT recurrence.[59] In patients with sarcoidosis and active inflammation, acute treatment with immunosuppressive agents and antiarrhythmics should be considered prior to ablation procedures.[3]

## MAGNETIC RESONANCE IMAGING-DEFINED CONDUCTION CHANNELS

Reentrant VT in structural heart disease is supported by strands of surviving myocardium within a larger scar architecture.[77] These channels consist of living myocardial cells interspersed with fibrotic tissue within regions of denser scar and these channels localize at border zone regions of DE-CMR-defined scar reflective of this heterogeneous tissue.[78–80] Numerous groups have used high-resolution DE-CMR to recreate the 3D structure of conduction channels and more precisely define critical VT targets.[81,82] Conduction channels with intramural or transmural paths are associated with higher rates of VT occurrence postablation, highlighting the importance of assessing arrhythmia substrate multidimensionally.[83]

Several clinical series have evaluated the efficacy and safety of ablation based on DE-CMR-defined conduction channels.[58,84] Andreu and colleagues examined 159 patients undergoing scar-related VT ablations, including 54 patients who underwent a scar dechanneling approach where DE-CMR identified conducting channels were targeted, followed by a more extensive ablation only if a patient remained inducible for arrhythmias.[85] Conducting channels identified on imaging were confirmed with electro-anatomical data. Compared to patients undergoing ablation without image guidance, a DE-CMR-guided approach resulted in fewer RF applications (28 ± 18 vs 36 ± 18) yet greater rates of acute noninducibility (68% vs 44%, P = 0.02) and lower arrhythmia recurrence (18.5% vs 43.8% over a 20 ± 19 months follow-up time, log-rank P = 0.027). Similarly, Soto-Iglesias compared an ablation strategy targeting DE-CMR-identified conduction channels to an EGM-based channel ablation approach in patients with scar-related VT.[86] Patients who underwent either imaging aided (ablation of conduction channels defined through the integration of imaging and electroanatomic mapping) or imaging guided (ablation based on imaging only) had shorter procedure and RF times with improved arrhythmia-free survival compared to the standard ablation group. These studies support the use of imaging to create tailored ablation plans that minimize excessive energy delivery yet have equal or improved outcomes compared to traditional approaches. Unfortunately, the spatial resolution of DE-CMR is limited and identification of these channels requires high-quality studies without artifacts limiting the applicability of this technique in patients with CIEDs.

## ADDITIVE VALUE OF IMAGING AND FUTURE DIRECTIONS

Multiple prospective reports support the use of imaging to improve ablation outcomes over traditional approaches.[45,58,86,87] Siontis and colleagues examined consecutive patients with NICM undergoing VT ablation to a historical cohort without image guidance.[88] The use of imaging resulted in shorter ablation procedures and was independently associated with improved procedural success. A meta-analysis by Henriks and colleagues examined 7748 patients with ischemic VT undergoing either imaging assisted or a traditional ablation approach.[89] Image-guided ablation was associated with a greater VT-

free survival (82% interquartile range (IQR)[75-87] vs 59% IQR[53-63]) over a mean follow-up of 35 months.

Despite progress in imaging quality and accuracy in identifying the arrhythmogenic substrate, there remain many areas for improvement. Specialized equipment and expertise are required both to attain high-quality images and to perform the postimaging reprocessing required for many of the techniques described above. Automated methods of scar reconstruction may help improve procedural workflow and increase the accessibility of these approaches.[90] Imaging incurs additional costs, risks, and inconvenience to patients and cost-benefit analysis of image-guided approaches are lacking. Critically, no randomized controlled trials comparing imaging versus standard ablation approaches have been performed, underscoring the need for further investigation. Future developments in high-resolution cross-sectional imaging may help to further define critical ablation targets prior to electroanatomic mapping. Finally, accurate identification of arrhythmogenic substrate of the RV remains challenging and is the subject of active research.

## SUMMARY

Multimodality imaging can readily identify arrhythmogenic substrate in patients with VT and aid in the planning and execution of ablation procedures. Beyond regional identification of scar, advanced imaging techniques can provide important prognostic information and help create tailored ablation approaches preprocedurally. While randomized controlled trials are lacking, prospective studies have shown that incorporating imaging into ablation workflow may improve safety, reduce procedural and ablation time, and improve ablation outcomes. Further work is needed to assess the widespread applicability of these techniques, and to reduce the time and expertise requirements these approaches require.

## CLINICS CARE POINTS

- Preprocedural imaging is beneficial for planning and executing ventricular tachycardia ablation procedures, particularly in patients with non-ischemic cardiomyopathy who can have complex arrhythmia substrates.

- It is critical to engage in a shared decision-making conversation with patients so they can understand the risks and benefits of these additional pre-procedural steps.

# REFERENCES

1. Tung R, Vaseghi M, Frankel DS, et al. Freedom from recurrent ventricular tachycardia after catheter ablation is associated with improved survival in patients with structural heart disease: an International VT Ablation Center Collaborative Group study. Heart Rhythm 2015;12:1997–2007.

2. Dinov B, Fiedler L, Schönbauer R, et al. Outcomes in catheter ablation of ventricular tachycardia in dilated nonischemic cardiomyopathy compared with ischemic cardiomyopathy. Circulation 2014;129:728–36.

3. Cronin EM, Bogun FM, Maury P, et al. 2019 HRS/EHRA/APHRS/LAHRS expert consensus statement on catheter ablation of ventricular arrhythmias: executive summary. J Arrhythmia 2020;36:1–58.

4. Beavers DL, Ghannam M, Liang J, et al. Diagnosis, significance, and management of ventricular thrombi in patients referred for VT ablation. J Cardiovasc Electrophysiol 2021;32:2473–83.

5. Picano E, Pelosi G, Marzilli M, et al. In Vivo quantitative ultrasonic evaluation of myocardial fibrosis in humans. Circulation 1990;81:58–64.

6. Bala R, Ren J-F, Hutchinson MD, et al. Assessing epicardial substrate using intracardiac echocardiography during VT ablation. Circ Arrhythm Electrophysiol 2011;4:667–73.

7. Hussein A, Jimenez A, Ahmad G, et al. Assessment of ventricular tachycardia scar substrate by intracardiac echocardiography. Pacing Clin Electrophysiol 2014;37:412–21.

8. Bunch TJ, Weiss JP, Crandall BG, et al. Image integration using intracardiac ultrasound and 3D reconstruction for scar mapping and ablation of ventricular tachycardia. J Cardiovasc Electrophysiol 2010;21:678–84.

9. Field ME, Gold MR, Reynolds MR, et al. Real-world outcomes of ventricular tachycardia catheter ablation with versus without intracardiac echocardiography. J Cardiovasc Electrophysiol 2020;31:417–22.

10. Pichler BJ, Wehrl HF, Judenhofer MS. Latest advances in molecular imaging instrumentation. J Nucl Med 2008;49:5S–23S.

11. Mahida S, Sacher F, Dubois R, et al. Cardiac imaging in patients with ventricular tachycardia. Circulation 2017;136:2491–507.

12. Dickfeld T, Lei P, Dilsizian V, et al. Integration of three-dimensional scar maps for ventricular tachycardia ablation with positron emission tomography-computed tomography. JACC Cardiovasc Imaging 2008;1:73–82.

13. Ghzally Y, Imanli H, Smith M, et al. Metabolic scar assessment with18F-FDG PET: correlation to ischemic ventricular tachycardia substrate and successful ablation sites. J Nucl Med Off Publ Soc Nucl Med 2021;62:1591–8.

14. Klein T, Abdulghani M, Smith M, et al. Three-dimensional 123I-meta-iodobenzylguanidine cardiac innervation maps to assess substrate and successful ablation sites for ventricular tachycardia: feasibility study for a novel paradigm of innervation imaging. Circ Arrhythm Electrophysiol 2015;8:583–91.

15. Komatsu Y, Cochet H, Jadidi A, et al. Regional myocardial wall thinning at multidetector computed tomography correlates to arrhythmogenic substrate in postinfarction ventricular tachycardia: assessment of structural and electrical substrate. Circ Arrhythm Electrophysiol 2013;6:342–50.

16. Ghannam M, Cochet H, Jais P, et al. Correlation between computer tomography-derived scar topography and critical ablation sites in postinfarction ventricular tachycardia. J Cardiovasc Electrophysiol 2018;29:438–45.

17. Takigawa M, Duchateau J, Sacher F, et al. Are wall thickness channels defined by computed tomography predictive of isthmuses of postinfarction ventricular tachycardia? Heart Rhythm 2019;16:1661–8.

18. Alyesh DM, Siontis KC, Sharaf Dabbagh G, et al. Postinfarction myocardial calcifications on cardiac computed tomography: implications for mapping and ablation in patients with nontolerated ventricular tachycardias. Circ Arrhythm Electrophysiol 2019;12:e007023.

19. Rodriguez-Granillo GA. Delayed enhancement cardiac computed tomography for the assessment of myocardial infarction: from bench to bedside. Cardiovasc Diagn Ther 2017;7:159–70.

20. Shiozaki AA, Senra T, Arteaga E, et al. Myocardial fibrosis detected by cardiac CT predicts ventricular fibrillation/ventricular tachycardia events in patients with hypertrophic cardiomyopathy. J Cardiovasc Comput Tomogr 2013;7:173–81.

21. Zhao L, Ma X, Feuchtner GM, et al. Quantification of myocardial delayed enhancement and wall thickness in hypertrophic cardiomyopathy: multidetector computed tomography versus magnetic resonance imaging. Eur J Radiol 2014;83:1778–85.

22. Esposito A, Palmisano A, Antunes S, et al. Cardiac CT with delayed enhancement in the characterization of ventricular tachycardia structural substrate: relationship between CT-segmented scar and electro-anatomic mapping. JACC Cardiovasc Imaging 2016;9:822–32.

23. Ustunkaya T, Desjardins B, Wedan R, et al. Epicardial conduction speed, electrogram abnormality, and computed tomography attenuation associations in arrhythmogenic right ventricular cardiomyopathy. JACC Clin Electrophysiol 2019;5:1158–67.

24. Aikawa T, Oyama-Manabe N, Naya M, et al. Delayed contrast-enhanced computed tomography in patients with known or suspected cardiac sarcoidosis: a feasibility study. Eur Radiol 2017;27:4054–63.

25. Yamashita S, Sacher F, Mahida S, et al. Role of high-resolution image integration to visualize left phrenic nerve and coronary arteries during epicardial ventricular tachycardia ablation. Circ Arrhythm Electrophysiol 2015;8:371–80.

26. van Huls van Taxis CF, Wijnmaalen AP, Piers SR, et al. Real-time integration of MDCT-derived coronary anatomy and epicardial fat: impact on epicardial electroanatomic mapping and ablation for ventricular arrhythmias. JACC Cardiovasc Imaging 2013;6:42–52.

27. Desjardins B, Morady F, Bogun F. Effect of epicardial fat on electroanatomical mapping and epicardial catheter ablation. J Am Coll Cardiol 2010;56:1320–7.

28. White JA, Fine NM, Gula L, et al. Utility of cardiovascular magnetic resonance in identifying substrate for malignant ventricular arrhythmias. Circ Cardiovasc Imaging 2012;5:12–20.

29. Faucon A-L, Bobrie G, Clément O. Nephrotoxicity of iodinated contrast media: from pathophysiology to prevention strategies. Eur J Radiol 2019;116:231–41.

30. Woolen SA, Shankar PR, Gagnier JJ, et al. Risk of nephrogenic systemic fibrosis in patients with stage 4 or 5 chronic kidney disease receiving a group II gadolinium-based contrast agent: a systematic review and meta-analysis. JAMA Intern Med 2020;180:223–30.

31. Weinreb JC, Rodby RA, Yee J, et al. Use of intravenous gadolinium-based contrast media in patients with kidney disease: consensus statements from the american college of radiology and the national kidney foundation. Radiology 2021;298:28–35.

32. Hennig A, Salel M, Sacher F, et al. High-resolution three-dimensional late gadolinium-enhanced cardiac magnetic resonance imaging to identify the underlying substrate of ventricular arrhythmia. Europace 2018;20:f179–91.

33. Indik JH, Gimbel JR, Abe H, et al. 2017 HRS expert consensus statement on magnetic resonance imaging and radiation exposure in patients with cardiovascular implantable electronic devices. Heart Rhythm 2017;14:e97–153.

34. Horwood L, Attili A, Luba F, et al. Magnetic resonance imaging in patients with cardiac implanted electronic devices: focus on contraindications to magnetic resonance imaging protocols. Europace 2017;19:812–7.

35. Mesubi O, Ahmad G, Jeudy J, et al. Impact of ICD artifact burden on late gadolinium enhancement cardiac MR imaging in patients undergoing ventricular tachycardia ablation. Pacing Clin Electrophysiol 2014;37:1274–83.

36. Ibrahim E-SH, Runge M, Stojanovska J, et al. Optimized cardiac magnetic resonance imaging inversion recovery sequence for metal artifact reduction and accurate myocardial scar assessment in patients with cardiac implantable electronic devices. World J Radiol 2018;10:100–7.

37. Runge M, Ibrahim E-SH, Bogun F, et al. Metal artifact reduction in cardiovascular MRI for accurate myocardial scar assessment in patients with cardiac implantable electronic devices. AJR Am J Roentgenol 2019;213:555–61.

38. Kim RJ, Fieno DS, Parrish TB, et al. Relationship of MRI delayed contrast enhancement to irreversible injury, infarct age, and contractile function. Circulation 1999;100:1992–2002.

39. Karamitsos TD, Francis JM, Myerson S, et al. The role of cardiovascular magnetic resonance imaging in heart failure. J Am Coll Cardiol 2009;54:1407–24.

40. Berruezo A, Penela D, Jáuregui B, et al. The role of imaging in catheter ablation of ventricular arrhythmias. Pacing Clin Electrophysiol 2021;44:1115–25.

41. Nelson T, Garg P, Clayton RH, et al. The role of cardiac MRI in the management of ventricular arrhythmias in ischaemic and non-ischaemic dilated cardiomyopathy. Arrhythmia Electrophysiol Rev 2019;8:191–201.

42. Bettencourt N, Ferreira ND, Leite D, et al. CAD detection in patients with intermediate-high pre-test probability. JACC Cardiovasc Imaging 2013;6:1062–71.

43. Aquaro GD, Pingitore A, Strata E, et al. Cardiac magnetic resonance predicts outcome in patients with premature ventricular complexes of left bundle branch block morphology. J Am Coll Cardiol 2010;56:1235–43.

44. Scott PA, Rosengarten JA, Curzen NP, et al. Late gadolinium enhancement cardiac magnetic resonance imaging for the prediction of ventricular tachyarrhythmic events: a meta-analysis. Eur J Heart Fail 2013;15:1019–27.

45. Ghannam M, Siontis KC, Kim HM, et al. Stepwise approach for ventricular tachycardia ablation in patients with predominantly intramural scar. JACC Clin Electrophysiol 2020;6:448–60.

46. Romero J, Cerrud-Rodriguez RC, Di Biase L, et al. Combined endocardial-epicardial versus endocardial catheter ablation alone for ventricular tachycardia in structural heart disease: a systematic review and meta-analysis. JACC Clin Electrophysiol 2019;5:13–24.

47. Bogun FM, Desjardins B, Good E, et al. Delayed-enhanced magnetic resonance imaging in nonischemic cardiomyopathy: utility for identifying the ventricular arrhythmia substrate. J Am Coll Cardiol 2009;53:1138–45.

48. Ghannam M, Siontis KC, Cochet H, et al. Value of mapping and ablation of ventricular tachycardia targets within the coronary venous system in patients

with nonischemic cardiomyopathy. Heart Rhythm 2020;17:520–6.

49. Chopra N, Tokuda M, Ng J, et al. Relation of the unipolar low-voltage penumbra surrounding the endocardial low-voltage scar to ventricular tachycardia circuit sites and ablation outcomes in ischemic cardiomyopathy. J Cardiovasc Electrophysiol 2014;25:602–8.

50. Spears DA, Suszko AM, Dalvi R, et al. Relationship of bipolar and unipolar electrogram voltage to scar transmurality and composition derived by magnetic resonance imaging in patients with nonischemic cardiomyopathy undergoing VT ablation. Heart Rhythm 2012;9:1837–46.

51. Benoit D, Miki Y, Good E, et al. Characteristics of intramural scar in patients with nonischemic cardiomyopathy and relation to intramural ventricular arrhythmias. Circ Arrhythm Electrophysiol 2013;6:891–7.

52. Park J, Desjardins B, Liang JJ, et al. Association of scar distribution with epicardial electrograms and surface ventricular tachycardia QRS duration in nonischemic cardiomyopathy. J Cardiovasc Electrophysiol 2020;31:2032–40.

53. Neira V, Santangeli P, Futyma P, et al. Ablation strategies for intramural ventricular arrhythmias. Heart Rhythm 2020;17(7):1176–84.

54. Tabib A, Loire R, Chalabreysse L, et al. Circumstances of death and gross and microscopic observations in a series of 200 cases of sudden death associated with arrhythmogenic right ventricular cardiomyopathy and/or dysplasia. Circulation 2003;108:3000–5.

55. Tandri H, Saranathan M, Rodriguez ER, et al. Noninvasive detection of myocardial fibrosis in arrhythmogenic right ventricular cardiomyopathy using delayed-enhancement magnetic resonance imaging. J Am Coll Cardiol 2005;45:98–103.

56. Kirubakaran S, Bisceglia C, Silberbauer J, et al. Characterization of the arrhythmogenic substrate in patients with arrhythmogenic right ventricular cardiomyopathy undergoing ventricular tachycardia ablation. EP Eur 2017;19:1049–62.

57. Marra MP, Leoni L, Bauce B, et al. Imaging study of ventricular scar in arrhythmogenic right ventricular cardiomyopathy: comparison of 3D standard electroanatomical voltage mapping and contrast-enhanced cardiac magnetic resonance. Circ Arrhythm Electrophysiol 2012;5:91–100.

58. Zghaib T, Ipek EG, Hansford R, et al. Standard ablation versus magnetic resonance imaging-guided ablation in the treatment of ventricular tachycardia. Circ Arrhythm Electrophysiol 2018;11:e005973.

59. Siontis KC, Santangeli P, Muser D, et al. Outcomes associated with catheter ablation of ventricular tachycardia in patients with cardiac sarcoidosis. JAMA Cardiol 2022;7:175–83.

60. Yokokawa M, Desjardins B, Crawford T, et al. Reasons for recurrent ventricular tachycardia after catheter ablation of post-infarction ventricular tachycardia. J Am Coll Cardiol 2013;61:66–73.

61. Tao S, Guttman MA, Fink S, et al. Ablation lesion characterization in scarred substrate assessed using cardiac magnetic resonance. JACC Clin Electrophysiol 2019;5:91–100.

62. Dabbagh GS, Ghannam M, Siontis KC, et al. Magnetic resonance mapping of catheter ablation lesions after post-infarction ventricular tachycardia ablation. JACC Cardiovasc Imaging 2021;14:588–98.

63. Vunnam R, Maheshwari V, Jeudy J, et al. Ventricular arrhythmia ablation lesions detectability and temporal changes on cardiac magnetic resonance. Pacing Clin Electrophysiol 2020;43:314–21.

64. Ghannam M, Liang J, Attili A, et al. Late gadolinium enhancement cardiac magnetic resonance imaging of ablation lesions after postinfarction ventricular tachycardia ablation: implications for ventricular tachycardia recurrence. J Cardiovasc Electrophysiol;n/a. doi:10.1111/jce.15386.

65. Soejima K, Stevenson WG, Maisel WH, et al. Electrically unexcitable scar mapping based on pacing threshold for identification of the reentry circuit isthmus: feasibility for guiding ventricular tachycardia ablation. Circulation 2002;106:1678–83.

66. Ilg K, Baman TS, Gupta SK, et al. Assessment of radiofrequency ablation lesions by CMR imaging after ablation of idiopathic ventricular arrhythmias. JACC Cardiovasc Imaging 2010;3:278–85.

67. Dickfeld T, Vunnam R. Chronic ablation lesions on CMR: is black a red herring? JACC Cardiovasc Imaging 2021;14:599–601.

68. Iles L, Pfluger H, Lefkovits L, et al. Myocardial fibrosis predicts appropriate device therapy in patients with implantable cardioverter-defibrillators for primary prevention of sudden cardiac death. J Am Coll Cardiol 2011;57:821–8.

69. Puntmann VO, Carr -White G, Jabbour A, et al. T1-mapping and outcome in nonischemic cardiomyopathy. JACC Cardiovasc Imaging 2016;9:40–50.

70. Gulati A, Jabbour A, Ismail TF, et al. Association of fibrosis with mortality and sudden cardiac death in patients with nonischemic dilated cardiomyopathy. JAMA 2013;309:896–908.

71. Iles L, Pfluger H, Phrommintikul A, et al. Evaluation of diffuse myocardial fibrosis in heart failure with cardiac magnetic resonance contrast-enhanced T1 mapping. J Am Coll Cardiol 2008;52:1574–80.

72. Muser D, Nucifora G, Castro SA, et al. Myocardial substrate characterization by CMR T1 mapping in patients with NICM and No LGE undergoing catheter ablation of VT. JACC Clin Electrophysiol 2021;7:831–40.

73. Messroghli DR, Moon JC, Ferreira VM, et al. Clinical recommendations for cardiovascular magnetic resonance mapping of T1, T2, T2* and extracellular volume: a consensus statement by the Society for Cardiovascular Magnetic Resonance (SCMR) endorsed by the European Association for Cardiovascular Imaging (EACVI). J Cardiovasc Magn Reson 2017;19:1–24.

74. Maccabelli G, Tsiachris D, Silberbauer J, et al. Imaging and epicardial substrate ablation of ventricular tachycardia in patients late after myocarditis. EP Eur 2014;16:1363–72.

75. Peretto G, Sala S, Basso C, et al. Inflammation as a predictor of recurrent ventricular tachycardia after ablation in patients with myocarditis. J Am Coll Cardiol 2020;76:1644–56.

76. Kaur D, Roukoz H, Shah M, et al. Impact of the inflammation on the outcomes of catheter ablation of drug-refractory ventricular tachycardia in cardiac sarcoidosis. J Cardiovasc Electrophysiol 2020;31:612–20.

77. de Bakker JM, van Capelle FJ, Janse MJ, et al. Slow conduction in the infarcted human heart. "Zigzag" course of activation. Circulation 1993;88:915–26.

78. Ashikaga H, Sasano T, Dong J, et al. Magnetic resonance-based anatomical analysis of scar-related ventricular tachycardia: implications for catheter ablation. Circ Res 2007;101:939–47.

79. Desjardins B, Crawford T, Good E, et al. Infarct architecture and characteristics on delayed enhanced magnetic resonance imaging and electroanatomic mapping in patients with postinfarction ventricular arrhythmia. Heart Rhythm 2009;6:644–51.

80. Piers SRD, Tao Q, de Riva Silva M, et al. CMR-based identification of critical isthmus sites of ischemic and nonischemic ventricular tachycardia. JACC Cardiovasc Imaging 2014;7:774–84.

81. Fernández-Armenta J, Berruezo A, Andreu D, et al. Three-dimensional architecture of scar and conducting channels based on high resolution ce-CMR. Circ Arrhythm Electrophysiol 2013;6:528–37.

82. Perez-David E, Arenal A, Rubio-Guivernau JL, et al. Noninvasive identification of ventricular tachycardia-related conducting channels using contrast-enhanced magnetic resonance imaging in patients with chronic myocardial infarction: comparison of signal intensity scar mapping and endocardial voltage mapping. J Am Coll Cardiol 2011;57:184–94.

83. Quinto L, Sanchez P, Alarcón F, et al. Cardiac magnetic resonance to predict recurrences after ventricular tachycardia ablation: septal involvement, transmural channels, and left ventricular mass. Europacer 2021;23:1437–45.

84. Roca-Luque I, Van Breukelen A, Alarcon F, et al. Ventricular scar channel entrances identified by new wideband cardiac magnetic resonance sequence to guide ventricular tachycardia ablation in patients with cardiac defibrillators. Europace 2020;22:598–606.

85. Andreu D, Penela D, Acosta J, et al. Cardiac magnetic resonance–aided scar dechanneling: influence on acute and long-term outcomes. Heart Rhythm 2017;14:1121–8.

86. Soto-Iglesias D, Penela D, Jáuregui B, et al. Cardiac magnetic resonance-guided ventricular tachycardia substrate ablation. JACC Clin Electrophysiol 2020;6:436–47.

87. Berte B, Cochet H, Dang L, et al. Image-guided ablation of scar-related ventricular tachycardia: towards a shorter and more predictable procedure. J Interv Card Electrophysiol Int J Arrhythm Pacing 2020;59:535–44.

88. Siontis KC, Kim HM, Sharaf Dabbagh G, et al. Association of preprocedural cardiac magnetic resonance imaging with outcomes of ventricular tachycardia ablation in patients with idiopathic dilated cardiomyopathy. Heart Rhythm 2017;14:1487–93.

89. Hendriks AA, Kis Z, Glisic M, et al. Pre-procedural image-guided versus non-image-guided ventricular tachycardia ablation-a review. Neth Heart J 2020;28:573–83.

90. Merino-Caviedes S, Gutierrez LK, Alfonso-Almazán JM, et al. Time-efficient three-dimensional transmural scar assessment provides relevant substrate characterization for ventricular tachycardia features and long-term recurrences in ischemic cardiomyopathy. Sci Rep 2021;11:18722.

# Techniques for Catheter Ablation of Idiopathic Ventricular Arrhythmias Originating from the Outflow Tract and Left Ventricular Summit

Takumi Yamada, MD, PhD

## KEYWORDS

- Left ventricular summit • Radiofrequency catheter ablation • Ventricular outflow tract
- Ventricular arrhythmia

## KEY POINTS

- The anatomy of the ventricular outflow tract is complex, and some ventricular arrhythmia (VA) origins are intramural and epicardial.
- Meticulous mapping in multiple different locations such as the right and left ventricular outflow tracts (RVOT/LVOT), endocardial and epicardial sites, and above and below the aortic and pulmonic valves may be required to achieve successful catheter ablation of VAs arising from this region.
- Sequential and simultaneous unipolar radiofrequency ablation from the LVOT and great cardiac vein (GCV) as well as endocardial ablation using an anatomic approach can improve the outcome of catheter ablation of intramural LVOT VAs and left ventricular summit VAs, respectively.
- Accurate recognition of the anatomy of this region is essential for the prevention of complications associated with catheter ablation.

## INTRODUCTION

The ventricular outflow tracts are the most common sites of origins of idiopathic ventricular arrhythmias (VAs).[1–11] The VAs arising from these regions are being increasingly recognized as targets for catheter ablation.[1–13] Advances in electrophysiology and the technologies of catheter ablation, combined with a better understanding of the complex cardiac anatomy of the ventricular outflow tracts, have improved the outcome of catheter ablation of these VAs.[1–13] In this article, techniques for catheter ablation of outflow tract VAs are discussed.

### Anatomic Background

The right and left ventricular outflow tracts (RVOT and LVOT) are located anatomically next to each other.[5,14] The right ventricular (RV) muscle extends epicardially above the pulmonary valves onto the pulmonary artery, and idiopathic VAs can originate from both the supravalvular and infravalvular regions in the RVOT. On the other hand, the superior end of the left ventricular (LV) muscle attaches to the aortic sinus of Valsalva (ASV), which is located between the aortic valve annulus and sinotubular ridge and never extends onto the aorta.[4,5] Therefore, idiopathic VAs

Cardiovascular Division, University of Minnesota, 420 Delaware Street SE, MMC 508, Minneapolis, MN 55455, USA
E-mail address: takumi-y@fb4.so-net.ne.jp

Card Electrophysiol Clin 14 (2022) 621–631
https://doi.org/10.1016/j.ccep.2022.07.008
1877-9182/22/© 2022 Elsevier Inc. All rights reserved.

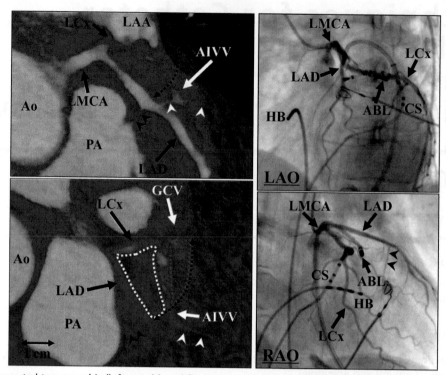

**Fig. 1.** Computed tomographic (left panels) and fluoroscopic (right panels) images exhibiting the summit of the LV. The LV summit was defined based on the fluoroscopy and coronary angiography as the region on the epicardial surface of the LV near the bifurcation of the left main coronary artery that is bounded by an arc (*black dotted line*) from the left anterior descending coronary artery (LAD), superior to the first septal perforating branch (*black arrowheads*), anteriorly to the left circumflex coronary artery (LCx), and then laterally along the LCx. The great cardiac vein (GCV) bisects the LV summit into the superior portion surrounded by the white dotted line (the inaccessible area) and the inferior portion surrounded by the red dotted line (the accessible area). The white arrowheads indicate the first diagonal branch of the LAD. The ablation catheter is positioned in the accessible area and a decapolar catheter in the GCV. ABL, ablation catheter; AIVV, anterior interventricular cardiac vein; Ao, aorta; CS, coronary sinus; HB, his bundle; LAA, left atrial appendage; LAO, left anterior oblique; LMCA, left main coronary artery; PA, pulmonary artery; RAO, right anterior oblique. (*Adapted from* Yamada T, McElderry HT, Doppalapudi H, Okada T, Murakami Y, Yoshida Y, Yoshida N, Inden Y, Murohara T, Plumb VJ, Kay GN. Idiopathic ventricular arrhythmias originating from the left ventricular summit: anatomic concepts relevant to ablation. Circ Arrhythm Electrophysiol 2010;3:616-623.; with permission.)

originating from the ASV can be ablated from the aortic sinus cusps (ASCs).

The muscle wall of the LVOT is thick, and idiopathic VAs can originate from the endocardial, intramural, and epicardial locations in the LVOT.[15] A region of the LV epicardial surface that lies anterior and superior to the aortic portion of the LV ostium occupies the most superior portion of the LV and has been termed the LV summit by McAlpine.[14] In clinical electrophysiology, the LV summit has been defined by Yamada and colleagues[9] based on fluoroscopy and coronary angiography as the region on the epicardial surface of the LV near the bifurcation of the left main coronary artery that is bounded by an arc from the left anterior descending coronary artery superior to the first septal perforating branch anteriorly, and extending to the left circumflex coronary artery laterally (**Fig. 1**).

Thus, the LV summit is fan-shaped with the distance from the bifurcation of the left coronary arteries to the first septal perforator being its radius. This region is one of the common sites of epicardial idiopathic VA origins. The main trunk of the great cardiac vein (GCV) bisects the LV summit into an upper portion that is not accessible to epicardial catheter ablation due to the close proximity to the proximal left coronary arteries and thick overlying epicardial fat (the *inaccessible area*) and a lower portion that may be accessible to epicardial catheter ablation (the *accessible area*).[9] The left atrial appendage may sometimes override the accessible area (see **Fig. 1**) and disturb the epicardial mapping in this area.[9] On the other hand, endocardial mapping within the left atrial appendage might provide a lot of useful information for identifying the sites of the VA origins in the accessible

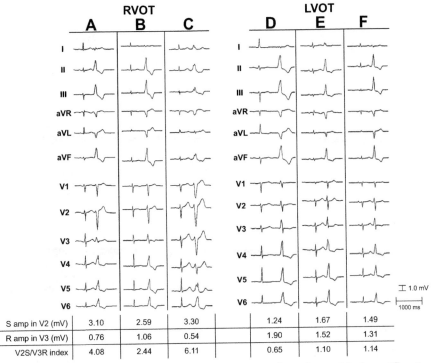

| | RVOT | | | LVOT | | |
| --- | --- | --- | --- | --- | --- | --- |
| | A | B | C | D | E | F |
| S amp in V2 (mV) | 3.10 | 2.59 | 3.30 | 1.24 | 1.67 | 1.49 |
| R amp in V3 (mV) | 0.76 | 1.06 | 0.54 | 1.90 | 1.52 | 1.31 |
| V2S/V3R index | 4.08 | 2.44 | 6.11 | 0.65 | 1.10 | 1.14 |

**Fig. 2.** Representative surface electrocardiograms of VAs originating from the ventricular outflow tract. The first beat is a sinus beat and the second is a premature ventricular contraction (PVC) in each panel (A–F). The S-wave amplitude in lead $V_2$, R-wave amplitude in lead $V_3$, and $V_2S/V_3R$ index are listed below each panel. All RVOT PVCs exhibited a $V_2S/V_3R$ index of greater than 1.5, whereas all LVOT PVCs exhibited a $V_2S/V_3R$ index of less than or equal to 1.5. The PVCs were successfully ablated in the RVOT septum (A and B), RVOT free wall (C), left coronary cusp (D), right coronary cusp (E), and aortomitral continuity (F). (*From* Yoshida N, Yamada T, McElderry HT, Inden Y, Shimano M, Murohara T, Kumar V, Doppalapudi H, Plumb VJ, Kay GN. A novel electrocardiographic criterion for differentiating a left from right ventricular outflow tract tachycardia origin: the V2S/V3R index. J Cardiovasc Electrophysiol 2014;25:747-753.; with permission.)

area of the LV summit by recording a far-field ventricular electrogram from that area.[16]

## Preprocedural Planning

Preprocedural planning of the mapping and catheter ablation approach is important to save procedural time and reduce costs and complications. The preprocedural planning is usually based on the electrocardiographic characteristics, which are helpful for predicting the site of the VA origins in these regions.[2–5,17,18] The most important diagnosis to make by an electrocardiogram may be whether the VAs originate from the right or left side. A right bundle branch block (RBBB) QRS morphology clearly suggests a VA origin on the left side. When a left bundle branch block (LBBB) QRS morphology is observed, it is often difficult to predict whether the VA originates from the right or left side. Because the LVOT is anatomically located posterior to the RVOT, LVOT VAs exhibit a taller and wider R wave in the right precordial leads than RVOT VAs. Therefore, the precordial

transition zone is helpful for predicting whether a VA originates from the RVOT or LVOT. A precordial transition of later than or equal to lead $V_4$ most likely predicts an RVOT VA origin, whereas a precordial transition of earlier than or equal to lead $V_2$ predicts an LVOT VA origin. When there is a precordial transition in lead $V_3$, it is the most difficult to predict whether it is an RVOT or LVOT VA origin. Several electrocardiographic algorithms to predict RVOT or LVOT VA origins have been proposed, and the $V_2S/V_3R$ ratio (**Fig. 2**)[18] seems to be the most accurate and useful among them, which is calculated by dividing the S wave amplitude in lead $V_2$ by the R wave amplitude in lead $V_3$ (see **Fig. 2**).[18] Ratios of the $V_2S/V_3R$ of greater than 1.5 and less than or equal to 1.5 predict RVOT and LVOT VA origins, respectively. This electrocardiographic algorithm has been proved to be useful in VAs with a precordial transition in lead $V_3$. The presence of "notching" in the middle of the QRS complex strongly suggests a VA origin on the RVOT free wall. The presence of S waves in lead $V_6$ may suggest a VA origin in the endocardial

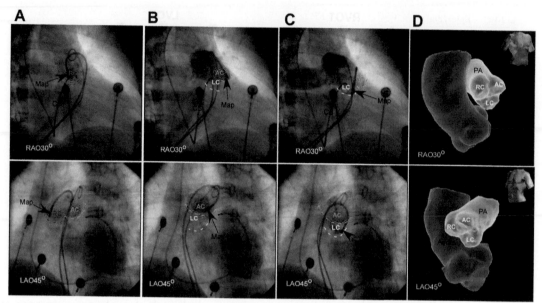

**Fig. 3.** Pulmonary sinus cusp anatomy and catheter positions. In the fluoroscopic images (*A–C*), the pulmonary artery angiograms demonstrated that the ablation catheter was looped and positioned within the pulmonary cusps with a "reversed U-curve technique." (*D*) Three-dimensional computed tomographic images of the pulmonary sinus cusps. AC, anterior cusp; CS, coronary sinus; LAO, left anterior oblique; Map, mapping catheter; PA, pulmonary artery; RAO, right anterior oblique; RC, right cusp. (*From* Liao Z, Zhan X, Wu S, Xue Y, Fang X, Liao H, Deng H, Liang Y, Wei W, Liu Y, Ouyang F. Idiopathic Ventricular Arrhythmias Originating From the Pulmonary Sinus Cusp: Prevalence, Electrocardiographic/Electrophysiological Characteristics, and Catheter Ablation. J Am Coll Cardiol. 2015;66:2633-2644.; with permission.)

LV below the aortic valve. A qrS pattern in the right precordial leads may be highly specific for a VA origin at the junction between the left and right ASCs.[3]

The electrocardiographic features for whether VAs can be successfully ablated from the endocardial or epicardial side are also important to recognize. The maximum deflection index (MDI), which is calculated by dividing the shortest time from the QRS onset to the maximum deflection in any precordial lead by the QRS duration and ratio of the Q wave amplitude in leads aVL to aVR (aVL/aVR ratio) may be helpful for making such a diagnosis.[9,17] An MDI of greater than 0.55 and aVL/aVR ratio of greater than 1.4 suggest that VAs may be ablated epicardially.

## Procedure

### Electrophysiological study

In patients with premature ventricular contractions (PVCs), the 12-lead surface electrocardiograms of clinical PVCs should be recorded before sedation is initiated because sedation may sometimes suppress PVCs. For mapping and pacing, a quadripolar catheter is positioned via the right femoral vein in the His bundle (HB) region, and a decapolar catheter in the coronary sinus (see **Fig. 1**). The decapolar catheter is advanced into the GCV as

far as possible until the proximal electrode pair records an earlier ventricular activation than the most distal electrode pair during the VAs. When this is impossible or further mapping within small branches of the GCV is required, a multielectrode microcatheter can be used for mapping within these veins. When PVCs are infrequent, induction of PVCs is attempted by burst ventricular pacing with the addition of an isoproterenol infusion.

### Mapping

Mapping catheters placed in the HB region and GCV can provide a lot of useful information for identifying the site of a VA origin before mapping with an ablation catheter. When the activation time during the VAs is compared between the HB region and GCV, an earlier ventricular activation in the HB or GCV would suggest that the VAs are likely to originate from the right or left side, respectively. When a presystolic ventricular activation is recorded from those mapping catheters during VAs, pace maps from those catheters can be performed and used as a reference for further mapping.

When VAs present with an RBBB QRS morphology, mapping in the LVOT and ASCs should be performed from the beginning. However, in patients with an LBBB QRS morphology,

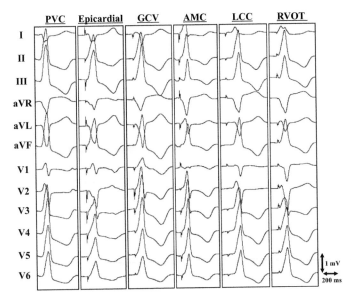

| PVC | Epicardial | GCV | AMC | LCC | RVOT |

I
II
III
aVR
aVL
aVF
V1
V2
V3
V4
V5
V6

1 mV
200 ms

**Fig. 4.** Comparison of the 12-lead electrocardiograms between the PVCs arising from the inaccessible area of the LV summit and pace maps from various right and left ventricular outflow tract locations. Note that pacing from any endocardial or epicardial sites never produced an excellent pace map especially with higher amplitudes of the R waves in the inferior leads. (*From* Yamada T, McElderry HT, Doppalapudi H, Okada T, Murakami Y, Yoshida Y, Yoshida N, Inden Y, Murohara T, Plumb VJ, Kay GN. Idiopathic ventricular arrhythmias originating from the left ventricular summit: anatomic concepts relevant to ablation. Circ Arrhythm Electrophysiol 2010;3:616-623.; with permission.)

mapping in the RV first should be recommended because a preprocedural electrocardiographic diagnosis is imperfect. Activation mapping seeking the earliest bipolar activity and/or a local unipolar QS pattern during VAs is the most reliable for identifying the site of the VA origin. When activation mapping reveals an early ventricular activation in the distal RVOT, mapping above the pulmonary valves should be performed to seek an earlier ventricular activation. The pulmonary sinus cusps can be mapped by a standard technique, but a "reversed U-curve technique" with an ablation catheter looped above the pulmonary valves may facilitate mapping within the pulmonary sinus cusps (**Fig. 3**).[19]

Pace mapping may be helpful for roughly localizing the site of the VA origin when VAs are infrequent. Pace mapping is especially helpful for RVOT VAs,[10,11] but may be less helpful for ASV VAs because pacing in the ASCs may not exactly reproduce the QRS morphology of the VAs because of preferential conduction[6] or the inability to obtain myocardial capture despite the use of a high pacing current. A comparison of the pace maps from the right and left side may predict whether a VA origin can be ablated from the RV or LV (**Fig. 4**). When an earlier precordial transition during VAs cannot be reproduced by pace mapping from the RV, the VA origin is likely to be located in the LV. A comparison of the pace maps from the ASCs, endocardial LVOT, and GCV by using the MDI as well as the pace map score may predict whether a VA origin can be ablated from the endocardial or epicardial side (see **Fig. 4**). When the MDI during VAs is closer to that during pace mapping

from the GCV than that during pace mapping from the ASCs and LVOT, the VA origin is likely to be located on the epicardial surface. The pace map score is determined as the number of leads with an identical height of the R wave/depth of the S wave (R/S) ratio match (12 represents a perfect R/S ratio match in all 12 leads), as well as the number of leads with a fine notching match in the 12-lead electrocardiogram as previously reported (a perfect pace mapping is equal to 24 points). An excellent pace map is defined as a pace map that obtains a score of greater than 20. The pace map score can also be automatically calculated with a computer software by comparing the paced QRS complex with a template of the spontaneous VA morphology. A greater than 90% overall match should usually be recorded at successful ablation sites. This computer software also can provide a matching score and display the detailed difference between the paced QRS complex and spontaneous VA morphology by overlaying them for each of the 12 leads. This information would be helpful for deciding where to map next to obtain a better matching score.

### Catheter ablation
When the earliest ventricular activation in the RV precedes the QRS onset by more than 20 milliseconds and is earlier than that recorded in the GCV, radiofrequency (RF) catheter ablation may be performed at that site when the pace map highly matches the QRS complex of the clinical VAs (**Fig. 5**). When there are no sites with early activation in the RV, or when RV catheter ablation is unsuccessful, mapping in the ASCs and LVOT should

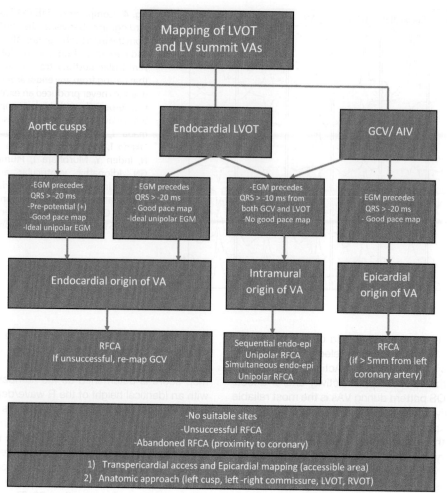

**Fig. 5.** Mapping and ablation of LVOT and LV summit VAs. EGM, electrogram; RFCA, radiofrequency catheter ablation.

follow. When the earliest ventricular activation preceding the QRS onset is recorded in the HB region, mapping in the right coronary and noncoronary cusps (NCCs) and LVOT below those ASCs should be performed before the ablation despite a highly matched pace map in the HB region.[7,10] A far-field presystolic ventricular electrogram recorded in the HB region during the VAs may suggest left-sided VA origins (**Fig. 6**).[7] If presystolic ventricular activation is recorded within those ASCs during the VAs, RF catheter ablation within those ASCs should be attempted first. Even when a ventricular activation within those ASCs is later than that in the HB region, RF catheter ablation within those ASCs is often successful with a much lower risk of damage to the atrioventricular conduction. Because the posterior portion of the RVOT is in close apposition to the LV near the aortic root, when catheter ablation has not been successful in the LVOT, the RVOT including

the pulmonary artery should be carefully remapped before determining that an epicardial approach is required.

Before mapping and catheter ablation above the aortic valve, selective angiography of the coronary artery and aorta should be performed to determine the coronary artery ostium in the ASCs, to precisely define the location of the ablation catheter and to avoid arterial injury (**Fig. 7**).[4,5] The 3 ASCs can be readily identified during biplane aortography or coronary angiography. The left coronary cusp (LCC) is most easily identified in the left anterior oblique (LAO) projection where this cusp is on the far lateral aspect of the aortic root, leftward and superior to the HB catheter (see **Fig. 7**A). The right coronary cusp (RCC) usually requires coronary angiography in both the right anterior oblique (RAO) and LAO projections for an accurate identification of the cusp relative to the right coronary artery (RCA) ostium (see **Fig. 7**B). In the RAO

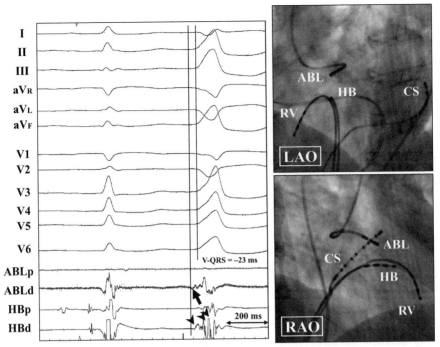

**Fig. 6.** Successful ablation site of a PVC within the right coronary cusp. During the PVC, a far-field electrogram (*single arrowhead*) preceding the QRS onset by 18 milliseconds and the following near-field electrogram (*double arrowheads*) were observed in the HB region. The local ventricular electrogram at the successful ablation site (*arrow*) preceded the QRS onset by 23 milliseconds. Note that the ablation catheter was located close to the HB catheter. ABL(HB) d(p), the distal (proximal) electrode pair of the ablation (His) catheter; RV, right ventricle; V-QRS, local ventricular activation time relative to QRS onset. (*From* Yamada T, McElderry HT, Doppalapudi H, Kay GN. Catheter Ablation of Ventricular Arrhythmias Originating from the Vicinity of the His Bundle: Significance of Mapping of the Aortic Sinus Cusp. Heart Rhythm 2008;5:37–42.; with permission.)

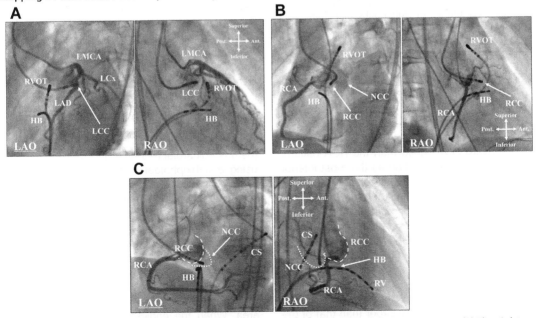

**Fig. 7.** Coronary angiograms and the catheter positions. (*A*) The left main coronary angiogram. (*B*) The right coronary angiograms. (*C*) The right coronary angiograms with the ablation catheter within the NCC. Note that the typical site of the catheter ablation of ventricular arrhythmias arising from the LCC and RCC is at the nadir of those cusps. LCC, left coronary cusp; NCC, noncoronary cusp; RCA, right coronary artery; RCC, right coronary cusp. (*From* Yamada T, Litovsky SH, Kay GN: The left ventricular ostium: an anatomic concept relevant to idiopathic ventricular arrhythmias. Circ Arrhythmia Electrophysiol 2008;1:396-404.; with permission.)

projection, the ablation catheter is typically located anterior and inferior to the RCA ostium. In the LAO projection, the typical ablation site is more leftward in the cusp than the RCA ostium. The NCC is readily identified as the most inferior of the 3 cusps and by its close relation to the HB catheter. In the RAO projection (see **Fig. 7**C), a catheter in the NCC is posterior and inferior to the RCA ostium, just above the HB catheter. In the LAO projection (see **Fig. 7**C), the NCC is just superior to the HB catheter. Intracardiac echocardiography may also be useful for identifying the site of the ablation catheter. Because the NCC overlies the atrial septum, the amplitude of the atrial electrogram is usually larger than that of the ventricular electrogram within the NCC.

When the earliest ventricular activation in the ASCs and endocardial LVOT precedes the QRS onset by more than 20 milliseconds and is earlier than that within the GCV, RF catheter ablation may be performed at that site. A ventricular prepotential preceding the QRS onset is often recorded within the ASCs during VAs, and it may suggest a successful ablation site (see **Fig. 6**). When endocardial catheter ablation is unsuccessful or the local ventricular activation during the VAs is earlier in the GCV than at any endocardial site, those VAs are suggested to originate from nonendocardial foci. When the local ventricular activation within the GCV precedes the QRS onset by more than 20 milliseconds and pacing from the earliest ventricular activation site within the GCV produces an excellent match to the QRS complex of the VAs, RF catheter ablation within the GCV is attempted if the left coronary angiogram assures a safe distance (>5 mm) between the presumed ablation site and left coronary artery.

When a presystolic ventricular activation preceding the QRS onset by greater than 10 milliseconds is recorded from both the endocardial LVOT and GCV, the VA origins may be suggested to be located in the middle between those structures (intramural LVOT origins).[20,21] Several specific electrophysiological features suggest intramural LVOT VA origins (**Box 1**).[20] Intramural LVOT VAs are usually eliminated by irrigated unipolar RF current applied sequentially from endocardial and epicardial sides.[20,21] However, when it is unsuccessful, a simultaneous delivery of an irrigated unipolar RF current to both the endocardial and epicardial sides using 2 ablation catheters and 2 RF generators may be considered (**Fig. 8**).[20,21]

When endocardial or transvenous epicardial mapping cannot identify a suitable site for catheter ablation of VAs or when the RF ablation within the GCV or anterior interventricular vein fails to eliminate the VAs or is abandoned due to close proximity to the coronary arteries and high impedance, alternative options should be considered to ablate those LV summit VAs.[9,15] One of them is epicardial mapping and catheter ablation using a subxiphoidal transpericardial approach. During this epicardial mapping, the mapping catheter within the GCV is helpful as a landmark, and epicardial mapping is performed around the site with the earliest ventricular activation within the GCV. Because the inaccessible area of the LV summit is covered with a thick fat pad, far-field electrograms are usually recorded, the local impedance is high, and pacing even with a maximal output may not capture the ventricular myocardium in this area. When the earliest ventricular activation is recorded in the inaccessible area, catheter ablation is usually abandoned because of the close proximity to the left coronary arteries or the efficacy of the RF energy delivery is usually limited because of an epicardial thick fat pad. When the earliest

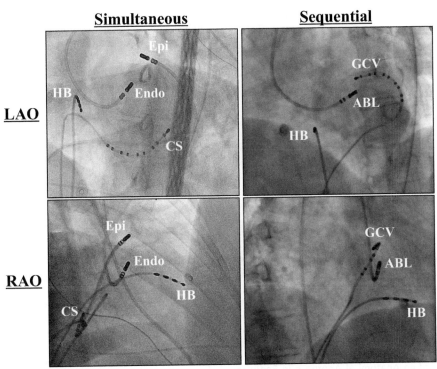

**Fig. 8.** Fluoroscopic images exhibiting the ablation sites. Note that the distance between the endocardial and epicardial ablation sites is greater in the case requiring a simultaneous ablation than in the case with a successful sequential ablation. Endo, endocardial ablation catheter; Epi, epicardial ablation catheter positioned within the GCV. (*From* Yamada T, Maddox WR, McElderry HT, Doppalapudi H, Plumb VJ, Kay GN. Radiofrequency catheter ablation of idiopathic ventricular arrhythmias originating from intramural foci in the left ventricular outflow tract: efficacy of sequential versus simultaneous unipolar catheter ablation. Circ Arrhythm Electrophysiol. 2015;8:344-352.; with permission.)

ventricular activation is recorded in the accessible area, catheter ablation should be attempted if the site is located more than 5 mm away from the coronary arteries. In the accessible area with lesser fat pad, catheter ablation may be effective even at the site with far-field electrograms.

The other option is a catheter ablation by an anatomic approach.[15,22] In this approach, RF catheter ablation at an endocardial site remote from the LV summit VA origins is expected to create an RF lesion large enough to reach those VA origins (**Fig. 9**). Anatomically, the endocardial structures adjacent to the LV summit include the LCC, junction between the LCC and RCC, LVOT including the aortomitral continuity, and RVOT (see **Fig. 1**). Endocardial catheter ablation of LV summit VAs by the anatomic approach can be successful at any of these locations, but the most successful location of this ablation should be determined based on the mapping results and anatomic consideration.

In the current practice, an irrigated ablation catheter may be routinely used for catheter ablation of VAs. Irrigated RF current is delivered in the power

control mode starting at 30 W for endocardial ablation, 20 W in the GCV, and 30 W on the epicardial surface with an irrigation flow rate of 15 to 30 mL/min. The RF power is titrated to as high as 50, 30, and 50 W, respectively, with the goal being to achieve a decrease in the impedance of 8 to 10 $\Omega$ and with care taken to limit the temperature to less than 41°C. High RF energy should not be applied to the RVOT or ASCs, because such an application could cause a perforation of the free wall of the RVOT or damage to the aortic valve. Selective angiography of the coronary artery should be performed before ablation within the ASCs and epicardial catheter ablation using transvenous and transpericardial approaches to ensure the location of the ablation catheter relative to the coronary arteries. Intracardiac echocardiography might also be helpful as a guide to keep the ablation catheter in a stable location, and to avoid complications, especially during ablation near the coronary arteries. Calcifications of the coronary arteries in older patients might also facilitate the delineation of the ostia of these vessels. RF ablation should never be delivered within 5 mm of any part of the

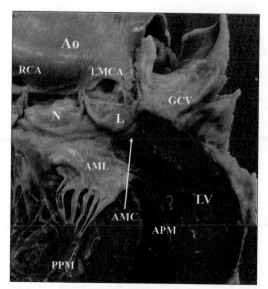

**Fig. 9.** An autopsy heart exhibiting the left ventricular outflow tract. AMC, aortomitral continuity; AML, anterior mitral leaflet; APM (PPM), anterolateral (posteromedial) papillary muscle; L, left coronary cusp; N, noncoronary cusp. (*From* Yamada T, Yoshida N, Doppalapudi H, Litovsky SH, McElderry HT, Kay GN. Efficacy of an Anatomical Approach in Radiofrequency Catheter Ablation of Idiopathic Ventricular Arrhythmias Originating From the Left Ventricular Outflow Tract. Circ Arrhythm Electrophysiol. 2017;10:e004959; with permission.)

coronary artery, because this could damage the vessel and lead to thrombus formation.[12,13]

When an acceleration or reduction in the frequency of the VAs is observed during the first 10 seconds of the application, the RF delivery is continued for 30 to 60 seconds. Otherwise, the RF delivery is terminated, and the catheter is repositioned. The end point of the catheter ablation is the elimination and noninducibility of VAs during isoproterenol infusion (2–4 μg/min) and burst pacing from the RV (to a cycle length as short as 240 milliseconds).

Cryothermal ablation may be a viable alternative to RF ablation in cases with a high impedance within the venous system or when the origin is located close to a coronary artery.[8]

## SUMMARY

Idiopathic VAs originating from the ventricular outflow tracts have been increasingly recognized as a target of catheter ablation. Because the anatomy of this region is complex and some VA origins are intramural and epicardial, it may sometimes be difficult to locate the site of the VA origin. Meticulous mapping of the RVOT, LVOT, ASCs, GCV, and

LV epicardial surface may be required to achieve a successful catheter ablation of VAs arising from this region. Sequential and simultaneous unipolar RF ablation from the LVOT and GCV and endocardial ablation by an anatomic approach can improve the outcome of catheter ablation of intramural LVOT VAs and LV summit VAs, respectively. Accurate recognition of the anatomy of this region is essential for the successful catheter ablation as well as the prevention of complications associated with catheter ablation.

## CLINICS CARE POINTS

- Preprocedural planning of the mapping and catheter ablation approach that is based on the electrocardiographic characteristics is important to save procedural time and to reduce cost and complications.

- Meticulous mapping in multiple different locations such as the RVOT and LVOT, endocardial and epicardial sites, and above and below the aortic and pulmonic valves may be required to locate the site of the VA origin in the ventricular outflow tract region.

- Sequential and simultaneous unipolar RF ablation from the endocardial LVOT and GCV and endocardial ablation by an anatomic approach can improve the outcome of catheter ablation of intramural LVOT VAs and LV summit VAs, respectively.

- Accurate recognition of the anatomy of this region is essential for the successful catheter ablation as well as the prevention of complications associated with catheter ablation.

## DISCLOSURE

None.

## REFERENCES

1. Callans DJ, Menz V, Schwartzman D, et al. Repetitive monomorphic tachycardia from the left ventricular outflow tract: electrocardiographic patterns consistent with a left ventricular site of origin. J Am Coll Cardiol 1997;29:1023–7.

2. Ouyang F, Fotuhi P, Ho SY, et al. Repetitive monomorphic ventricular tachycardia originating from the aortic sinus cusp: electrocardiographic characterization for guiding catheter ablation. J Am Coll Cardiol 2002;39:500–8.

3. Yamada T, Yoshida N, Murakami Y, et al. Electrocardiographic characteristics of ventricular arrhythmias

originating from the junction of the left and right coronary sinuses of Valsalva in the aorta: the activation pattern as a rationale for the electrocardiographic characteristics. Heart Rhythm 2008;5:184–92.

4. Yamada T, McElderry HT, Doppalapudi H, et al. Idiopathic ventricular arrhythmias originating from the aortic root: prevalence, electrocardiographic and electrophysiological characteristics, and results of the radiofrequency catheter ablation. J Am Coll Cardiol 2008;52:139–47.

5. Yamada T, Litovsky SH, Kay GN. The left ventricular ostium: an anatomic concept relevant to idiopathic ventricular arrhythmias. Circ Arrhythmia Electrophysiol 2008;1:396–404.

6. Yamada T, Murakami Y, Yoshida N, et al. Preferential conduction across the ventricular outflow septum in ventricular arrhythmias originating from the aortic sinus cusp. J Am Coll Cardiol 2007;50:884–91.

7. Yamada T, McElderry HT, Doppalapudi H, et al. Catheter ablation of ventricular arrhythmias originating from the vicinity of the His bundle: significance of mapping of the aortic sinus cusp. Heart Rhythm 2008;5:37–42.

8. Obel OA, d'Avila A, Neuzil P, et al. Ablation of left ventricular epicardial outflow tract tachycardia from the distal great cardiac vein. J Am Coll Cardiol 2006;48:1813–7.

9. Yamada T, McElderry HT, Doppalapudi H, et al. Idiopathic ventricular arrhythmias originating from the left ventricular summit: anatomic concepts relevant to ablation. Circ Arrhythm Electrophysiol 2010;3: 616–23.

10. Yamada T, Plumb VJ, McElderry HT, et al. Focal ventricular arrhythmias originating from the left ventricle adjacent to the membranous septum. Europace 2010;12:1467–74.

11. Yamada T, Lau YR, Litovsky SH, et al. Prevalence and clinical, electrocardiographic, and electrophysiologic characteristics of ventricular arrhythmias originating from the noncoronary sinus of Valsalva. Heart Rhythm 2013;10:1605–12.

12. Stevenson WG, Soejima K. Catheter ablation for ventricular tachycardia. Circulation 2007;115: 2750–60.

13. Yamada T, Kay GN. Optimal ablation strategies for different types of ventricular tachycardias. Nat Rev Cardiol 2012;9:512–25.

14. McAlpine WA. Heart and coronary arteries. New York: Springer-Verlag; 1975. p. 9–26.

15. Yamada T, Yoshida N, Doppalapudi H, et al. Efficacy of an anatomical approach in radiofrequency catheter ablation of idiopathic ventricular arrhythmias originating from the left ventricular outflow tract. Circ Arrhythm Electrophysiol 2017;10:e004959.

16. Benhayon D, Cogan J, Young M. Left atrial appendage as a vantage point for mapping and ablating premature ventricular contractions originating in the epicardial left ventricular summit. Clin Case Rep 2018;6:1124–7.

17. Daniels DV, Lu YY, Morton JB, et al. Idiopathic epicardial left ventricular tachycardia originating remote from the sinus of Valsalva: electrophysiological characteristics, catheter ablation, and identification from the 12-lead electrocardiogram. Circulation 2006;113:1659–66.

18. Yoshida N, Yamada T, McElderry HT, et al. A novel electrocardiographic criterion for differentiating a left from right ventricular outflow tract tachycardia origin: the V2S/V3R index. J Cardiovasc Electrophysiol 2014;25:747–53.

19. Liao Z, Zhan X, Wu S, et al. Idiopathic ventricular arrhythmias originating from the pulmonary sinus cusp: prevalence, electrocardiographic/electrophysiological characteristics, and catheter ablation. J Am Coll Cardiol 2015;66:2633–44.

20. Yamada T, Maddox WR, McElderry HT, et al. Radiofrequency catheter ablation of idiopathic ventricular arrhythmias originating from intramural foci in the left ventricular outflow tract; efficacy of sequential vs. simultaneous unipolar catheter ablation. Circ Arrhythm Electrophysiol 2015;8:344–52.

21. Yamada T, Doppalapudi H, Maddox WR, et al. Prevalence and electrocardiographic and electrophysiological characteristics of idiopathic ventricular arrhythmias originating from intramural foci in the left ventricular outflow tract. Circ Arrhythm Electrophysiol 2016;9:e004079.

22. Shirai Y, Santangeli P, Liang JJ, et al. Anatomical proximity dictates successful ablation from adjacent sites for outflow tract ventricular arrhythmias linked to the coronary venous system. Europace 2019;21: 484–91.

# Catheter Ablation for Ventricular Tachycardia Involving the His-Purkinje System
## Fascicular and Bundle Branch Reentrant Ventricular Tachycardia

Akihiko Nogami, MD, PhD[a],*, Wipat Phanthawimol, MD[a],
Tetsuya Haruna, MD, PhD[b]

## KEYWORDS

- Catheter ablation • Fascicular • Purkinje • Ventricular tachycardia • Reentry • Automaticity
- Bundle branch reentry

## KEY POINTS

- Fascicular ventricular tachycardia (VT) includes verapamil-sensitive idiopathic left fascicular VT (reentrant), Purkinje-mediated VT post myocardial infarction (reentrant), and nonreentrant fascicular VT.
- Idiopathic verapamil-sensitive fascicular VT can be classified into 3 types: 1) left posterior fascicular VT (right bundle branch block [RBBB] configuration and superior axis), 2) left anterior fascicular VT (RBBB configuration and inferior axis), and 3) upper septal fascicular VT (similar QRS as sinus rhythm). The reentrant circuit of VT often involves the Purkinje network around the papillary muscles. Furthermore, a reverse-type left posterior fascicular VT can occur.
- A Purkinje-mediated monomorphic VT after myocardial infarction is a macroreentrant VT that includes the surviving muscle bundles and Purkinje fiber as a part of the VT circuit.
- Nonreentrant fascicular VT is caused by abnormal automaticity of the distal Purkinje tissue, and it cannot be distinguished from reentrant fascicular VT on surface ECG. The successful ablation site is the earliest site of Purkinje activation during the VT. The recurrence rate after ablation for nonreentrant fascicular VT is much higher than that for reentrant fascicular VT.
- Bundle branch reentry VT, a unique form of macroreentrant VT involving the His-Purkinje system, occurs in patients with His-Purkinje conduction disease. It responds poorly to antiarrhythmic drugs and can be cured with catheter ablation. However, even after ablation, patients may remain at risk of mortality and sudden cardiac death and may require further therapies, including cardiac resynchronization therapy with defibrillators.

 Video content accompanies this article at http://www.cardiacep.theclinics.com.

[a] Department of Cardiology, Faculty of Medicine, University of Tsukuba, 1-1-1 Tennodai, Tsukuba, Ibaraki 305-8575, Japan; [b] Department of Cardiology, Kitano Hospital, 2-4-20 Ohgimachi, Kita-ku, Osaka 530-8480, Japan
* Corresponding author. Department of Cardiology, Faculty of Medicine, University of Tsukuba, 1-1-1 Tennodai, Tsukuba, Ibaraki 305-8575, Japan.
E-mail address: anogami@md.tsukuba.ac.jp

Card Electrophysiol Clin 14 (2022) 633–656
https://doi.org/10.1016/j.ccep.2022.06.003
1877-9182/22/© 2022 Elsevier Inc. All rights reserved.

## INTRODUCTION

Purkinje-related monomorphic ventricular tachycardias (VTs) include fascicular VT and bundle branch reentrant (BBR) VTs. Recently, we reported a new type of verapamil-sensitive left ventricle (LV) fascicular VT with distinctive surface ECG and electrophysiological characteristics that seems to share a reentrant circuit with the frequently seen left posterior (LP) fascicular VT, in the reverse direction.[1] Careful and detailed analysis of this reverse-type LP fascicular VT might clarify unanswered questions about the circuit underlying LP fascicular VT. Although the circuitry underlying reentrant fascicular VTs remains unsolved, the circuits underlying BBR-VTs have already been elucidated. In this article, we focus on the latest updates of the mechanisms underlying LV fascicular VTs and BBR-VTs as well as the latest catheter ablation techniques.

## FASCICULAR VENTRICULAR TACHYCARDIA
### Classification of Fascicular Ventricular Tachycardias

Verapamil-sensitive idiopathic left fascicular VT is the most common form of idiopathic left VT. It was first reported in 1979 by Zipes and colleagues,[2] who identified the diagnostic triad: (1) induction by atrial burst pacing, (2) a right bundle branch block (RBBB) and left axis configuration, and (3) no apparent structural heart disease. In 1981, Belhassen and colleagues[3] demonstrated that VTs are sensitive to verapamil, which became a fourth identifying feature. In 1988, Ohe and colleagues[4] reported another type of VT, with an RBBB and a right-axis configuration. We previously reported yet another type of VT, upper septal fascicular VT.[5–7] Based on the QRS morphology, we first classified verapamil-sensitive left fascicular VT into 3 groups[5]: (1) LP fascicular VTs, in which the QRS morphology exhibits an RBBB configuration and a superior axis[8], (2) left anterior (LA) fascicular VTs, in which the QRS morphology exhibits an RBBB configuration and inferior axis[9], and (3) upper septal fascicular VT, in which the QRS morphology is similar to that during sinus rhythm.[5–7] Importantly, studies show that LP fascicular VTs are common, although LA fascicular VTs are uncommon, and left upper septal fascicular VT is rare. Notably, left upper septal fascicular VT can sometimes seem after a catheter ablation in other types of fascicular VTs.[6,7,10,11]

The reentrant circuit underlying left fascicular VT often involves the Purkinje network around the papillary muscles. Therefore, we divided LP/LA fascicular VTs into septal and papillary muscle subtypes.[12] Recently, we reported a new type of verapamil-sensitive LV fascicular VT with distinctive surface ECG and electrophysiological characteristics that seem to share a reentrant circuit with the reverse direction of the common LP fascicular VT.[1]

A Purkinje-mediated monomorphic VT after myocardial infarction (MI) is a macroreentrant VT that includes the surviving muscle bundles and Purkinje fibers as part of the VT circuit.[13] The VT has a relatively narrow QRS and can be suppressed by radiofrequency (RF) energy delivered to the presystolic/diastolic Purkinje potential.

Another type of fascicular VT is nonreentrant fascicular VT, which originates from the Purkinje system. The mechanism underlying VT involves abnormal automaticity. Although VT is usually observed in patients with ischemic heart disease, it can also occur in patients without signs of structural heart disease.[14]

In addition to the previous classification, we propose a new classification of LV fascicular VTs, including recent subtypes (**Box 1**).

---

**Box 1**
**Classification of fascicular ventricular tachycardias**

I. Idiopathic verapamil-sensitive fascicular VTs

  1. Left posterior fascicular VT

    i. Left posterior septal fascicular VT

    ii. Left posterior papillary muscle fascicular VT

    iii. Reverse type of left posterior fascicular VT

  2. Left anterior fascicular VT

    i. Left anterior septal fascicular VT

    ii. Left anterior papillary muscle fascicular VT

  3. Upper septal fascicular VT

II. Purkinje-mediated VT post myocardial infarction

III. Nonreentrant fascicular VT

  1. Nonreentrant fascicular VT with structural heart disease

    (eg, ischemic cardiomyopathy, myocarditis, sarcoidosis)

  2. Idiopathic nonreentrant fascicular VT

*Abbreviation:* VT, ventricular tachycardia

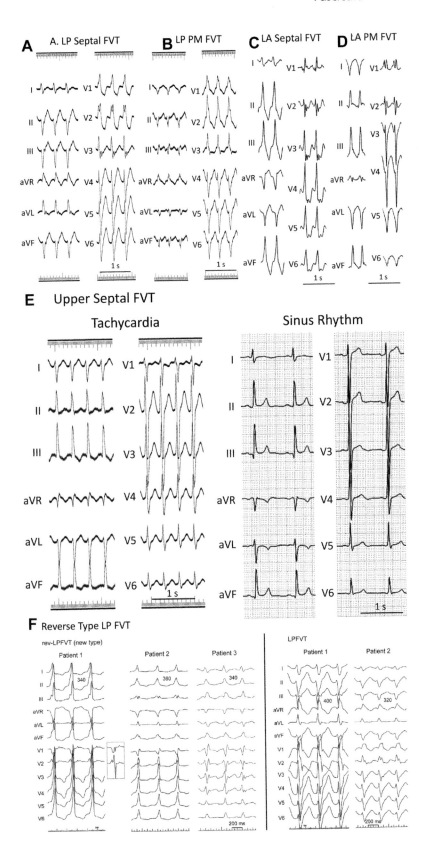

A. LP Septal FVT
B LP PM FVT
C LA Septal FVT
D LA PM FVT

E Upper Septal FVT

Tachycardia    Sinus Rhythm

F Reverse Type LP FVT

rev-LPFVT (new type)    LPFVT

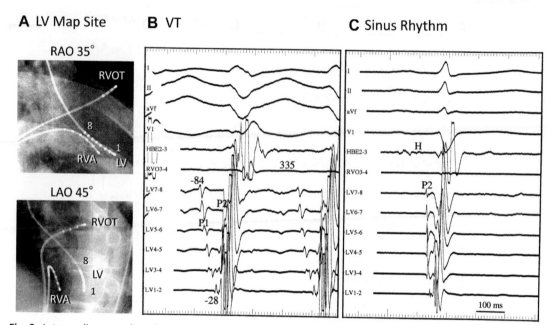

**Fig. 2.** Intracardiac recording during left posterior septal fascicular VT. (*A*) Octapolar electrode catheter position in the left ventricular septum. (*B*) During the left posterior fascicular VT, diastolic P1 and presystolic P2 were recorded. (*C*) During sinus rhythm, recording at the same site demonstrated P2, which was recorded before the onset of the QRS complex. H, His; HBE, His bundle electrogram; LV, left ventricle; RVA, right ventricular apex; RVOT, right ventricular outflow tract. (*Adapted from* Nogami A, et al. Demonstration of diastolic and presystolic Purkinje potential as critical potentials on a macroreentry circuit of verapamil-sensitive idiopathic left ventricular tachycardia. J Am Coll Cardiol. 2000;36:812,813; with permission.)

### Left Posterior Septal Fascicular Ventricular Tachycardia

LP fascicular VT is the most common form of verapamil-sensitive LV fascicular VT. The 12-lead ECG of the LP fascicular VT exhibits an RBBB configuration and left-axis deviation (**Fig. 1**A). The mechanism for this is reentry. Importantly, it can be induced, entrained, or terminated by ventricular or atrial pacing. We previously confirmed the reentry circuit after performing left ventricular septal mapping using an octapolar electrode catheter.[8] In 75% of patients, 2 distinct potentials, P1 and P2, were recorded during VT at the midseptum (**Fig. 2**). Although the mid-diastolic potential (P1) was recorded earlier from the proximal than the distal electrodes, the presystolic Purkinje potential (P2) was recorded earlier from the distal electrodes. During sinus rhythm, recordings at

the same site revealed that the P2 potential occurred before the QRS (LP fascicular potential). Entrainment pacing from the atrium or ventricle captures P1 orthodromically and resets the VT. These findings demonstrate that P1 is a critical potential in the circuit of verapamil-sensitive LP fascicular VT and suggest the presence of a macroreentry circuit involving abnormal Purkinje tissue. Although P1 has proven to be a critical potential in the VT circuit, whether the LP fascicle or Purkinje fiber (P2) is involved in the retrograde limb of the reentrant circuit is controversial.[15–18] For example, Morishima and colleagues[17] reported a case wherein proximal P2 was not part of the LP fascicular VT circuit. Selective capture of P2 by a sinus beat did not reset the VT, suggesting that proximal P2 was a bystander (**Fig. 3**). Maeda and colleagues[18] also reported a case in which P2 was recorded as the bystander of the

**Fig. 1.** Twelve-lead electrocardiograms of verapamil-sensitive left fascicular VTs. (*A*) Left posterior septal fascicular VT. (*B*) Left posterior papillary muscle fascicular VT. (*C*) Left anterior septal fascicular VT. (*D*) Left anterior papillary muscle fascicular VT. (*E*) Upper septal fascicular VT (tachycardia on the left and sinus rhythm on the right). (*F*) Reverse-type left posterior fascicular VT. FVT, fascicular VT; LA, left anterior; LP, left posterior; PM, papillary muscle; VT, ventricular tachycardia. (*F panel adapted from* Phanthawimol W, et al. Reverse-type left posterior fascicular ventricular tachycardia: a new electrocardiographic entity. JACC Clin. Electrophysiol. 2021;7:845, with permission.)

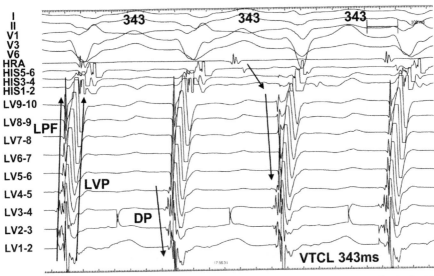

**Fig. 3.** Negative participation of the proximal left posterior fascicle to the left posterior fascicular VT circuit. Selective capture of the proximal left posterior fascicle (P2) by sinus beat did not affect the cycle length of the VT. CL, cycle length; HRA, high right atrium; LPF, left posterior fascicle; LVP, left ventricular myocardium potential; PCL, pacing cycle length; S, pacing stimulus. (*Adapted from* Morishima I, et al. Negative participation of the left posterior fascicle in the reentry circuit of verapamil-sensitive idiopathic left ventricular tachycardia. J Cardiovasc Electrophysiol. 2012;23:557; with permission.)

LP fascicular VT circuit. Although RF energy delivery at the site with P1 and P2 changed the activation sequence of P2 and the surface QRS morphology, the VT did not terminate, and the activation sequence of P1 and cycle length of the VT remained unchanged (**Fig. 4**).

The reason why P1 was not always recorded during VT remained unclear until a hypothesis was proposed by Liu and colleagues.[19] They proposed a new schematic diagram of LP fascicular VT (**Fig. 5**). They suggested that a slow conduction zone connects the ventricular myocardium and P1, and in cases where a P1 is recorded during VT, the P1 fiber is parallel and adjacent to the LP fascicle. In contrast, in cases without a P1 recording, the P1 fiber is likely shorter in length or nonparallel in orientation to the LP fascicle, or both.

### Left Posterior Papillary Muscle Fascicular Ventricular Tachycardia

Although LP septal fascicular VT exhibits a left-axis deviation, LP papillary muscle fascicular VT exhibits a superior right-axis deviation (or northwest axis; **Fig. 1**B).[12] A diastolic P1 potential during VT can be recorded around the papillary muscles but not on the septum. Notably, the ablation of diastolic P1 is highly effective in suppressing this type of VT. **Fig. 6** shows an example of a catheter ablation for an LP papillary muscle fascicular

VT.[12] The VT exhibited an RBBB configuration and superior right-axis deviation. After ablation in the posterior papillary muscle region, the VT exhibiting RBBB configuration and horizontal axis recurred (see **Fig. 6**A). In the second session, both the diastolic P1 and presystolic P2 potentials were recorded during VT at the successful ablation site around the posterior papillary muscles, which was confirmed by intracardiac ultrasonography (see **Fig. 6**B, C).

### Left Anterior Septal Fascicular Ventricular Tachycardia

**Fig. 1**C shows the 12-lead ECG of a verapamil-sensitive LA septal fascicular VT, which exhibits an RBBB configuration, inferior-axis, right-axis deviation, and Rs pattern in V5-6.[9] In this subtype, the earliest ventricular activation is recorded at the left anterolateral wall but RF energy application does not suppress the VT. **Fig. 7**A shows intracardiac recordings at the VT exit. The fused Purkinje potential was recorded, and pace mapping at this site produced a similar QRS configuration, with an interval of 25 ms between the pacing stimulus and QRS, which is equal to the P-QRS interval during VT. RF energy application at this site terminated the VT; however, a VT was still induced. **Fig. 7**B shows intracardiac recordings at the successful ablation site at the anterior midseptum,

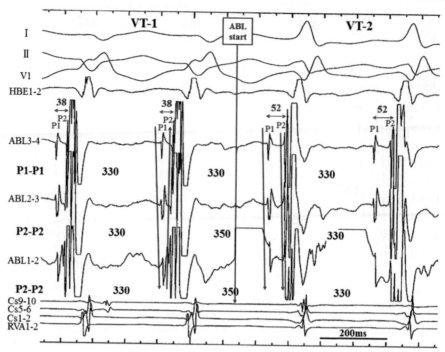

**Fig. 4.** Left posterior fascicle as a bystander circuit of left posterior fascicular VT. During VT-1, the diastolic P1 and presystolic P2 potentials were recorded in the midseptal area. Immediately after RF energy delivery at this site, VT–1 changed to VT-2 with the same tachycardia cycle length. During VT-2, the activation sequence of P2 changed, whereas the activation sequence of P1 remained unchanged (*arrows*). The P1-P1 interval also remained unchanged during VT-1 and VT-2. Cs, coronary sinus; HBE, His-bundle electrogram; RVA, right ventricular apex. (*Adapted from* Maeda S, et al. First case of left posterior fascicle in a bystander circuit of idiopathic left ventricular tachycardia. Can J Cardiol. 2014;30:e12; with permission.)

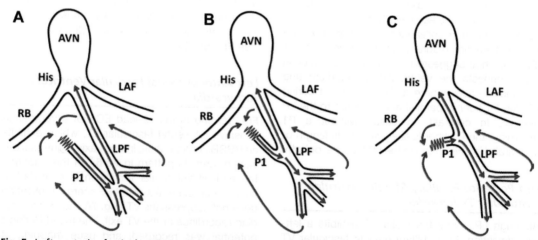

**Fig. 5.** Left posterior fascicular VT reentry circuit. (*A*) In cases with a recorded P1 during the left posterior fascicular VT, the P1 fiber is parallel and adjacent to the LPF, and the connection between P1 and P2 is at the distal site of the LPF. (*B*) The P1 fiber is parallel and adjacent to the LPF but short, and the connection between P1 and P2 is located at the proximal site of the LPF. (*C*) In cases without a recorded P1, the P1 fiber may be short in length or nonparallel in orientation to the LPF, or both. AVN, atrioventricular node; LAF, left anterior fascicle; LPF, left posterior fascicle; RB, right bundle. (*Adapted from* Liu Q, et al. Macroreentrant loop in ventricular tachycardia from the left posterior fascicle: new implications for mapping and ablation. Circ Arrhyth Electrophysiol. 2016; 9:e004272; with permission.)

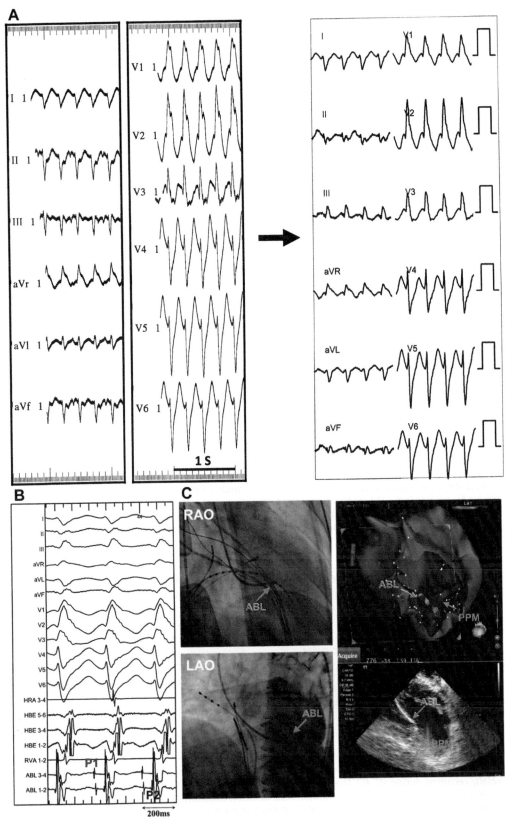

**Fig. 6.** Catheter ablation of posterior papillary muscle fascicular VT. (*A*) A VT exhibiting an RBBB configuration, superior right-axis deviation, and left posterior fascicular and posterior papillary muscle regions were ablated during the initial procedure. The patient had recurrent VT with an RBBB configuration and a horizontal axis.

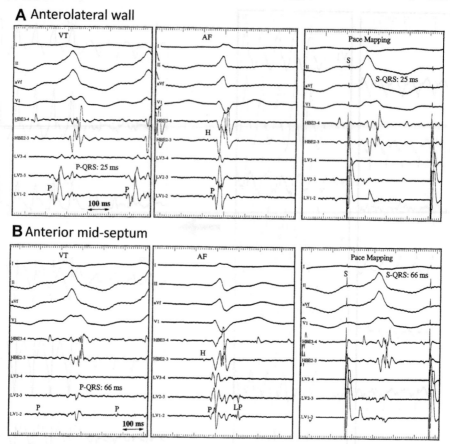

**Fig. 7.** Intracardiac electrograms during left anterior septal fascicular VT. (*A*) The fused Purkinje potential was recorded at the anterolateral wall (exit) during the VT. Radiofrequency energy application at this site terminated VT; however, the VT remained inducible. (*B*) At the anterior midseptum, the diastolic Purkinje potential preceded the QRS by 66 milliseconds. The application of radiofrequency energy at this site terminated the VT, and VT became noninducible. H, His; HBE, His bundle electrogram; LV, left ventricle. (*Adapted from* Nogami A, et al. Verapamil-sensitive left anterior fascicular ventricular tachycardia: Results of radiofrequency ablation in six patients. J Cardiovasc Electrophysiol. 1998;9:1275-6; with permission.)

where the diastolic P potential was recorded (−66 ms). Pace mapping at that site reproduced a similar QRS configuration with an S–QRS interval of 66 ms.

### Left Anterior Papillary Muscle Fascicular Ventricular Tachycardia

**Fig. 1**D shows the 12-lead ECG of a verapamil-sensitive LA papillary muscle fascicular VT, which exhibits an RBBB configuration, inferior axis, right axis deviation, and deep S-waves in V5-6.[9,12] LV endocardial mapping during LA fascicular VT identified the earliest ventricular activation in the anterolateral wall of the LV (**Fig. 8**).[9] RF energy application at this site has been found to suppress the VT and the fused Purkinje potential has been found to exhibit excellent pace mapping.

---

(*B*) At the successful ablation site in the repeat procedure, both the diastolic P1 and presystolic P2 potentials were sequentially recorded during VT. (*C*) The successful ablation site was located on the posterior papillary muscles, which was confirmed by intracardiac ultrasound. ABL, ablation catheter; LAO, left oblique projection; RAO, right oblique projection. (*Adapted from* Komatsu Y, et al. Fascicular ventricular tachycardia originating from papillary muscles: Purkinje network involvement in the reentrant circuit. Circ Arrhythm Electrophysiol. 2017;10. pii: e004549 with permission.)

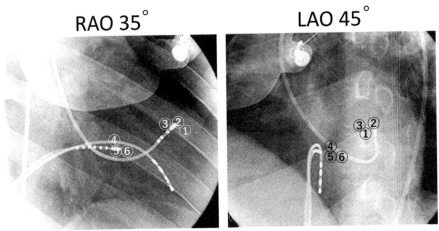

## RAO 35°            LAO 45°

**Fig. 8.** Successful ablation sites of left anterior septal and papillary muscle fascicular VTs. Patients 1 to 3 had a left anterior papillary muscle fascicular VT and patients 4 to 6 had a left anterior septal fascicular VT. In the left anterior septal fascicular VT (patients 4–6), ablation at the VT exit site was unsuccessful, and ablation was successful at the midanterior septum of the left ventricle. LAO, left oblique projection; RAO, right oblique projection. (*Adapted from* Nogami A, et al. Verapamil-sensitive left anterior fascicular ventricular tachycardia: results of radiofrequency ablation in six patients. J Cardiovasc Electrophysiol. 1998;9:1277; with permission.)

Based on the above findings, we modified Liu's schematic diagrams[19] and hypothesized the potential circuits underlying LP and anterior fascicular VTs, as in **Fig. 9**A, B.

### Left Upper Septal Fascicular Ventricular Tachycardia

Left upper septal fascicular VT exhibits a narrow QRS configuration and a normal or right-axis deviation (**Fig. 1**E).[5–7] The QRS configurations during VT is similar to the QRS in sinus rhythm. This type of fascicular VT is very rare and sometimes occurs after a previous catheter ablation for some other type of LV fascicular VT.[6,7,10,11]

**Fig. 10** shows the intracardiac electrograms during upper septal fascicular VT for previously ablated LP septal fascicular VT.[6] During a common LP fascicular VT, a diastolic P1 potential and presystolic P2 potential are observed (see **Fig. 10**A). Although the P1 potential is recorded earlier from the proximal electrodes than from the distal electrodes, the P2 potential is recorded earlier from the distal electrodes than from the proximal electrodes, and the His-bundle potential is recorded after the QRS onset (negative H-V interval). During an upper septal fascicular VT, the P1 potential is recorded earlier from the distal than from the proximal electrodes, whereas the P2 potential is recorded earlier

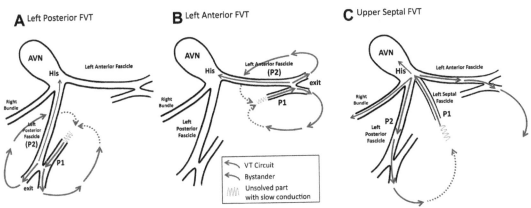

**Fig. 9.** Reentrant fascicular VTs. (*A*) Left posterior fascicular VT. The antegrade limb was P1, and the retrograde limb was the septal myocardium. P2 (left posterior fascicle) is a bystander. The reentrant circuit of VT can involve the Purkinje network around the papillary muscles. (*B*) Left anterior fascicular VT. (*C*) Upper septal fascicular VT. In this circuit, the left septal branch is the retrograde limb and the antegrade limb is the left posterior fascicle. AVN, atrioventricular node; LAF, left anterior fascicle; LPF, left posterior fascicle; RB, right bundle.

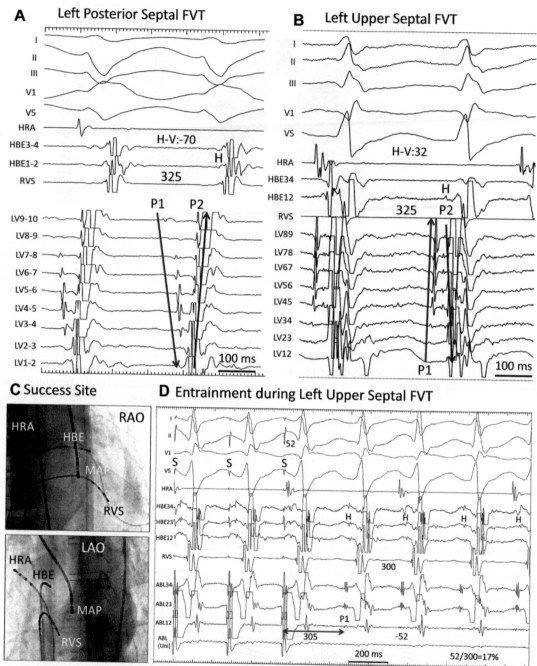

**Fig. 10.** Upper septal fascicular VT after the ablation of posterior septal fascicular VT. Intracardiac recordings of the left posterior septal fascicular VT (*A*) and upper septal fascicular VT (*B*) demonstrating the activation sequence of the diastolic potential (P1) (*red arrows*) and presystolic Purkinje potential (P2) (*blue arrows*) during each rhythm. At the successful ablation site (*C*), the diastolic P1 preceded the onset of the QRS by 52 milliseconds, and entrainment from this site resulted in a concealed fusion as well as a postpacing interval–ventricular tachycardia cycle length difference of 5 milliseconds and an interval between the pacing stimulus and QRS onset of 52 milliseconds, equal to the P1-QRS interval during VT (*D*). ABL, ablation catheter; FVT, fascicular VT; H, His-bundle potential; HBE, His-bundle electrogram; HRA, high right atrium; LV, left ventricle; RVS, right ventricular septum; S, stimulation artifact. (*Adapted from* Talib AK, et al. Verapamil-sensitive upper septal idiopathic left ventricular tachycardia: Prevalence, mechanism and electrophysiological characteristics. J Am Coll Cardiol EP. 2015;1:374, 376; with permission.)

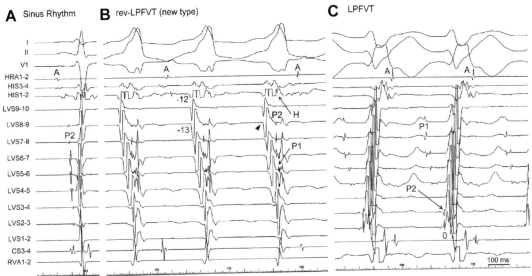

**Fig. 11.** Intracardiac recording in a patient with reverse type left posterior fascicular VT. (*A*) During sinus rhythm. (*B*) During reverse-type left posterior fascicular VT. (*C*) During left posterior fascicular VT. During reverse-type LP fascicular VT, the earliest ventricular activation was recorded at the LV and RV superior-middle septa (*arrowhead*). The paced QRS morphology from the LV septum produced a similar QRS configuration to the VT but not identical. During the reverse-type LP fascicular VT, although no diastolic Purkinje potentials were recorded, there were 2 spiky potentials, P2 and P1, within the local ventricular electrogram. A, atrial potential; H, His bundle potential; HIS, his bundle electrogram; LPFVT, left posterior fascicular VT; LVS, left ventricular septum. (*Adapted from* Phanthawimol W, et al. Reverse-type left posterior fascicular ventricular tachycardia: a new electrocardiographic entity. JACC Clin. Electrophysiol. 2021;7:847 with permission.)

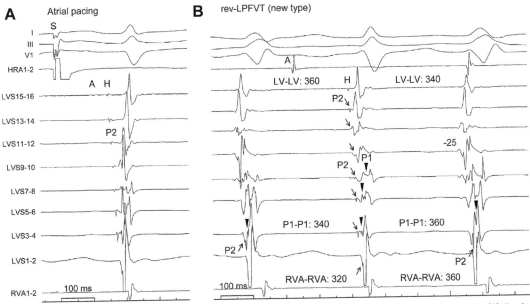

**Fig. 12.** Reset of reverse type left posterior fascicular VT by sinus rhythm. (*A*) During atrial pacing. (*B*) During reverse-type LPFVT, the spiky P2 potential (*arrows*) and fragmented P1 potential (*arrowheads*) were recorded within the local ventricular electrogram. When the sinus rhythm captured the QRS (middle beat), the His and P2 potentials advanced and appeared before the QRS complex. The P1 potential was advanced by 20 milliseconds. The subsequent QRS complex was also advanced, indicating that the VT had been reset. A, atrial potential; H, His bundle potential; LPFVT, left posterior fascicular VT; LVS, left ventricular septum; RVA, right ventricular apex. (*Adapted from* Phanthawimol W, et al. Reverse-type left posterior fascicular ventricular tachycardia: a new electrocardiographic entity. JACC Clin. Electrophysiol. 2021;7:851, with permission.)

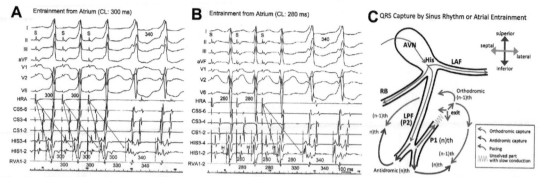

**Fig. 13.** Atrial entrainment during reverse type left posterior fascicular VT. (*A*) Atrial entrainment pacing (300 milliseconds) showing constant fusion of the QRS complex. Although atrial pacing directly captured the right ventricular apex (*red arrows*), it also captured the anterior ventricular septum (HIS1-2) of the subsequent QRS complex (*blue arrows*). Red arrows indicate antidromic capture, and blue arrows indicate orthodromic capture. The final captured QRS complex exhibited no fusion. (*B*) During atrial entrainment pacing (280 milliseconds), His potential appeared before the QRS complex, and the QRS complex became narrower (progressive fusion). (*C*) Sinus capture and atrial entrainment. CS, coronary sinus; HIS, His-bundle electrogram; HRA, high right atrium; RVA, right ventricular apex; S, pacing stimulus. (*Adapted from* Phanthawimol W, et al. Reverse-type left posterior fascicular ventricular tachycardia: a new electrocardiographic entity. JACC Clin. Electrophysiol. 2021;7:846; with permission.)

from the proximal than from the distal electrodes (see **Fig. 10**B). Furthermore, the His-bundle potential typically precedes the onset of the QRS complex by 32 ms, which is shorter than that during the sinus rhythm. Importantly, this can be used for the differentiation of supraventricular tachycardia. In fact, entrainment pacing from the upper-middle ventricular septum where the diastolic P1 preceded the QRS by 52 ms has been found to result in concealed fusion and a post-pacing interval–VT cycle length difference of 5 ms as well as an S-QRS interval of 52 ms, which is equal to the P1-QRS interval during VT (see **Fig. 10**C, D). RF energy application at this

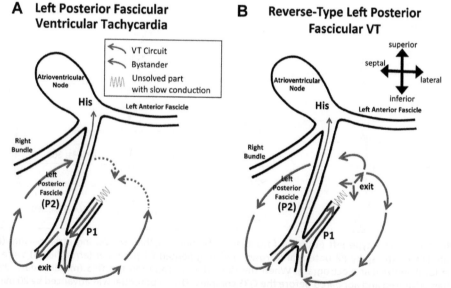

**Fig. 14.** Hypothesized circuit of reverse type left posterior fascicular VT. (*A*) Left posterior fascicular VT. (*B*) Reverse-type left posterior fascicular VT. (*Adapted from* Phanthawimol W, et al. Reverse-type left posterior fascicular ventricular tachycardia: a new electrocardiographic entity. JACC Clin. Electrophysiol. 2021;7:852, with permission.)

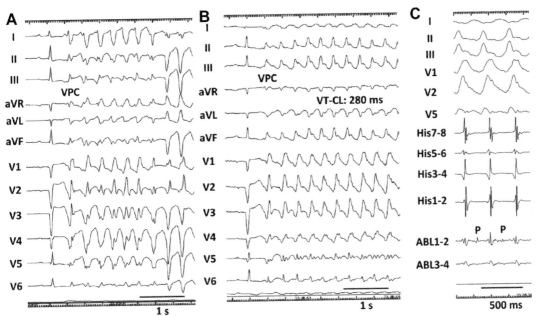

**Fig. 15.** Conversion from VF to rapid sustained monomorphic VT shortly after the VF ablation. (*A*) A 12-lead ECG was performed during the first ablation session. VF was initiated by the trigger of a premature ventricular contraction. (*B*) A 12-lead ECG during the second ablation session was performed the next day. A sustained mono-morphic VT was initiated. (*C*) At the successful ablation site of monomorphic VT, diastolic Purkinje potentials (P) were recorded on the left ventricular septum. ABL, ablation catheter; His, His bundle electrogram; VPC, ventric-ular premature contraction; VT-CL, cycle length of VT. (*Adapted from* Masuda K, et al. Conversion to Purkinje-related monomorphic ventricular tachycardia after ablation of ventricular fibrillation in ischemic heart disease. Circ Arrhythm Electrophysiol. 2016;9:e004224; with permission.)

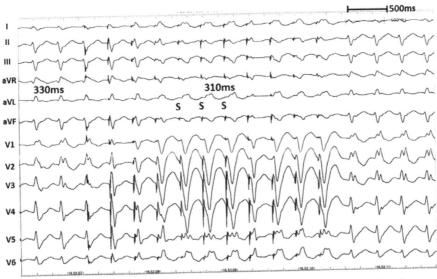

**Fig. 16.** Burst pacing during nonreentrant fascicular VT. A surface 12-lead ECG showing the absence of constant fusion by right ventricular overdrive pacing during nonreentrant fascicular VT. (*Adapted from* Talib AK, et al. Non-reentrant fascicular tachycardia: clinical and electrophysiological characteristics of a distinct type of idio-pathic ventricular tachycardia. Circ Arrhythm Electrophysiol. 2016; 9. pii:e004177; with permission.)

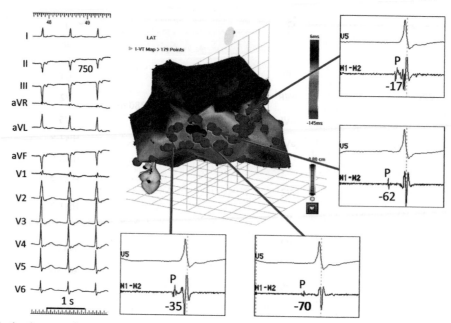

**Fig. 17.** Activation map during nonreentrant fascicular VT with right bundle branch block and left-axis deviation. The earliest Purkinje potential was recorded at the basal inferior wall. The Purkinje potential preceded the QRS during VT by 70 milliseconds, and radiofrequency energy allocation at this site suppressed the VT.

site can slow and terminate the VT, and the VT becomes noninducible.

We hypothesized the potential VT circuits that mediate the left upper septal fascicular VT, as shown in **Fig. 9**C. We propose the existence of a left septal fascicle in this circuit where P1 represents retrograde conduction within the left septal fascicle, whereas P2 represents activation of the LP fascicle. LP fascicle is the anterograde limb of the reentrant circuit for this VT. Although His and RBB are the bystanders, they are activated almost at the same time as the LA and LP fascicules, which explains why VT exhibits an almost similar QRS configuration to that during sinus rhythm. Therefore, P1 is the common retrograde limb of the VT circuit and represents an important ablation target. This left septal fascicle might exclusively conduct retrogradely, because most patients do not exhibit septal q-waves before ablation, and there is typically no change in QRS morphology after successful RF ablation.[7]

## Reverse Type of Left Posterior Fascicular Ventricular Tachycardia

Recently, we reported on 3 patients with a new type of verapamil-sensitive LV fascicular VT with distinctive surface ECG and electrophysiological characteristics that seem to share a reentrant circuit in the reverse direction of the common LP

fascicular VT.[1] The 12-lead ECG of this new type exhibited rSr morphology in V1 with an early precordial transition and inferior-axis (**Fig. 1**F). All 3 VTs showed verapamil sensitivity, and 2 of the 3 patients had a common-type LP fascicular VT as well.

**Fig. 11** shows intracardiac recordings during sinus rhythm, reverse-type LP fascicular VT, and during typical LP fascicular VT. **Fig. 12** shows the importance of the P1 potential in the circuit because this potential needs to be captured to reset the VT. Entrainment pacing from the atrium during reverse-type LP fascicular VT captures the conduction system and exhibits constant and progressive fusion (**Fig. 13**). The hypothesized VT circuit in reverse-type LP fascicular VT is depicted in **Fig. 14**. During a reverse-type LP fascicular VT, the LV superior-middle septum is activated first displaying a centrifugal activation pattern. Importantly, the ventricular septal propagation is the antegrade limb of the reentrant circuit while the fragmented P1 potential buried in the local ventricular electrogram is the retrograde limb of the reentrant circuit (see **Fig. 14**B). Among LP fascicular VTs, although the inferior turnaround of the circuit in the LP fascicular VT has been clearly demonstrated, the superior turnaround is still unsolved (see **Fig. 14**A). If the circuits of LP fascicular VT and reverse-type LP fascicular VT are completely reversed, the intramural site at

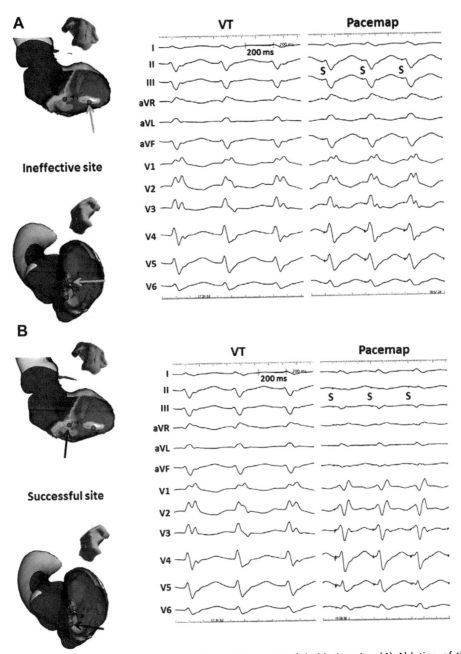

**Fig. 18.** Discrepancy between a good pacemap site and the successful ablation site. (*A*) Ablation of the apical third of the inferior left ventricular septum, where an excellent pacemap was obtained, could not suppress the VT. (*B*) Ablating the mid-third of the left ventricular septum eliminated the VT in 4 seconds, despite a poor pacemap at that site. VT, ventricular tachycardia; S, stimulus. (*Adapted from* Talib AK, et al. Non-reentrant fascicular tachycardia: clinical and electrophysiological characteristics of a distinct type of idiopathic ventricular tachycardia. Circ Arrhythm Electrophysiol. 2016; 9. pii:e004177; with permission.)

the earliest activation during reverse-type LP fascicular VT may be the superior turnaround of the LP fascicular VT circuit. Nevertheless, further electrophysiological investigation is needed to confirm this.

## Purkinje-Mediated Ventricular Tachycardia After Myocardial Infarction

Purkinje-mediated monomorphic VT post-MI is a macroreentrant VT that includes the surviving muscle bundles and Purkinje fibers as a part of

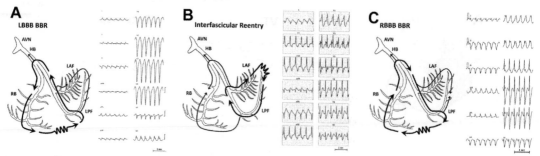

**Fig. 19.** Reentrant circuit and 12-lead ECG for bundle branch reentrant VT and interfascicular reentrant VT. (*A*) Type A. Typical BBR-VT in which retrograde conduction occurs via the left bundle branch and anterograde conduction over the right bundle branch. (*B*) Type B. Interfascicular reentrant VT with anterograde and retrograde conduction over the opposing fascicles of the left bundle branch. (*C*) Type C. Reversal of the circuit depicted in Type A. AVN, atrioventricular node; BBR, bundle branch reentry; HB, His bundle; LAF, left anterior fascicle; LPF, left posterior fascicle; RB, right bundle. (*Adapted from* Nogami A: Purkinje-related arrhythmias. Part I: Monomorphic ventricular tachycardias. Pacing Clin Electrophysiol 2011;34:643; with permission.)

the VT circuit.[13] VT has a relatively narrow QRS and can be suppressed by RF energy delivery to the presystolic/diastolic Purkinje potential. Hayashi and colleagues first reported 4 post-MI patients who presented with LP fascicular VT.[20] Later, Morishima and colleagues described a verapamil-sensitive LA fascicular VT that exhibited an RBBB configuration and right-axis deviation in a prior anteroseptal MI.[21] These VTs have several characteristic differences compared with the usual scar-related VT post-MI: (1) a relatively narrow QRS duration, (2) verapamil sensitivity, and (3) termination by a single or a few RF energy applications to the presystolic/diastolic Purkinje potential sites. We have previously reported that Purkinje-mediated VT post-MI can occur after ablation of ischemic ventricular fibrillation (VF).[22] In fact, more than one-fifth of patients experience newly emergent Purkinje-related monomorphic VT after ablation for primary ischemic VF. The circuit underlying monomorphic VTs is thought to be the Purkinje network, which is located in the same low-voltage area as the Purkinje tissue. This network has been shown to trigger VF, and it can be suppressed by additional ablation. **Fig. 15**

shows the conversion from VF to rapid sustained monomorphic VT shortly after VF ablation. VF was initiated by triggering a ventricular premature contraction (VPC; see **Fig. 15**A). The day after VF ablation, sustained monomorphic VPC was initiated by a similar, but not identical, VPC (see **Fig. 15**B). During VT, the diastolic Purkinje potential was recorded at the left ventricular septum, and a single RF energy application suppressed the VT.

## Nonreentrant Fascicular Ventricular Tachycardia

Although reentry is a common mechanism of fascicular VT, a nonreentrant mechanism also exists. Nonreentrant fascicular VT is usually observed in patients with structural heart diseases such as ischemic cardiomyopathy,[23] myocarditis,[24] and sarcoidosis[25]; however, it can occur in patients without structural heart disease.[14] For example, we previously reported that 2.8% of patients with an idiopathic VT that were referred for ablation had a nonreentrant fascicular VT.[14] Idiopathic nonreentrant fascicular

**Table 1**
**Types of bundle branch reentrant tachycardias**

|  | Type A | Type B (Interfascicular Reentrant VT) | Type B |
|---|---|---|---|
| ECG morphology | LBBB configuration | RBBB configuration with left anterior or posterior fascicular hemiblock | RBBB configuration |
| Antegrade limb | RBB | LAF or LPF | LBB |
| Retrograde limb | LBB | Contraleft fascicle | RBB |

*Abbreviations:* LAF, left anterior fascicle; LBB, left bundle branch; LBBB, left bundle branch block; LPF, left posterior fascicle; RBB, right bundle branch; RBBB, right bundle branch block; VT, ventricular tachycardia.

**Table 2**
**Diagnostic criteria for bundle branch reentrant and interfascicular ventricular tachycardias**

|  | Bundle Branch Reentrant VT | Interfascicular Reentrant VT |
|---|---|---|
| ECG morphology | Typical LBBB or RBBB configuration | RBBB with LA or LP fascicular hemiblock configuration |
| Induction | Depends on His–Purkinje conduction delay | Depends on left fascicular conduction delay |
| His potential | His potential precedes each QRS complex. H–V during VT usually ≥ H–V during sinus rhythm | His potential precedes each QRS complex. H–V during VT usually < H–V during sinus rhythm |
| Termination | Terminates with block in His-Purkinje system | Terminates with block in left fascicular system |
| Activation sequence | His, RBB, and LBB activation sequences during an LBBB morphology tachycardia; or His, LBB, and RBB activation sequences during an RBBB morphology tachycardia | LAF, ventricle, and LPF activation sequences during an LP hemiblock morphology tachycardia; or LPF, ventricle, and LAF activation sequences during an LA hemiblock morphology tachycardia |
| Changes in V–V and H–H intervals | Variations in the V–V interval are preceded by similar changes in the H–H interval | Variations in the V–V interval are preceded by similar changes in the H–H interval |
| Entrainment from RVA | Postpacing interval—VT cycle length <30 ms with entrainment from RVA | Postpacing interval—VT cycle length >30 ms with entrainment from RVA |
| Atrial entrainment | QRS morphology during atrial entrainment is similar to QRS morphology during VT | Atrial entrainment exhibits similar left fascicular hemiblock morphology; however, RBBB configuration might be changed |

*Abbreviations:* LA, left anterior; LAF, left anterior fascicle; LBB, left bundle branch; LBBB, left bundle branch block; LP, left posterior; LPF, left posterior fascicle; RBB, right bundle branch; RBBB, right bundle branch block; RVA, right ventricular apex; VT, ventricular tachycardia.

VT usually originates from the LP fascicle and less commonly from the LA fascicle and right Purkinje network. The 12-lead ECG of idiopathic nonreentrant fascicular VT exhibits RBBB and, less commonly, left bundle branch block (LBBB) morphology, depending on the site of origin with a relatively narrow QRS complex. Importantly, it cannot be distinguished from reentrant fascicular VT on a surface ECG. Furthermore, although nonreentrant fascicular VT cannot be induced by programmed ventricular stimulation, VT or PVC with the same morphology is sometimes induced by intravenous isoproterenol infusion and burst ventricular stimulation. Because the mechanism does not involve reentry, it cannot be entrained (**Fig. 16**). Catheter ablation is effective at the earliest presystolic Purkinje potential (**Fig. 17**), whereas the pacemap-guided approach is less efficacious (**Fig. 18**).[14] The recurrence rate after ablation for nonreentrant fascicular VT has been found to be much higher than that for reentrant fascicular VTs.

## BUNDLE BRANCH REENTRANT VENTRICULAR TACHYCARDIA

### Classification of Bundle Branch Reentrant-Ventricular Tachycardia

BBR VT is a unique, fast (200–300 bpm) monomorphic VT associated with hemodynamic collapse, syncope, and cardiac arrest.[26] It is caused by a macroreentry circuit involving the right bundle branch (RBB), left bundle branch (LBB), and septal ventricular muscle.[26–33] BBR-VT occurs in patients with structural heart diseases, such as cardiomyopathy, coronary artery disease, valvular heart

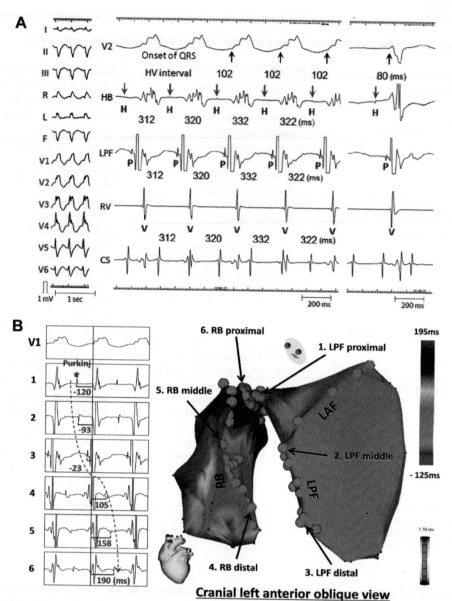

**Fig. 20.** Mapping during bundle branch reentrant VT (BBR-VT). (*A*) During type C BBR-VT, His (H) activation precedes ventricular (V) depolarization. Changes in the H–H interval precede changes in the V–V interval. The H–V interval during the BBR-VT is longer than the H–V interval during sinus rhythm. (*B*) Three-dimensional activation map of type C BBR-VT descending the left posterior fascicle (LPF) and ascending the right bundle branch (RB), with the earliest activation displayed in red (LPF proximal) and the latest in violet (RB proximal). See Supplemental Video 1. CS, coronary sinus; HB, His bundle electrogram; LPH, left posterior fascicle; P, Purkinje potential; RV, right ventricle. (*From* Machino T, et al. Three-dimensional visualization of the entire reentrant circuit. Heart Rhythm 2013;10:459-60; with permission.)

disease, congenital heart disease, sarcoidosis, and muscular dystrophy. Furthermore, BBR-VT can occur in patients with associated His-Purkinje system disease but no structural heart disease.[34–37] The incidence of sustained BBR-VT has been reported to be 6% in sustained

monomorphic VTs[38] and 19% in a series of patients with nonischemic cardiomyopathy.[39] Furthermore, a high incidence of BBR-VT has been reported in patients receiving ventricular assist device support.[40,41] Therefore, it is likely that BBR-VT is underrecognized.

**Table 3**
**Targets for ablation of bundle branch reentrant ventricular tachycardia and interfascicular reentrant ventricular tachycardia**

| Bundle Branch Reentrant VT | Interfascicular Reentrant VT | Bundle Branch Reentrant VT and Interfascicular Reentrant VT |
|---|---|---|
| • RBB, usual primary target or<br>• LBB | • LAF or LPF or<br>• Distal Purkinje network between LAF and LPF | • RBB and LAF or<br>• RBB and LPF or<br>• LAF and LPF |

*Abbreviations:* LAF, left anterior fascicle; LBB, left bundle branch; LPF, left posterior fascicle; RBB, right bundle branch; VT, ventricular tachycardia.

BBR-VT can present with a typical LBBB pattern or a typical RBBB pattern (**Fig. 19**).[33] Some patients have both a counterclockwise BBR-VT (LBBB morphology) and clockwise BBR-VT (RBBB morphology). In fact, Tchou and colleagues[42] described 3 types of BBR-VT (see **Fig. 19**; **Table 1**). Types A and C are classic counterclockwise and clockwise BBR-VT circuits, respectively, whereas type B is an interfascicular reentrant VT and reentry within the LA and LP fascicles. An RBBB configuration and left hemiblock pattern is more consistent with interfascicular reentrant VTs. Notably, the most common type of BBR-VT is type A (98%).[43]

### Diagnosis and Mapping

The diagnostic criteria for BBR-VT and interfascicular VT are summarized in **Table 2**. Although atrioventricular (AV) dissociation may be present, there is a persistent 1:1 His–QRS activation with the H–V interval during tachycardia equal to or longer than the H–V interval in sinus rhythm.[44]

In type A and type C BBR-VTs, the onset of ventricular depolarization is preceded by His bundle, RBB, or LBB potentials with a sequence of His bundle > RBB > LBB or His bundle > LBB > RBB activation. Spontaneous variations in V–V intervals have been shown to be preceded by similar changes in the H–H/RBB–RBB/LBB–LBB or H–H/LBB–LBB/RBB–RBB intervals (**Fig. 20**A). Therefore, recordings from both sides of the septum may help identify the mechanism(s) underlying BBR-VT. Additionally, 3-dimensional electroanatomical mapping may prove to be valuable for revealing the entire macroreentrant circuit (**Fig. 20**B; Supplemental Video 1).[45]

Interfascicular reentrant VT is less common.[28] In VT, one of the LBB fascicles serves as the anterograde limb and the other as the retrograde circuit. Importantly, the distal link between fascicles occurs through the ventricular myocardium and the LA fascicle is usually the anterograde limb, whereas the LP fascicle is the retrograde limb.[23,35] The H–V interval during interfascicular reentrant VT is usually shorter than that recorded in sinus rhythm by more than 40 ms,[46] which occurs because the upper turnaround point of the circuit (the LB branching point) is relatively far from the His bundle activation in the retrograde direction (see **Fig. 19**B).

### Catheter Ablation

Pharmacologic therapy has been shown to be ineffective. In contrast, RF catheter ablation of a bundle branch can cure BBR-VTs (**Table 3**) and is currently regarded as the first-line therapy.[28,38] As the underlying structural abnormalities remain unchanged, concomitant placement of an implantable cardioverter-defibrillator should be strongly considered.[47] The technique of choice is typically ablation of the RBB.[28] Importantly, BBR-VT can be suppressed by ablation of the right or left main bundle branch.[34,42] RBBs are typically targeted for ablation since ablation of the RBB is technically easier than that of the LBB. In sinus rhythm, a complete RBBB or LBBB develops after successful ablation, although QRS changes may be subtle in patients with preexisting conduction abnormalities (**Fig. 21**).[48] Additionally, the elimination of retrograde V–H conduction has also been used as a marker of successful ablation.[28] Notably, the incidence of a significant conduction block requiring a permanent pacemaker has been reported to range from 0% to 30%.[28,31,32]

For many patients with BBR-VT who have "LBBB" during sinus rhythm, anterograde slow conduction over the LBB is present[45] or the LBB is activated retrogradely (**Fig. 22**).[35] However, in patients with a complete LBBB pattern during sinus rhythm, anterograde ventricular activation occurs solely via the RBB. Patients with the latter pattern are at risk of developing a complete AV block with RBB ablation. Therefore, to avoid the

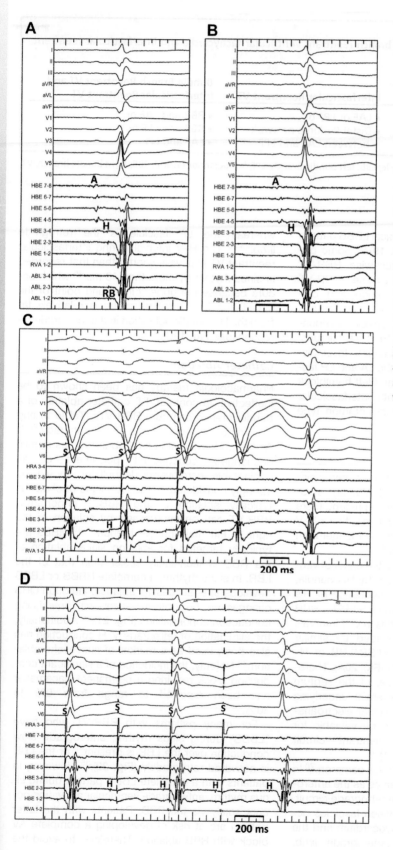

**Fig. 21.** Recordings before and after right bundle ablation during sinus rhythm and atrial pacing. (*A*) Before ablation of the right bundle branch block (RBBB). The RBB recording occurred 10 milliseconds after the His potential. The RBB-V interval was 32 milliseconds. (*B*) After ablation of the RBB, the surface ECG showed a complete RBBB, and the RBB potential disappeared. (*C*) Before ablation, burst atrial pacing at a cycle length of 400 milliseconds exhibited a complete LBBB configuration identical to clinical BBR-VT. (*D*) After ablation of the RBB, the burst atrial pacing showed a 2:1 H–V block. H, His potential; HBE, His bundle electrogram; RB, right bundle; RVA, right ventricular apex. (*Adapted from* Nogami A, Olshansky B. Bundle branch reentry tachycardia. In: Zipes DP, Jalife J, Stevenson WG, eds. Cardiac Electrophysiology: From Cell to Bedside. 7th ed. Philadelphia, PA: Elsevier; 2018, pp 809-810; with permission.)

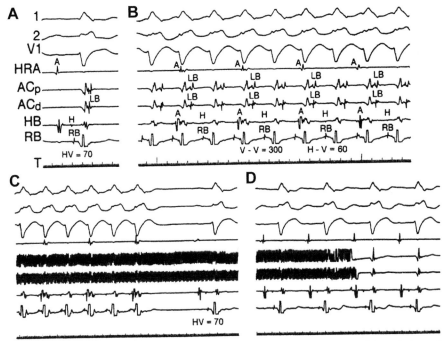

**Fig. 22.** Termination of bundle branch reentrant VT (BBR-VT) by the ablation of the left bundle branch. (*A*) Retrograde (transseptal) activation of the LBB recorded during sinus rhythm. (*B*) During BBR-VT, activation propagated down the right bundle branch and up the LBB. The sequence of activation of the LBB recordings during sinus rhythm and BBR-VT was identical. (*C*) Catheter ablation of the LBB terminated the tachycardia. (*D*) After ablation, the QRS duration and configuration remained unchanged, but retrograde activation of the LBB disappeared. A, atrial potential; AC, ablation catheter; H, His potential; HB, His bundle electrogram; HRA, high right atrium; LB, left bundle; RB, right bundle. (Blanck Z, et al. Catheter ablation of the left bundle branch for the treatment of sustained bundle branch reentrant ventricular tachycardia. J Cardiovasc Electrophysiol 1995; 6: 40–3; with permission.)

creation of a complete AV block, retrograde conduction of the LBB may be a better target in such patients.[35,49]

In interfascicular reentrant VT, creation of an RBBB will not cure the tachycardia because the RBB is a bystander. Similarly, ablation of the main LBB would not terminate tachycardia because the turnaround of the circuit is distal to the main LBB. In this case, a catheter ablation of the LA fascicle or the LP fascicle results in termination of tachycardia.[23]

Two previous large studies reported that acute success rates for BBR-VT and interfascicular reentrant VT were 100%.[23,28] Furthermore, after ablation, BBR-VT recurrence is uncommon. Despite the success of ablation of the RBB branch in eliminating BBR-VT, patients with cardiomyopathy and heart failure continue to have high mortality rates. In fact, even with the impressive success rates of BBR-VT ablation, progressive heart failure remains a common cause of death.[28,31,38,43,47,49] However, a recent study

observed no heart blocks in patients with a normal H–V interval and no deaths in patients with normal LV systolic function during a long-term follow-up.[50]

Nevertheless, following ablation, the indication for cardiac resynchronization therapy with a defibrillator should be considered based on the status of the residual conduction system and severity of heart failure. Furthermore, myocardial VT may be induced in 36% to 60% of patients after successful ablation of BBR-VT.[23,43]

## SUMMARY

Previous studies have revealed that monomorphic VTs involving the His-Purkinje system are composed of multiple discrete subtypes that are best differentiated by their mechanism, drug effect, VT morphology, and successful ablation site. Recognition of the heterogeneity of VTs and their unique characteristics should facilitate appropriate diagnosis and therapy.

## CLINICS CARE POINTS

- Idiopathic verapamil-sensitive fascicular VT can be classified into 3 types: 1) left posterior fascicular VT, 2) left anterior fascicular VT, and 3) upper septal fascicular VT. The reentrant circuit of VT often involves the Purkinje network around the papillary muscles. Furthermore, a reverse-type left posterior fascicular VT can occur.

- Nonreentrant fascicular VT cannot be distinguished from reentrant fascicular VT on surface ECG. Because the mechanism is not reentry, it cannot be entrained. Catheter ablation is effective at the earliest presystolic Purkinje potential, whereas the pacemap-guided approach is less efficacious. The recurrence rate after ablation for nonreentrant fascicular VT is much higher than that for reentrant fascicular VT.

- BBR-VT responds poorly to antiarrhythmic drugs and can be cured with catheter ablation, it currently regarded as the first-line therapy. However, even after ablation, patients may remain at risk of mortality and sudden cardiac death and may require further therapies, including cardiac resynchronization therapy with defibrillators.

## DISCLOSURE

Dr A. Nogami received honoraria from Abbott and Biosense Webster; and an endowment from Medtronic and DVx. The other authors report no conflicts.

## SUPPLEMENTARY DATA

Supplementary data related to this article can be found online at https://doi.org/10.1016/j.ccep.2022.06.003.

## REFERENCES

1. Phanthawimol W, Nogami A, Haruna T, et al. Reverse-Type left posterior fascicular ventricular tachycardia: a new electrocardiographic entity. JACC Clin Electrophysiol 2021;7:843–54.

2. Zipes DP, Foster PR, Troup PJ, et al. Atrial induction of ventricular tachycardia: reentry versus triggered automaticity. Am J Cardiol 1979;44:1–8.

3. Belhassen B, Rotmensch HH, Laniado S. Response of recurrent sustained ventricular tachycardia to verapamil. Br Heart J 1981;46:679–82.

4. Ohe T, Shimomura K, Aihara N, et al. Idiopathic sustained left ventricular tachycardia: clinical and electrophysiological characteristics. Circulation 1988;77:560–8.

5. Nogami A. Idiopathic left ventricular tachycardia: assessment and treatment. Card Electrophysiol Rev 2002;6:448–57.

6. Nishiuchi S, Nogami A, Naito S. A case with occurrence of antidromic tachycardia after ablation of idiopathic left fascicular tachycardia: mechanism of left upper septal ventricular tachycardia. J Cardiovasc Electrophysiol 2013;24:825–7.

7. Talib AK, Nogami A, Nishiuchi S, et al. Verapamil-sensitive upper septal idiopathic left ventricular tachycardia: Prevalence, mechanism, and electrophysiological characteristics. J Am Coll Cardiol EP 2015;1:369–80.

8. Nogami A, Naito S, Tada H, et al. Demonstration of diastolic and presystolic Purkinje potential as critical potentials on a macroreentry circuit of verapamil-sensitive idiopathic left ventricular tachycardia. J Am Coll Cardiol 2000;36:811–23.

9. Nogami A, Naito S, Tada H, et al. Verapamil-sensitive left anterior fascicular ventricular tachycardia: results of radiofrequency ablation in six patients. J Cardiovasc Electrophysiol 1998;9:1269–78.

10. Liu Y, Fang Z, Yang B, et al. Catheter ablation of fascicular ventricular tachycardia: long-term clinical Outcomes and mechanisms of recurrence. Circ Arrhythm Electrophysiol 2015;8:1443–51.

11. Guo XG, Liu X, Zhou GB, et al. Clinical, electrocardiographic, and electrophysiological characteristics of left upper septal fascicular ventricular tachycardia. Europace 2018;20:673–81.

12. Komatsu Y, Nogami A, Kurosaki K, et al. Fascicular ventricular tachycardia originating from papillary muscles: Purkinje network involvement in the reentrant circuit. Circ Arrhythm Electrophysiol 2017;10: e004549.

13. Bogun F, Good E, Reich S, et al. Role of Purkinje fibers in post-infarction ventricular tachycardia. J Am Coll Cardiol 2006;48:2500–7.

14. Talib AK, Nogami A, Morishima I, et al. Non-reentrant fascicular tachycardia: clinical and electrophysiological characteristics of a distinct type of idiopathic ventricular tachycardia. Circ Arrhythm Electrophysiol 2016;9:e004177.

15. Maruyama M, Terada T, Miyamoto S, et al. Demonstration of the reentrant circuit of verapamil-sensitive idiopathic left ventricular tachycardia: direct evidence for macroreentry as the underlying mechanism. J Cardiovasc Electrophysiol 2001;12:968–72.

16. Kuo JY, Tai CT, Chiang CE, et al. Is the fascicle of left bundle branch involved in the reentrant circuit of verapamil-sensitive idiopathic left ventricular tachycardia? Pacing Clin Electrophysiol 2003;26: 1986–92.

17. Morishima I, Nogami A, Tsuboi H, et al. Negative participation of the left posterior fascicle in the reentry

circuit of verapamil-sensitive idiopathic left ventricular tachycardia. Heart Rhythm 2012;23:556–9.

18. Maeda S, Yokoyama Y, Nogami A, et al. First case of left posterior fascicle in a bystander circuit of idiopathic left ventricular tachycardia. Can J Cardiol 2014;30:e11–3.

19. Liu Q, Shehata M, Jiang R, et al. Macroreentrant loop in ventricular tachycardia from the left posterior fascicle: new implications for mapping and ablation. Circ Arrhythmia Electrophysiol 2016;9:e004272.

20. Hayashi M, Kobayashi Y, Iwasaki YK, et al. Novel mechanism of postinfarction ventricular tachycardia originating in surviving left posterior Purkinje fibers. Heart Rhythm 2006;3:908–18.

21. Morishima I, Nogami A, Tsuboi H, et al. Verapamil-sensitive left anterior fascicular ventricular tachycardia associated with a healed myocardial infarction: changes in the delayed Purkinje potential during sinus rhythm. J Interv Card Electrophysiol 2008;22:233–7.

22. Masuda K, Nogami A, Kuroki K, et al. Conversion to Purkinje-related monomorphic ventricular tachycardia after ablation of ventricular fibrillation in ischemic heart disease. Circ Arrhythm Electrophysiol 2016;9:e004224.

23. Lopera G, Stevenson WG, Soejima K, et al. Identification and ablation of three types of ventricular tachycardia involving the His-Purkinje system in patients with heart disease. J Cardiovasc Electrophysiol 2004;15:52–8.

24. Zeppenfeld K, Blom NA, Bootsma M, et al. Incessant ventricular tachycardia in fulminant lymphocytic myocarditis: evidence for origin in the Purkinje system and successful treatment with ablation. Heart Rhythm 2007;4:88–91.

25. Naruse Y, Sekiguchi Y, Nogami A, et al. Systematic treatment approach to ventricular tachycardia in cardiac sarcoidosis. Circ Arrhythm Electrophysiol 2014;7:407–13.

26. Guerot C, Valere PE, Castillo-Fenoy A, et al. [Tachycardia by branch-to-branch reentry]. Arch Mal Coeur Vaiss 1974;67:1–11.

27. Akhtar M, Damato AN, Batsford WP, et al. Demonstration of re-entry within the His-Purkinje system in man. Circulation 1974;50:1150–62.

28. Blanck Z, Dhala A, Deshpande S, et al. Bundle branch reentrant ventricular tachycardia: cumulative experience in 48 patients. J Cardiovasc Electrophysiol 1993;4:253–62.

29. Lloyd EA, Zipes DP, Heger JJ, et al. Sustained ventricular tachycardia due to bundle branch reentry. Am Heart J 1982;104:1095–7.

30. Touboul P, Kirkorian G, Atallah G, et al. Bundle branch reentry: a possible mechanism of ventricular tachycardia. Circulation 1983;67:674–80.

31. Narasimhan C, Jazayeri MR, Sra J, et al. Ventricular tachycardia in valvular heart disease: facilitation of sustained bundle-branch reentry by valve surgery. Circulation 1997;96:4307–13.

32. Merino JL, Carmona JR, Fernandez-Lozano I, et al. Mechanisms of sustained ventricular tachycardia in myotonic dystrophy: implications for catheter ablation. Circulation 1998;98:541–6.

33. Nogami A. Purkinje-related arrhythmias part I: monomorphic ventricular tachycardias. Pacing Clin Electrophysiol 2011;34:624–50.

34. Blanck Z, Jazayeri M, Dhala A, et al. Bundle branch reentry: a mechanism of ventricular tachycardia in the absence of myocardial or valvular dysfunction. J Am Coll Cardiol 1993;22:1718–22.

35. Blanck Z, Deshpande S, Jazayeri MR, et al. Catheter ablation of the left bundle branch for the treatment of sustained bundle branch reentrant ventricular tachycardia. J Cardiovasc Electrophysiol 1995;6:40–3.

36. Phlips T, Ramchurn H, De Roy L. Reverse BBRVT in a structurally normal heart. Acta Cardiol 2012;67:603–7.

37. Chen H, Shi L, Yang B, et al. Electrophysiological characteristics of bundle branch reentry ventricular tachycardia in patients without structural heart disease. Circ Arrhythm Electrophysiol 2018;11:e006049.

38. Caceres J, Jazayeri M, McKinnie J, et al. Sustained bundle branch reentry as a mechanism of clinical tachycardia. Circulation 1989;79:256–70.

39. Delacretaz E, Stevenson WG, Ellison KE, et al. Mapping and radiofrequency catheter ablation of the three types of sustained monomorphic ventricular tachycardia in nonischemic heart disease. J Cardiovasc Electrophysiol 2000;11:11–7.

40. Moss JD, Flatley EE, Beaser AD, et al. Characterization of ventricular tachycardia after left ventricular assist device implantation as destination therapy: a single-center ablation experience. JACC Clin Electrophysiol 2017;3:1412–24.

41. Dallaglio PD, Aceña M, Canals OA, et al. Double bundle branch reentrant ventricular tachycardia ablation in a patient on ventricular assist device support. Heartrhythm Case Rep 2019;5:452–6.

42. Tchou P, Mehdirad AA. Bundle branch reentry ventricular tachycardia. Pacing Clin Electrophysiol 1995;18:1427–37.

43. Blanck Z, Akhtar M. Ventricular tachycardia due to sustained bundle branch reentry: diagnostic and therapeutic considerations. Clin Cardiol 1993;16:619–22.

44. Fisher JD. Bundle branch reentry tachycardia: why is the HV interval often longer than in sinus rhythm? The critical role of anisotropic conduction. J Interv Card Electrophysiol 2001;5:173–6.

45. Machino T, Tada H, Sekiguchi Y, et al. Three-dimensional visualization of the entire reentrant circuit of bundle branch reentrant tachycardia. Heart Rhythm 2013;10:459–60.

46. Crijns HJ, Kingma JH, Gosselink AT, et al. Comparison in the same patient of aberrant conduction and bundle branch reentry after dofetilide, a new selective class III antiarrhythmic agent. Pacing Clin Electrophysiol 1993;16:1006–16.

47. Tchou P, Jazayeri M, Denker S, et al. Transcatheter electrical ablation of right bundle branch: a method of treating macroreentrant ventricular tachycardia attributed to bundle branch reentry. Circulation 1988;78:246–57.

48. Nogami A, Olshansky B. Bundle branch reentry tachycardia. In: Zipes DP, Jalife J, Stevenson WG, editors. Cardiac Electrophysiology: from Cell to Bedside. 7th edition. Philadelphia, (PA): Elsevier; 2018. p. 799–819.

49. Schmidt B, Tang M, Chun KR, et al. Left bundle branch-Purkinje system in patients with bundle branch reentrant tachycardia: lessons from catheter ablation and electroanatomic mapping. Heart Rhythm 2009;6:51–8.

50. Pathak RK, Fahed J, Santangeli P, et al. Long-term outcome of catheter ablation for treatment of bundle branch re-entrant tachycardia. JACC Clin Electrophysiol 2018;4:331–8.

# Patient Selection, Techniques, and Complication Mitigation for Epicardial Ventricular Tachycardia Ablation

Timothy Maher, MD[a,b], John-Ross Clarke, MD[a,b], Zain Virk, MD[b,c],
Andre d'Avila, MD, PhD[a,b],*

## KEYWORDS

• Epicardial access • Ventricular tachycardia • Radiofrequency ablation

## KEY POINTS

• Epicardial ventricular tachycardia ablation can improve the efficacy of ventricular tachycardia ablation procedures but with an increased risk of procedural complications.
• Epicardial ablation is most helpful when prior endocardial ablation fails, in certain nonischemic cardiomyopathy substrates, and when the electrocardiogram or advanced imaging suggests the presence of an epicardial ventricular tachycardia origin.
• Careful laboratory preparation, meticulous technique, and an awareness of the potential complications are necessary to improve the safety of epicardial access and ablation.
• Not all patients can undergo percutaneous epicardial access, and not all nonendocardial ventricular tachycardia origins are best ablated from the epicardial space.
• Adjunct techniques may be effective alternatives to percutaneous epicardial access.

## INTRODUCTION

Pioneered in the late 1990s by Brazilian electrophysiologists seeking to better treat ventricular arrhythmias caused by Chagas heart disease,[1,2] percutaneous epicardial ventricular tachycardia (VT) mapping and ablation expanded worldwide over the subsequent 2 decades, and quickly relocated epicardial arrhythmia treatment from the operating room to the electrophysiology (EP) laboratory. Epicardial ablation has since emerged as a fundamental technique to improve the success of VT ablation procedures in properly selected patients.[3] Initially adopted by high-volume and expert centers, epicardial VT ablation is now performed in approximately 25% of VT cases in EP laboratories across the world.[4,5] The technique should be available to any institution where complex ablations are performed as long as there is a commitment to the preparation and resources required to execute the procedure safely.

Advances in high-density mapping of the epicardial surface of the heart has enhanced the understanding of the 3-dimensional (3D) properties of VT circuits within the myocardial wall and the distribution of scar and VT substrate among different cardiomyopathies. Any patient with a cardiomyopathy causing scar-related VT can have

[a] Harvard Thorndike Electrophysiology Institute and Arrhythmia Service, Beth Israel Deaconess Medical Center, 185 Pilgrim Road, Palmer 4, Boston, MA 02215, USA; [b] Harvard Medical School, Boston, MA, USA; [c] Department of Medicine, Vanderbilt University Medical Center, 1161 21st Avenue South, Nashville, TN, USA
* Corresponding author.
E-mail address: tmaher@bidmc.harvard.edu

Card Electrophysiol Clin 14 (2022) 657–677
https://doi.org/10.1016/j.ccep.2022.07.007

epicardial substrate; however, in certain cardio-myopathies the need for epicardial ablation is more likely, including those with arrhythmogenic right ventricular cardiomyopathy (ARVC), idio-pathic dilated cardiomyopathy, myocarditis, sarcoidosis, Brugada syndrome, and hypertrophic cardiomyopathy (HCM). Although the use of epicardial access to map and ablate patients after a failed endocardial procedure is the common indication,[6] the use of VT electrocardiogram (ECG) QRS morphology assessment and prepro-cedure advanced imaging can help to determine whether up-front epicardial access should be ob-tained. The appropriate inclusion of epicardial ac-cess reduces recurrent VT and implanted cardioverter defibrillator (ICD) shocks in system-atic meta-analyses of observational cohorts.[7,8] However, the benefits of epicardial ablation in increasing the likelihood of a successful procedure are tempered by the risk of significant complica-tions beyond endocardial procedures, including serious intrathoracic or intra-abdominal bleeding, coronary vessel injury, and phrenic nerve injury.[9]

Recent innovations and developments to improve the safety and success of percutaneous epicardial VT ablation stand to further expand its use. In this review we will describe the best prac-tices to maximize the chance of a safe and effica-cious procedure in a modern EP laboratory, including:

- When to attempt epicardial access
- How to safely perform percutaneous epicar-dial access
- How to minimize and manage complications from epicardial access
- How to map and ablate VT in the epicardial space
- How to make use of alternatives to percuta-neous access

## BEST PRACTICE: WHEN TO ATTEMPT PERCUTANEOUS EPICARDIAL ACCESS

The decision to attempt epicardial access is consequential, with the increased risk of bleeding complications and collateral organ damage dur-ing access and need for the resources required to manage such complications, the benefits anticipated in treating the arrhythmia must exceed the possible risks compared with endocardial-only access. To maximize the antici-pated benefits, there should be reasonable suspi-cion that the patient has potential epicardial VT substrate such that mapping and ablation will improve the procedural outcome. Meta-analyses of observation and registry-based studies have

shown that, although combined endocardial–epicardial ablation can decrease VT recurrence and ICD shocks, particularly in patients with ischemic cardiomyopathy (ICM) and ARVC, there is a nearly 3-fold increase in significant acute complications.[7,8,10]

Therefore, instead of routine up-front epicardial access for VT ablation, we propose a serious of questions to ask in whether deciding on obtaining epicardial access.

1. Has the patient had a failed endocardial VT ablation?
2. Does the 12-lead ECG suggest an epicardial exit?
3. Does the patient have a cardiomyopathy with an increased odds of critical epicardial VT substrate?
4. Is there imaging evidence of abnormal subepi-cardial or free wall midmyocardial substrate?

If the answer to any of these questions is yes, then epicardial access is reasonable; if the answer to multiple questions is yes, then epicardial access is recommended if the patient has not had prior cardiac surgery or pericarditis, both of which can make epicardial access more difficult or dangerous. Each of these questions involves nuance that is worth discussion. **Fig. 1** graphically depicts this approach to choosing when to obtain epicardial access.

### Has the Patient Failed Endocardial VT Ablation?

If a patient experiences recurrent VT after a previ-ous endocardial ablation, the prospect of surviving critical midmyocardial or subepicardial substrate must be considered, regardless of the cardiomy-opathy etiology. Although patients with ICM have predominantly subendocardial VT circuits,[11,12] it has long been demonstrated that in patients with ICM, approximately 14% to 33% of VTs involve subepicardial critical substrate, and particularly right coronary or left circumflex territory infarctions can require epicardial ablation to render them non-inducible.[13–16] Most ICM VTs can be treated suc-cessfully with endocardial ablation, but after recurrence, combined endocardial–epicardial ablation on the repeat procedure significantly im-proves freedom from VT.[17]

Although nonischemic cardiomyopathies (NICM)—a heterogenous collection of diseases including idiopathic dilated cardiomyopathies, Chagas disease, myocarditis, and sarcoidosis—are more likely to have subepicardial substrate, the benefit of combined endocardial–epicardial ablation is less clear based on systematic

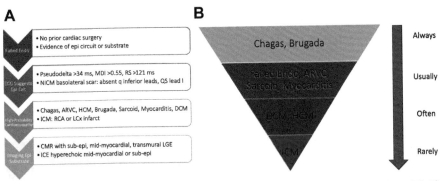

**Fig. 1.** Schema to help guide decision on when to obtain epicardial access for VT ablation. (**A**) Algorithm to decide on epicardial access. (**B**) Approximate frequency of need for epicardial access by cardiomyopathy type. CMR, cardiac MRI; DCM, dilated cardiomyopathy; ENDO, endocardial; EPI, epicardial; ICM, infarct cardiomyopathy; LCx, left circumflex artery; MDI, maximum deflection index; RCA, right coronary artery.

meta-analyses, with higher risks of recurrence regardless of the approach taken.[7,8] As a result, we do not advocate for routine up-front epicardial access during a first-time procedure in patients with NICM, unless there are other convincing clues to important subepicardial substrate based on the 12-lead ECG or imaging (see **Fig. 1**A). With repeat procedures after failed endocardial ablation for NICM VT, obtaining epicardial access is often necessary, barring contraindication.

Additionally, the endocardial map can provide clues as to whether epicardial access can be helpful. Endocardial activation maps of VT that show a pseudofocal pattern centrifugal activation around the earliest endocardial exit, or activation maps with missing diastolic cycle length may represent 3D circuits with critical portions either midmyocardial or subepicardial that can best be treated with epicardial ablation.[18] In the presence of no or minimal scar appreciated on bipolar voltage endocardial mapping, low unipolar voltage (indicative of far-field abnormal tissue), has been demonstrated to correlate well with epicardial substrate in both patients with ICM and patients with NICM. Exact unipolar voltage cut-offs can vary by cardiomyopathy and were initially validated with 3.5- to 4.0-mm tip ablation catheters; 8.3 mV in the left ventricle (LV) and 5.5 mV in the right ventricular (RV) free wall are commonly used.[19,20] The presence of these clues during endocardial mapping should prompt consideration of epicardial access after a failed procedure, or even during the index procedure.

## Is There 12-Lead Electrocardiogram Evidence of an Epicardial Exit?

Multiple groups have proposed ECG criteria to predict epicardial origins based on either measured QRS intervals or QRS morphologies in specific leads (**Fig. 2**). The accuracy of these methods depends on the etiology of the cardiomyopathy and the location of scar substrate.[21] In 2004, Berruezo et al[22] proposed QRS interval criteria for VTs with right bundle branch block morphology from a cohort of both patients with ICM and patients with NICM using both pacemapping and clinical VT mapping. They proposed epicardial origins of VT when there is pseudodelta wave of 34 ms or greater, an intrinsicoid deflection in V2 of 85 ms or more, or shortest RS complex of 121 ms or more. In contrast, morphologic criteria make use of the frontal plane axis in a site-specific fashion, noting that epicardial exit sites will produce q-waves in the corresponding nearest ECG lead, because all myocardial depolarization forces will point away from that lead, including epicardial to endocardial transmural activation. The presence of transmural infarct–related q-waves limits the applicability of these criteria to patients with ICM, and both ECG interval and morphologic criteria overall poorly predict an epicardial VT origin in patients with prior infarcts during external validation.[23]

ECG criteria have been more predictive with patients with NICM. Vallès et al[24] combined morphologic and interval criteria and assessed patients with NICM with basal anterior or lateral substrate and showed excellent specificity (95%) but poor sensitivity (20%) using as the criteria a lack of inferior q-waves, q-wave in lead I, a pseudodelta wave of 75 ms or more, and a maximum deflection index of 0.59 or higher. **Fig. 2**B shows an example of an ECG satisfying this morphologic criteria. A more sensitive but slightly less specific 4-step algorithm using these criteria for patients with NICM with basal anterior or lateral substrate demonstrated 93% sensitivity and 86% specificity. Bazan et al[21] later extended these criteria to other scar regions in patients with NICM with approximately

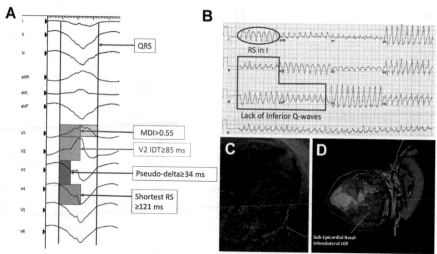

**Fig. 2.** ECG and imaging clues to an epicardial origin of a ventricular arrhythmia. (*A*) An example QRS from a VT fulfilling proposed ECG interval criteria for epicardial origin. (*B*) Twelve-lead ECG of a patient with epicardial VT with evidence of lateral subepicardial scar fulfilling proposed QRS morphology criteria for NICM. The same patient had scar seen on MRI 4-chamber view (*C*) with 3D reconstruction (*D*) noting the dense (*dark blue*) and border zone (*light blue*) LGE segmentation. IDT, intrinsicoid deflection time; MDI, maximum deflection index; QRS, QRS duration.

84% accuracy and widely variable sensitivity and specificity by LV location.

Given the imperfect sensitivity and specificity of published ECG criteria for epicardial arrhythmias,[23] we do not advocate for basing the decision to obtain epicardial access solely on satisfying a set of criteria, but recommend incorporating this information with other factors (such as cardiomyopathy type, imaging, history of failed endocardial ablation) if the decision is otherwise equivocal.

### Does the Patient Have a Cardiomyopathy with Increased Odds of Critical Epicardial Ventricular Tachycardia Substrate?

In patients with structural heart disease leading to scar-related VT, certain NICM etiologies are more likely to have subepicardial substrate requiring epicardial access for mapping and ablation—and with ARVC, Chagas disease, and Brugada syndrome, a first-line epicardial access approach is advisable (see **Fig. 1**B). With other types of NICM, including dilated cardiomyopathy, HCM, myocarditis, and sarcoidosis, the location of scar can be patchy with critical portions of VT circuits either endocardial, midmyocardial, or epicardial. We briefly discuss the motivation for epicardial access in these different groups.

Chagas cardiomyopathy, a disease endemic to Latin America caused by *Trypanosoma cruzi* leading to transmural and subepicardial fibrotic substrate predominantly in the inferolateral LV, represented the prototypical substrate requiring epicardial access for successful treatment of the VT.[25,26] Sosa et al,[1,2] motivated by the poor effectiveness with endocardial ablation with many patients with Chagas disease, developed the technique for percutaneous transthoracic pericardial puncture to facilitate epicardial mapping and ablation. With voltage mapping, patients with Chagas disease have significantly more epicardial scar than endocardial scar, and a randomized controlled trial has demonstrated greater acute procedural success and improved long-term freedom from VT recurrence without a difference in complication rates.[27] Therefore, we recommend up-front epicardial access during VT ablation for Chagas cardiomyopathy.

Patients with ARVC possess fibrofatty dysplasia of the RV, leading to predominantly reentrant arrhythmias. Despite the thin wall of the RV, the arrhythmogenic substrate of the RV in ARVC can be compartmentalized into endocardial and epicardial layers. Although critical isthmuses can be present in either layer, most patients with ARVC have predominantly epicardial substrate as defined by either areas of low-voltage or wavefront discontinuities during sinus rhythm activation mapping.[28–30] Although a staged procedure starting with an endocardial ablation followed by epicardial mapping and ablation at the time of recurrence can lead to reasonable long-term suppression of VT,[31] a combined endocardial–epicardial approach is associated with superior freedom from recurrent VT.[32,33] High-density multielectrode simultaneous endocardial–epicardial mapping of VTs in patients with ARVC has shown that significantly more cycle length of the VTs were epicardial as opposed to endocardial, 71% had entirely epicardial circuits, and most successful ablation sites were epicardial (70%).[30] As a result, we favor a very low threshold for epicardial mapping in patients with ARVC.

Brugada syndrome, a channelopathy associated with the risk of sudden death from ventricular arrhythmias has been demonstrated on epicardial mapping to show areas of low-voltage, conduction delay, and long, fragmented electrograms (EGMs) in the epicardial RV outflow tract. The epicardial substrate in Brugada syndrome is thought be functional, because areas of abnormal EGMs and voltage expand from the RV outflow tract to the free wall with sodium channel blockade via ajmaline infusion.[34] Ablation of this substrate in high-risk patients can in some cases nearly normalize a type 1 Brugada ECG pattern, promote noninducibility on programmed stimulation, and is associated with a low incidence of recurrent VT or ventricular fibrillation (VF).[34,35] It has not yet been proven if ablation improves long-term outcomes in Brugada syndrome patients; a randomized controlled trial, the Ablation in Brugada Syndrome for the Prevention of VF, is currently in progress and will randomize patients to continued ICD (control arm) or continued ICD and ablation therapy (NCT02704416).[36] Based on the observational data to date, if ablation is pursued to decrease VT or VF in high-risk patients with Brugada syndrome, then up-front epicardial access is appropriate.

HCM is associated with VT and VF owing to myocyte disarray and resultant fibrosis. ICDs prevent sudden death in high-risk patients, although a small number of patients can experience recurrent monomorphic VT that can benefit from catheter ablation. Studies have shown that epicardial scar and epicardial successful VT ablation sites are more common than endocardial, illustrating the need for epicardial access as an important tool in VT ablation in patients with HCM.[37] With an excessively thick myocardium, a combined endocardial–epicardial substrate is commonly required; VT circuits can be predominantly endocardial, midmyocardial, epicardial, or a combination of each. Particular attention should be paid to an aneurysmal neck with the common apical aneurysms formed in patients with HCM, although epicardial access may be especially helpful in patients with scarring in other LV regions.[38] Epicardial access is reasonable, and possibly necessary, in patients with HCM, especially if there is a failed prior endocardial ablation, especially thick myocardial tissue near the VT origin, or endocardial VT mapping suggesting the participation of epicardial tissue.

Sarcoidosis and myocarditis can lead to cardiomyopathies, with inflammation and scarring leading to ventricular arrhythmias, often in a patchy pattern of scar noted on cardiac MRI (CMR) in a noncoronary pattern and thus often involving the LV midmyocardium or epicardium. Myocarditis often involves the LV free wall and sarcoidosis can occasionally involve the RV. Active myocarditis and healed myocarditis can both be associated with ventricular arrhythmias, with the active inflammatory phase more likely to have polymorphic VT or VF, and the healed phase more likely to have monomorphic VT, likely reentry from fibrosis.[39] Patients with myocarditis can have extensive epicardial low-voltage areas, and epicardial ablation is often necessary for acute procedural success, although a systematic assessment of endocardial vs combined endocardial–epicardial first-line approaches has not been performed.[40]

Similarly, there are few data on epicardial ablation in patients with sarcoidosis. Observational cohorts of patients with sarcoidosis show that VT ablation in drug-refractory patients can decrease the VT burden in a majority of patients, although epicardial mapping and ablation were performed in a minority of patients.[41] Active inflammation is associated with poor outcomes with VT ablation in both myocarditis and sarcoidosis.[40,42] For myocarditis and sarcoidosis, we recommend epicardial access in the setting of failed endocardial ablation, endocardial mapping supporting an epicardial origin, or adjunct data from the 12-lead or imaging suggesting significant epicardial substrate.

Dilated cardiomyopathies, often idiopathic or genetic, are heterogenous, and outcomes with catheter ablation for VT, when adjusted for comorbidities, are similar to those of other causes of NICM, including ARVC and myocarditis, and superior to sarcoid cardiomyopathy, valvular cardiomyopathy, or HCM, although they seem to be inferior to the results for patients with ICM.[43,44] Epicardial mapping and ablation are common in dilated cardiomyopathy patients ($\leq$37% involved epicardial ablation in a large registry), who can often have septal striae or patchy perivalvular, basal anterior or lateral midmyocardial or subepicardial scar.[44–46] We recommend epicardial access in the setting of failed endocardial ablation, endocardial mapping suggesting an epicardial origin, or adjunct data from the 12-lead or imaging suggest significant epicardial substrate.

Finally, in patients without structural heart disease, epicardial access is rarely effective in improving the ablation outcome.[17] Idiopathic ventricular arrhythmias, even when originating from midmyocardial or subepicardial sources of the outflow tracts and LV summit, are not typically accessible from a catheter in the pericardial space owing to the proximity to the coronary vessels and overlying epicardial fat, rendering ablation at worst unsafe and at best ineffective.[47] Elsewhere in this review, we discuss alternative methods of approaching epicardial VTs when percutaneous access is not suitable.

### Is There Imaging Evidence of Abnormal Subepicardial or Free Wall Midmyocardial Substrate?

Advanced cardiac imaging techniques, including CMR, cardiac computed tomography (CT) scans, and intracardiac echocardiography (ICE) can assess for the extent and distribution of myocardial scar or wall thinning that can predict if epicardial access may be necessary during VT ablation. Additionally, 3D segmentations of cross-sectional imaging (CMR and CT scans) can be coregistered with the electroanatomic mapping system to help focus mapping and ablation on areas of known scar or wall thinning, as well as demonstrate the relationship of critical nearby structures, including the coronary vessels, valves, phrenic nerves, and ICD leads to avoid complications (see **Fig. 2**C, D). **Fig. 3** demonstrates the correlation between coregistered CT angiography and invasive coronary angiography during epicardial VT mapping.

Late gadolinium enhancement (LGE) and the heterogenous border zone between dense LGE and normal tissue are associated with both low-voltage areas on mapping and VT isthmuses.[48,49] Transmural, free wall–midmyocardial, and subepicardial distributions of LGE should raise the suspicion that epicardial access may be needed for mapping and ablation.[50–53] Corridors of border zone between denser scar may harbor surviving myocardial bundles that can promote reentry, and CMR-guided ablation strategies targeting these areas after coregistration with the electroanatomic mapping system are associated with excellent freedom from VT.[54–56]

Cardiac CT scanning has a high spatial resolution with excellent demarcation of anatomic structures and accurate assessment of myocardial wall thickness. Although wall thinning predicts endocardial low-voltage areas well in patients with ICM, it is not well-correlated with epicardial scar.[57] However, severe wall thinning on a CT scan is associated with transmural substrate (abnormal EGMs both endocardially and epicardially) in both ICM and NICM, and ablation of endocardial local abnormal ventricular activity in areas of wall thinning on a CT scan can eliminate epicardial local abnormal ventricular activity in patients with ICM.[58,59] The use of late iodine enhancement (>8 minutes after injection) may correlate with LGE and VT isthmuses, although its use remains investigational and a decreased signal-to-noise ratio on most CT scanners precludes its reliability at the moment.[60] At this juncture, wall thinning alone on a CT scan should not prompt epicardial access; however, obtaining preprocedure CT angiography can provide significant value by improving coregistration with CMR, demarcating critical structures, showing patency of coronary arteries, and excluding intracardiac thrombus.

Although coregistration can help catheter navigation around important structures, the small

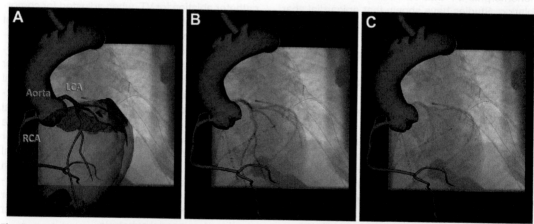

**Fig. 3.** Real-time integration of a cardiac CT scan registered to electroanatomic map and coronary angiography during ablation of a basal anterior epicardial focal VT. (*A*) Epicardial activation map with segmented aortic root and coronary arteries to assess proximity of coronary arteries to the ablation target site. (*B*) LCA segmentation partially transparent to show accuracy of co-registration with coronary angiography. (*C*) Transparent LCA. LCA, left coronary artery; RCA, right coronary artery.

but unavoidable errors in registration (approximately 5 mm) do not obviate the need for fluoroscopy, angiography, or ICE to verify that an ablation location is safe. As compared with the traditional technique for image coregistration with electroanatomic maps (which require sample anatomy from the aortic arch, LV apex, mitral annulus, coronary sinus, or RV outflow tract–pulmonary trunk), ICE integration into the mapping system can allow rapid and accurate segmentation of these structures to be used as fiducial markers. ICE can additionally be used to identify echogenic subepicardium or midmyocardium that has been shown to correlate with scar during mapping.[61,62]

## BEST PRACTICE: HOW TO SAFELY OBTAIN EPICARDIAL ACCESS
### EP Laboratory and Patient Preparation

Given the risk for major complications, we recommend epicardial access be performed in centers with in-house access to cardiac surgery, urgent echocardiography, blood products, as well as intensive care unit–level care.[3] We perform epicardial access with the patient under general anesthesia in the EP laboratory with a wide field sterilized and draped around the subxiphoid region with the patient in the supine position.

### Pericardial Puncture

The dry pericardial puncture remains largely unchanged since its description by Sosa et al in 1996.[1] To facilitate access to the virtual space between the parietal and visceral pericardium while minimizing the chance of lacerating adjacent structures, Sosa et al used the Tuohy needle with its spoon-shaped tip that can help separate planes of tissue on its trajectory with minimal trauma. Most operators still use the 17G to 18G Tuohy needle, although other approaches are discussed elsewhere in this article. To find the puncture site, the xiphoid process should first be palpated. The entry site should be lateral to the xiphoid below the margin of the left-sided rib cage (**Fig. 4**A). The needle should then be pointed toward the patient's left shoulder, and the stylet can be removed once under the skin. The needle should be advanced under live fluoroscopy during an inspiratory breath hold or apnea.[63] The authors favor an inspiratory breath hold because this technique results in maximum separation of the heart and the abdominal organs.

Both inferiorly and anteriorly directed puncture approaches can safely be used to access the epicardial space. For an inferior puncture, the skin is punctured 2 to 3 cm below the rib cage margin at a roughly 30° to 45° angle, which allows the needle to pass through the space of Larrey just superior to the diaphragm. An anterior puncture requires a shallow angle of 20° to 30° and requires skin entry 1 to 2 cm more caudally and a more medial trajectory to ensure the needle trajectory is not impeded by the underside of the sternum or passes too close to the internal mammary artery.[64] Many providers prefer bevel down for the inferior approach and bevel up for the anterior approach to prevent inadvertent damage to the epicardial coronary vessels (**Fig. 5**).

For an inferior approach, we recommend using fluoroscopy with either in anteroposterior or right anterior oblique orientation. A right anterior oblique orientation can help to ensure the puncture is directed toward the base of the heart. With the anterior approach, a left lateral fluoroscopic view can help to guide the needle approach over the diaphragm and under the sternum toward the pericardium.[65] A comparison of the anterior and inferior approaches has suggested higher rates of puncture complications with the inferior approach, driven by the risk of coronary, diaphragmatic, and abdominal structure injury, whereas the rates of tamponade are similar.[66] The inferior approach may be helpful in certain circumstances, such as in the presence of anterior adhesions from prior cardiac surgery or the need to manipulate the catheter to the lateral wall.

Once the needle advances to the edge of the pericardium, the operator can often feel the pulsation of the heartbeat transmitted by the needle if there is no preexisting pericardial effusion. With further gentle advancement of the needle as it tents the pericardium toward the RV, the pericardium will be entered, often with the sensation of a pop or slight loss of resistance. At this point, a small amount of contrast (0.5–1.0 mL is typically sufficient) can be injected through the needle to confirm pericardial access. If the pericardium has been accessed, the contrast will layer along the inferior border and then rapidly diffuse into the pericardial space. If the needle is still in the mediastinum, there will be staining at the needle tip without washout. If the needle is in the RV, there will be rapid washout without the layering at the pericardial border. It is best to avoid excessive contrast injection because the staining can obscure the fluoroscopic view. An RV puncture during epicardial access is common, occurring in 17% of attempts in 1 series,[67] and rarely causes major bleeding if the needle is retracted before laceration because the myocardium can contract around the tract. Pulsating bleeding through the needle will be observed. If RV puncture occurs, slowly pull the needle back a few

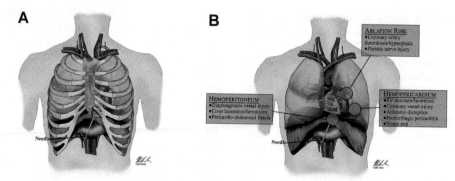

**Fig. 4.** Epicardial access anatomy and complications. (*A*) Bony landmarks and the sternocostal triangle where the needle will puncture the skin. (*B*) Complications from epicardial access and ablation. (*Courtesy of John-Ross Clarke, MD, Boston, MA.*)

millimeters and advance the guidewire into the pericardial space and continue with the procedure, checking periodically on ICE for a new pericardial effusion.

We recommend next advancing a long 0.032/0.035″ guidewire through the needle around the border of the heart under fluoroscopy. Anteroposterior or right anterior oblique views are insufficient

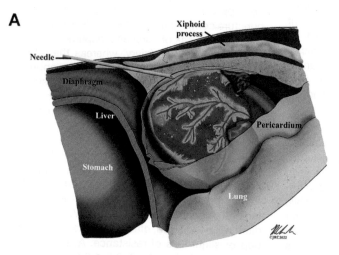

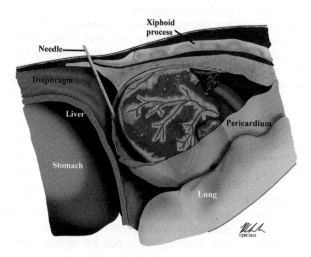

**Fig. 5.** Needle approach with inferior and anterior techniques for epicardial puncture. The inferior approach requires a deeper angle (*A*) than the shallower anterior approach (*B*). (*Courtesy of John-Ross Clarke, MD, Boston, MA.*)

to confirm that the wire is in the pericardial space versus passing through the RV outflow tract into the pulmonary arteries. Instead, the left anterior oblique projection must be used to show the wire passing around both the left and right heart borders as it traverses the cardiac chambers (**Fig. 6**).[63] The guidewire can also often be visualized on ICE passing in the pericardial space with the probe in the RV. ICE can also be used for real-time monitoring for effusion after the puncture.

Once intrapericardial access is confirmed, the needle is removed while maintaining guidewire position. We recommend a small skin nick at the puncture site and predilation with an 8F dilator followed by the advancement of a long sheath. The Agilis EPI Steerable Introducer (Abbott Vascular, Abbott Park, IL) is designed specifically for facile manipulation of intrapericardial catheters. No long sheath should be left in the pericardial space without either a blunt-tipped catheter (such as an ablation or mapping catheter) or pigtail catheter, because the hollow tip can lacerate intrapericardial structures. Aspiration from the sheath should reveal only serous or serosanginous fluid with a nontraumatic puncture.

## Anticoagulation Management

Conventional practice has held that hemopericardium, hemothorax, and hemoperitoneum complications from pericardial access can be best managed or avoided if the patient is not anticoagulated at the time of pericardial puncture. The feasibility of obtaining epicardial access on oral anticoagulation or while heparinized is well-documented.[68,69] We feel it remains the best practice to hold oral anticoagulation for 48 hours before

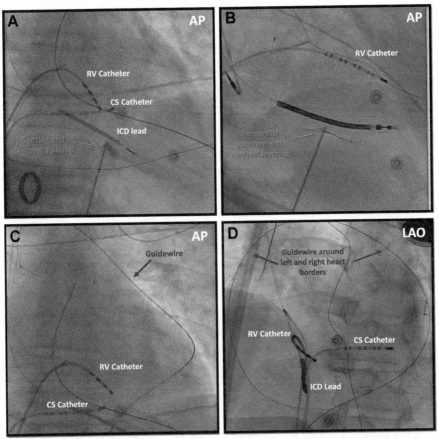

**Fig. 6.** Fluoroscopic guidance of percutaneous pericardial puncture. (*A*) AP view of tenting of the Touhy needle at the edge of the pericardial border and small contrast injection showing local staining. (*B*) After successful pericardial puncture, a small contrast injection will show layer along the pericardial border and rapid washout into the rest of the pericardial space. (*C*) In the AP view after the guidewire is advanced it is not definitive that the wire passes within the pericardial space or is in the RV outflow tract and pulmonary artery branches. (*D*) In the LAO view, the guidewire passes along the left and right heart borders, confirming the wire is in the pericardial space. AP, anteroposterior; CS, coronary sinus; LAO, left anterior oblique view.

the procedure and to obtain epicardial access before systemic heparinization when the probability of needing to map or ablate on the epicardial surface is high (see **Fig. 1**). If the operator decides to obtain epicardial access after systemic heparinization, then we recommend protamine reversal. Ultimately, accidental cardiac puncture seems to be the main predictor of significant pericardial bleeding.[70] If there is a high risk for stroke owing to a history of prior embolic stroke or atrial fibrillation, then heparin bridging is reasonable, or transesophageal echocardiography should be obtained before the procedure to exclude intracardiac thrombus in case electrical cardioversion is necessary during the procedure.

### Imaging-guided access approaches

Cross-sectional imaging obtained before the procedure can reveal atypical or anomalous anatomy, including pectus, sternal, or xiphoid abnormalities; situs inversus; and pericardial thickening. In patients with prior coronary artery bypass grafting, CT angiography can identify the graft anastomoses to allow extra care in those areas during mapping and ablation. Rarely, patients can have a congenital absence of the pericardium, which is typically an incidental finding and has been noted in up to 1 in 10,000 to 14,000 people.[71] Congenital pericardial cysts, also very rare, typically measure less than 5 cm and can be incidental or cause symptoms, or uncommonly, complications from rupture, and can preclude safe epicardial access.[72,73] Subramanian et al[74] recently showed that a preprocedural cardiac CT scan can be used to identify an optimal needle entry location and angle to avoid nearby viscera to decrease complications.

### Ending the Procedure

At the conclusion of the procedure, the pigtail catheter can be replaced inside the long sheath after removal of the mapping and/or ablation catheters. Any remaining intrapericardial fluid can be aspirated. If radiofrequency is performed, we recommend intrapericardial injection of steroids through the pigtail (either triamcinolone 2 mg/kg or methylprednisolone 125 mg) to limit the risk of postprocedural pericarditis.[75] Through the long sheath, the guidewire should be readvanced into the pericardial space, after which the sheath can be removed. In the event of a double RV puncture (caused by occult entry of the needle into RV and exiting back into the pericardial space during the puncture), an immediate effusion accumulation and tamponade will occur and the presence of the guidewire will allow the long sheath to be readvanced to plug the RV punctures to stabilize the

patient, drain the effusion, and prepare the operating room for repair.

If no effusion is noted on ICE after sheath removal and vital signs are stable, the guidewire may be removed and dressing applied. We recommend monitoring the patient in a recovery area or telemetry floor for at least 4 to 6 hours after the procedure or overnight observation before discharge. If accidental cardiac puncture or limited effusion were noted during the procedure then we recommend obtaining a focused transthoracic echocardiogram to check for effusion before discharge.

### Obtaining Access in Special Populations

Obesity can make epicardial access more challenging owing to difficulty palpating landmarks, difficult fluoroscopy, and the need to use steeper angles. An anterior approach can be particularly difficult with an obese abdomen. However, epicardial access in patients with elevated body mass index can be obtained with similar success and complication rates as normal weight individuals and is not a contraindication.[76]

In patients with prior cardiac surgery or pericarditis, it is possible that pericardial adhesions can prevent epicardial access or adequate catheter movement. Difficulty manipulating the guidewire can be a clue as to the presence of adhesions, which are more common anteriorly. The reported success rate of epicardial access is variable in the literature, ranging from 15% to 90%, although restriction of catheter movement was uniform in all cases and meticulous dissection of adhesions may be necessary.[77,78] To dissect adhesions percutaneously, we recommend the use of a deflective catheter, preferably with contact force sensing to manipulate the adhesions; the use of a steerable sheath directly for lysing adhesions can lead to laceration of the myocardium, coronary vessels, or bypass grafts. An alternative approach if percutaneous access fails in patients with prior cardiac surgery is obtaining epicardial access via a surgical window, typically via a subxiphoid window (best for inferior or inferolateral access) or anterior thoracotomy (best for anterior, anterolateral, and apical access).[79,80] The surgeon can then place the long sheath in the epicardial space, and further blunt dissection of adhesions can be performed by both the surgeons finger and/or the steerable catheter. The hybrid surgical approach is best accomplished in a hybrid operating room with the availability of EP recording, mapping, and ablation systems, although in some centers this procedure is performed in the EP laboratory as well. Although only 36% of the epicardial surface on average is accessible via the hybrid surgical approach, results from propensity matching to percutaneous epicardial VT ablations are similar.[80]

## Other Percutaneous Puncture Techniques

Alternative techniques for pericardial puncture have been explored that can offer distinct advantages over the traditional and widely used Sosa/Tuohy approach. The needle-in-needle approach makes use of an 18G Cook (Cook Medical, Bloomington, IN) needle for support, and a smaller profile 21G micropuncture needle inside it for the puncture. This strategy decreases the risk of bleeding, especially in the case of RV entry, while using. However, the shorter micropuncture wire may be inadequate to confirm an intrapericardial location and may not provide enough support in the presence of adhesions. Observational cohorts suggest lower rates of major pericardial bleeding and other acute complications with the needle-in-needle approach.[81,82]

An additional technique includes the use of a pressure sensor needle (EpiAccess System, EpiEP, Inc., New Haven, CT), which makes use of real-time pressure frequency signal analysis to determine which tissue the needle is currently passing through based on the differing waveform characteristics in each tissue. A small multicenter experience showed 100% success in access with no complications directly attributed to epicardial access.[83] In contrast with pressure waveform analysis, near-field impedance differences in thoracic tissues has also been proposed as a tool to determine the location of the needle tip and shown to be feasible in a preclinical model.[84]

Other preclinical investigational techniques to improve the safety of epicardial access include the use of video endoscopy coupled with forceps[85] or suction (PeriCardioScope, Perifect, Herzliya, Israel). Alternatively, separating the parietal and visceral pericardium with carbon dioxide insufflation after intentional exit from a distal coronary sinus branch with a microcatheter has been demonstrated in a multicenter patient registry to be not only feasible, but associated with very low rates of major bleeding.[86]

## BEST PRACTICE: HOW TO MINIMIZE AND MANAGE COMPLICATIONS FROM EPICARDIAL ACCESS

Decreasing complications with epicardial access requires proper procedural preparation, acute recognition, and rapid mobilizing of the necessary resources to treat the patient. Attention to safe and precise technique for access, mapping, and ablation (discussed elsewhere in this article) will minimize the risk of complications. Despite this finding, complications from epicardial VT ablation are common even in expert centers (approximately 7%–9%).[17,67] See **Fig. 4**B, which outlines common complications.

## Hemopericardium

Major intrapericardial bleeding (often described as >80 mL of blood) is the most common major complication of epicardial VT ablation. Causes of acute hemopericardium during epicardial VT ablation procedures includes:[87]

1. RV laceration from the access needle or intrapericardial sheath, advancement of a sheath or dilator into the ventricle if the guidewire was advanced into or through the RV
2. Coronary vessel laceration by the access needle, sheath, or catheters
3. Shearing of myocardium after disruption of adhesions.
4. Steam pop or disruption of epicardial bleb from epicardial ablation
5. Postprocedure acute pericarditis

Preprocedurally, we recommend holding anticoagulation when possible (discussed elsewhere in this article) and obtaining a blood type and screen to ensure preparedness for transfusion if necessary. Baseline blood counts and coagulation parameters are advisable as well. Hemopericardium can most easily be recognized via aspiration of sanguineous contents from the pericardium or by noting an enlarging pericardial effusion on ICE. ICE also can monitor for reaccumulation after an intervention, such as reversal of anticoagulation, and even help to ensure that the guidewire has advanced in the pericardial space after the puncture; as such, we recommend the use of ICE for all epicardial VT ablation procedures. Proper sheath management is paramount—no intrapericardial sheath should be left empty—instead, a mapping, ablation, or pigtail catheter should occupy the sheath to prevent the hollow tip from causing a laceration.

In the event of major pericardial bleeding, we recommend reversing anticoagulation, mobilizing blood products, and autotransfusion via a cell-saver system, which can allow drained pericardial blood to be immediately retransfused back into the patient and can assist in patient stabilization as a bridge to hemostasis or definitive cardiac surgery.[88] Acute drainage of the hemopericardium can be accomplished by placing a multihole pigtail in the pericardial space along the inferior heart border. The cardiac surgery team should be alerted, and an operating room prepared in case the bleeding cannot be controlled. If a sheath or dilator has been advanced into the ventricle, it is important to not remove it because the sheath acts as a plug and rapid tamponade will commence if it removed before emergent surgery.

Beyond persistent bleeding, situations in which hemopericardium may require surgical intervention include the presence of an intrapericardial clot causing tamponade or bleeding within inaccessible adhesions after access attempt not amenable to drainage.[87]

### Hemoperitoneum

More common with an inferior epicardial access approach, the needle may pass through the diaphragm or liver before entering the thorax, and this may not be appreciated initially. Resistance or difficulty advancing the sheath after puncture may be a sign the needle course went through the muscular diaphragm. An inspiratory hold to depress the diaphragm or using a left lateral fluoroscopic projection to visualize the needle course over the diaphragm may be helpful to ensure an intrathoracic trajectory. Injury to the diaphragmatic blood vessels, hepatic puncture, or, less commonly, an RV–abdominal fistula can cause hemoperitoneum.[89] Hypotension during or shortly after an epicardial VT ablation without a pericardial effusion should raise the suspicion for hemoperitoneum or abdominal organ damage. Pulling the ICE catheter back to the IVC may reveal intraabdominal fluid which should prompt a surgical evaluation and potential laparotomy in the setting of hemodynamic compromise. After the procedure, minor abdominal bleeding from an infradiaphragmatic puncture can cause abdominal pain and a plain-film standing X-ray may note air below the diaphragm indicative of pneumoperitoneum. We recommend close observation and initial conservative management.

### Coronary Injury

Direct traumatic damage to the coronary arteries and vessels can occur from both the puncture itself, as well as owing to manipulation of the sheath and catheters. Laceration of the vessels can lead to hemopericardium, although coronary vasospasm has also been described.[89] Although epicardial fat can provide some protection, radiofrequency ablation of less than 5 mm from a coronary artery can lead to hyperplasia of the intima and media chronically and possible risk of acute coronary thrombosis.[90,91] We recommend coronary angiography to determine the distance between the ablation catheter tip and nearby major coronary arteries before ablation. Delayed hemopericardium or ischemic ECG changes should also prompt coronary angiography.

### Phrenic Nerve Injury

The course of the left phrenic nerve passes across the pericardium over the left atrial appendage and then across the lateral margin of the LV in most patients or more anteriorly or inferiorly in some patients. Radiofrequency ablation in close proximity to the phrenic nerve can lead to phrenic injury and diaphragmatic paralysis.[92] A preprocedure cardiac CT scan can approximate the location when registered to the mapping system, although we always recommend high output pacing (at least 10 mA at 2 ms) to map the course of the phrenic nerve. Paralytics, if used, must be reversed for this maneuver. Ablations should occur at sites without phrenic capture, and, after ablation pacing, the phrenic nerve more superiorly should be performed to ensure preservation of phrenic nerve function. In cases where the critical ablation site coincides with sites of phrenic capture, the phrenic nerve can be separated away from the myocardium using a large-diameter vascular balloon, which requires double wiring of the epicardial access and advancement of a second steerable sheath to the appropriate site for insufflation, which can be difficult to maneuver.[93]

Alternatively, intrapericardial infusion of air and/or saline can be used to separate the layers of the pericardium to move the phrenic nerve farther away; however, these techniques risk tamponade or higher defibrillation thresholds.[94,95]

### Pericarditis

Pericarditis is a common complication of epicardial ablation owing to a local inflammatory reaction and, in our experience, is more dramatic after radiofrequency application than mapping alone. Symptoms can range from mild positional pain to tamponade.[89] In addition to intrapericardial instillation of steroids after the procedure (discussed elsewhere in this article), symptomatic treatment with oral steroids and colchicine can improve symptoms.

Rarer described complications to be aware of include ventricular pseudoaneurysm owing to contained rupture after puncture attempts in the presence of adhesions, contained subcapsular liver hematoma from a hepatic puncture, or ventriculoabdominal, pericardioabdominal, or pleuropericardial fistulas.[9,89] An index of suspicion, prompt imaging, and access to emergency surgery are critical to optimizing patient outcomes in the setting of complications.

## BEST PRACTICE: HOW TO MAP AND ABLATE VENTRICULAR TACHYCARDIA IN THE EPICARDIAL SPACE

In contrast with the endocardial mapping of the ventricle where intracavitary structures including valves, papillary muscles, chordae tendineae, and trabeculations can impede catheter movement and stable contact, the epicardial surface is smooth with few impediments. Multispline mapping catheters with 3D profiles such as the Pentaray, Octaray (Biosense Webster, Irvine, CA) or Orion (Boston Scientific, Marlborough, MA) can be difficult or unsafe to manipulate in the intrapericardial space, so we recommend the use of linear multipolar catheters or the flat, fixed grid-shaped multipolar catheters including the Advisor HD Grid (Abbott Vascular), or Optrell (Biosense Webster, Irvine, CA).[96]

Epicardial mapping in sinus rhythm may show areas of low voltage, late potentials, isochronal crowding, and fractionated EGMs to identify substrate for VT ablation. High-density simultaneous endocardial and epicardial mapping of VT circuits has shown that the majority of reentrant VTs in both ICM and patients with NICM are 3D, with only 17% of VTs possessing the entire cycle length and critical isthmus on either the endocardial or epicardial surface (so-called planar VTs).[18] There is no agreed upon definition of an epicardial VT, and Tung et al[18] have noted that a 3D circuit can have an epicardial exit, a critical isthmus partially or wholly present on the epicardium, a majority of the tachycardia cycle length, or be terminated with epicardial ablation. Based on the definition of epicardial VT, the prevalence ranges widely from 21% to 80% in patients with ICM and 28% to 77% in patients with NICM. See **Fig. 7** for an example of a 3D reentrant VT.[18]

While analyzing EGMs in the epicardium, it is important to factor in the epicardial fat distribution and thickness. Epicardial fat is most prominent in the atrioventricular and interventricular grooves as well as the RV margin and free wall, with less fat over the left lateral wall and diaphragmatic surface. Women and those ages more than 65 years tend to have more epicardial fat.[97] Fat thickness of more than 4 to 5 mm can significantly influence EGMs, and in areas of thick fat overlying normal tissue the bipolar voltage area can be low (<0.5 mV) and mistaken for scar on a bipolar voltage map.[98] As a result, it is critical to examine the EGM morphologies, with preclinical work showing that, with high-density mapping, bipolar voltage is similar between scar and fat, although the scar EGMs were longer and more fractionated than fat EGMs. Late potentials were highly specific for scarring.[99]

Radiofrequency ablation on the epicardial surface requires an understanding of the catheter tip orientation to create durable safe lesions. The contact force required in the epicardial space for good contact is less than that of the endocardial space, but the operator must ensure the force vector is directed toward the myocardium because the tip can instead be pointed at the parietal pericardium and mapped EGMs may be less accurate or ablation lesions less effective despite apparently good contact force. In contrast with endocardial ablation, where the direction of force is more likely to point toward myocardium given distal electrode tissue contact at the catheter tip, with epicardial ablation the catheter contacts the myocardium with the lateral aspect of the distal electrode. This leads to broad, shallow lesions with on average less measured contact force than with endocardial ablation.[100] This finding makes the proper orientation of the ablation catheter tip paramount when ablating from the epicardium.

In areas of thick epicardial fat (>10 mm), temperature-controlled nonirrigated RF is ineffective, so we recommend ablating in the epicardium with irrigated catheters. A relatively low flow rate of 5 to 7 mL/min is recommended, which limits the accumulation of intrapericardial fluid (which can reduce lesions size) while limiting the risk of steam pops or char formation.[101] Periodic aspiration of the intrapericardial space through the sheath will prevent the irrigant from causing tamponade or acting as a current sink. We typically start at 30 W and titrate up the power as needed to achieve a current of 650 to 700 Ω.

## BEST PRACTICE: HOW TO MAKE USE OF ALTERNATIVES TO PERCUTANEOUS ACCESS

Not all patients in whom epicardial mapping and ablation would otherwise be indicated can have the pericardial space accessed percutaneously owing to abnormal body habitus or prohibitive adhesions owing to cardiac surgery or pericarditis. Furthermore, not all VT critical sites that are inaccessible from the endocardial surface are best approached by obtaining epicardial access. One-third of epicardial VTs may require ablation from a nonepicardial site.[102] Patients with NICM in particular often have a midseptal substrate that is ill-suited for epicardial ablation, or a basal periannular VT substrate for which thick epicardial fat or the proximity of critical structures, including the coronary arteries, phrenic nerve, or left atrial appendage, making ablation challenging from these regions.

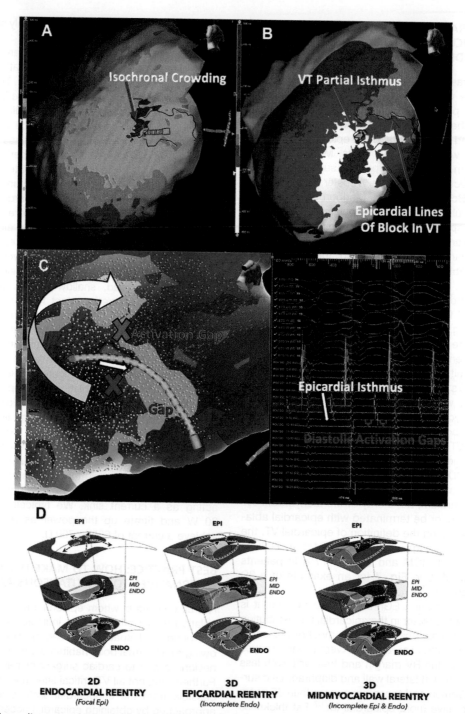

**Fig. 7.** Three-dimensional VT circuit mapped on the inferolateral epicardial surface. (*A*) Isochronal late activation mapping showing a deceleration zone at the basal inferolateral wall demonstrated by isochronal crowding. This area correlated with the epicardial portion of the critical isthmus of the VT circuit as shown by the VT activation map in (*B*) with noted missing cycle length. (*C*) The isthmus enlarged with mid-diastolic activation with epicardial diastolic activation gaps consistent with midmyocardial or endocardial portions of a 3D circuit. (*D*) Schema of patterns of VT reentry activation on the endocardial and epicardial surfaces with pure planar endocardial reentry, pure planar epicardial reentry, or 3D reentry that can be appreciated with simultaneous endocardial and epicardial activation mapping. (*D adapted from Tung R, Raiman M, Liao H, et al. Simultaneous Endocardial and Epicardial Delineation of 3D Reentrant Ventricular Tachycardia. Journal of the American College of Cardiology. 2020;75(8):884-897; with permission.*)

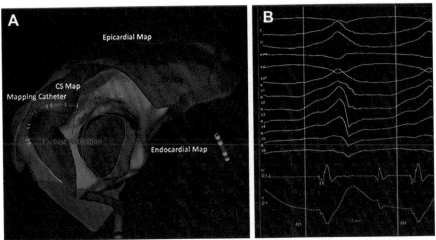

**Fig. 8.** Activation map of a focal midmyocardial basal anterolateral VT. (*A*) Surgeon's view of the endocardial, epicardial and distal coronary sinus maps with the distal mapping catheter in the great cardiac vein at the site of earliest activation, which was earlier than both the adjacent endocardial and epicardial sites, suggesting a mid-myocardial VT best accessed via the coronary sinus. (*B*) shows the corresponding bipolar (D 1–2) and unipolar (D 1) EGMs.

Several alternative techniques to approach difficult-to-reach substrates are possible, although these second-line approaches can be associated with up to a 25% risk of complications.[103] As discussed elsewhere in this article, prior adhesions, particularly on the inferior and lateral wall, can be overcome with a surgical epicardial window and manual lysis of adhesions. The coronary venous system is an important nonpericardial alternative for epicardial mapping and ablation. Particularly in patients the outflow tract, LV summit or cardiac crux, idiopathic VT or premature ventricular contractions, the distal coronary venous system and its branches can be explored with 2F and 4F multi-electrode mapping catheters and, in some cases, ablated within the coronary venous system if the ablation catheter can be advanced distally enough.[104,105] **Fig. 8** shows an example of a mid-myocardial VT successfully treated with ablation in the great cardiac vein. Often the ablation catheter cannot be advanced far enough into the distal branches to reach the best site for ablation, and in these cases selective ethanol infusion into a coronary venous branch can ablate the relevant territory.[106] Minimally invasive robot-assisted epicardial ablation of LV summit premature ventricular contractions with dissection of epicardial fat and isolation of coronary vessels has also been shown to be feasible.[107]

Can epicardial substrate be successfully ablated from the endocardial surface? This option an attractive if epicardial access is contraindicated or in some cases when the patient is already anticoagulated. Komatsu et al[59] showed that ablating

from the endocardium can eliminate abnormal EGMs on the opposite epicardial surface, especially in areas of thin myocardium in infarcted tissue or patients with ARVC; however, the majority of the abnormal epicardial EGMs were unaffected. With the use of half-normal saline as an irrigant during radiofrequency ablation to increase the impedance surrounding the catheter tip in the blood pool owing to lower ionic content and thus divert more current toward the myocardium, larger lesions can be delivered, although at the expense of an increased risk of steam pops. This adjunct technique may successfully treat ventricular arrhythmias refractory to a standard radiofrequency approach with normal saline irrigation.[108] Given the increased risk, we reserve half-normal saline as a second-line approach only. Finally, in cases of refractory VT despite endocardial and epicardial approaches, stereotactic radiation therapy for noninvasive ablation may be effective, although the long-term safety is still being established.[109]

## SUMMARY

With the risk of major complications greater than that of endocardial-only ablation, the choice of when to obtain epicardial access is as important as impeccable epicardial technique. In cases with a failed prior endocardial ablation, an endocardial map or 12-lead ECG suggesting an epicardial VT origin, advanced imaging suggesting epicardial abnormal substrate, or certain high-probability cardiomyopathies, the benefits of epicardial access outweigh the risks in well-prepared EP laboratories. With burgeoning advancements in methods to obtain epicardial access, including carbon dioxide insufflation, pressure tipped wires, pericardioscopy, and advanced imaging guidance, the technique may eventually progress to a point where the risk benefit profile favors more routine use. In the meantime, an appreciation and understanding of the unique anatomic and biophysical considerations of mapping and ablation in the epicardial space will allow for a safe and efficacious procedure.

## CLINICS CARE POINT

- Despite proper technique for the pericardial puncture, complication rates are approximately 5-10% driven by hemopericardium.
- Given the risk of complication, proper patient selection is necessary based on history of prior ablation, ECG or mapping suggesting epicardial source, ECG QRS clues, cardiomyopathy etiology, or imaging evidence of epicardial or mid-myocardial substrate.
- Proper EP lab preparation and access to a cardiac surgeon are prerequisites for attempting epicardial access in case of a major complication.
- In patients with a contraindication to epicardial access adjunctive techniques may be requires such as a hybrid surgical approach, coronary vessel access, half-normal saline irrigation, or stereotactic radiation therapy may be necessary.

## ACKNOWLEDGMENTS

The authors thank Dr Andrew Locke for his thoughtful comments on this article and Madison Tracey, BS, for her assistance with figure preparation.

## DISCLOSURE

Andre d'Avila receives research funding from Medtronic, Inc, Medtronic, Inc, Biosense Webster, Inc, and Abbott, Inc. All other authors have no relationships to disclose.

## REFERENCES

1. Sosa E, Scanavacca M, D'avila A, et al. A new technique to perform epicardial mapping in the electrophysiology laboratory. J Cardiovasc Electrophysiol 1996;7(6):531–6. https://doi.org/10.1111/j.1540-8167.1996.tb00559.x.

2. Sosa E, Scanavacca M, D'avila A, et al. Endocardial and epicardial ablation guided by nonsurgical transthoracic epicardial mapping to treat recurrent ventricular tachycardia. J Cardiovasc Electrophysiol 1998;9(3):229–39. https://doi.org/10.1111/j.1540-8167.1998.tb00907.x.

3. Cronin EM, Bogun FM, Maury P, et al. 2019 HRS/EHRA/APHRS/LAHRS expert consensus statement on catheter ablation of ventricular arrhythmias. Heart Rhythm 2020;17(1):e2–154.

4. Tung R, Vaseghi M, Frankel D. Freedom from recurrent ventricular tachycardia after catheter ablation is associated with improved survival in patients with structural heart disease: an International VT Ablation Center Collaborative Group study. Heart Rhythm 2015;12:1997–2007.

5. Tilz RR, Lenarczyk R, Scherr D, et al. Management of ventricular tachycardia in the ablation era: results of the European Heart Rhythm Association Survey. Europace 2018;20(1):209–13. https://doi.org/10.1093/europace/eux332.

6. Schweikert RA, Saliba WI, Tomassoni G, et al. Percutaneous pericardial instrumentation for endo-epicardial mapping of previously failed ablations. Circulation 2003;108(11):1329–35. https://doi.org/10.1161/01.CIR.0000087407.53326.31.

7. Cardoso R, Assis FR, D'Avila A. Endo-epicardial vs endocardial-only catheter ablation of ventricular tachycardia: a meta-analysis. J Cardiovasc Electrophysiol 2019;30(9):1537–48. https://doi.org/10.1111/jce.14013.

8. Romero J, Cerrud-Rodriguez RC, Di Biase L, et al. Combined endocardial-epicardial versus endocardial catheter ablation alone for ventricular tachycardia in structural heart disease. JACC: Clin Electrophysiol 2019;5(1):13–24. https://doi.org/10.1016/j.jacep.2018.08.010.

9. Aryana A, Tung R, d'Avila A. Percutaneous epicardial approach to catheter ablation of cardiac arrhythmias. JACC: Clin Electrophysiol 2020;6(1):1–20. https://doi.org/10.1016/j.jacep.2019.10.016.

10. Di Biase L, Santangeli P, Burkhardt DJ, et al. Endo-epicardial homogenization of the scar versus limited substrate ablation for the treatment of electrical storms in patients with ischemic cardiomyopathy. J Am Coll Cardiol 2012;60(2):132–41. https://doi.org/10.1016/j.jacc.2012.03.044.

11. Josephson ME, Simson MB, Harken AH, et al. The incidence and clinical significance of epicardial late potentials in patients with recurrent sustained ventricular tachycardia and coronary artery disease. Circulation 1982;66(6):1199–204. https://doi.org/10.1161/01.CIR.66.6.1199.

12. Horowitz LN, Harken AH, Kastor JA, et al. Ventricular resection guided by epicardial and endocardial mapping for treatment of recurrent ventricular tachycardia. N Engl J Med 1980;302(11):589–93. https://doi.org/10.1056/NEJM198003133021101.

13. Svenson RH, Littmann L, Gallagher JJ, et al. Termination of ventricular tachycardia with epicardial laser photocoagulation: a clinical comparison with patients undergoing successful endocardial photocoagulation alone. J Am Coll Cardiol 1990;15(1):163–70. https://doi.org/10.1016/0735-1097(90)90194-T.

14. Kaltenbrunner W, Cardinal R, Dubuc M, et al. Epicardial and endocardial mapping of ventricular tachycardia in patients with myocardial infarction. Is the origin of the tachycardia always subendocardially localized? Circulation 1991;84(3):1058–71. https://doi.org/10.1161/01.CIR.84.3.1058.

15. Hayashi T, Liang JJ, Muser D, et al. Epicardial ventricular tachycardia in ischemic cardiomyopathy: prevalence, electrophysiological characteristics, and long-term ablation outcomes. J Cardiovasc Electrophysiol 2018;29(11):1530–9. https://doi.org/10.1111/jce.13739.

16. Izquierdo M, Sánchez-Gómez JM, Ferrero de Loma-Osorio A, et al. Endo-epicardial versus only-endocardial ablation as a first line strategy for the treatment of ventricular tachycardia in patients with ischemic heart disease. Circ Arrhythm Electrophysiol 2015;8(4):882–9. https://doi.org/10.1161/CIRCEP.115.002827.

17. Tung R, Michowitz Y, Yu R, et al. Epicardial ablation of ventricular tachycardia: an institutional experience of safety and efficacy. Heart Rhythm 2013;10(4):490–8. https://doi.org/10.1016/j.hrthm.2012.12.013.

18. Tung R, Raiman M, Liao H, et al. Simultaneous endocardial and epicardial delineation of 3D reentrant ventricular tachycardia. J Am Coll Cardiol 2020;75(8):884–97. https://doi.org/10.1016/j.jacc.2019.12.044.

19. Hutchinson MD, Gerstenfeld EP, Desjardins B, et al. Endocardial unipolar voltage mapping to detect epicardial VT substrate in patients with nonischemic left ventricular cardiomyopathy. Circ Arrhythm Electrophysiol 2011;4(1):49–55. https://doi.org/10.1161/CIRCEP.110.959957.

20. Polin GM, Haqqani H, Tzou W, et al. Endocardial unipolar voltage mapping to identify epicardial substrate in arrhythmogenic right ventricular cardiomyopathy/dysplasia. Heart Rhythm 2011;8(1):76–83. https://doi.org/10.1016/j.hrthm.2010.09.088.

21. Bazan V, Gerstenfeld EP, Garcia FC, et al. Site-specific twelve-lead ECG features to identify an epicardial origin for left ventricular tachycardia in the absence of myocardial infarction. Heart Rhythm 2007;4(11):1403–10. https://doi.org/10.1016/j.hrthm.2007.07.004.

22. Berruezo A, Mont L, Nava S, et al. Electrocardiographic Recognition of the Epicardial Origin of Ventricular Tachycardias. Circulation 2004;109(15):1842–7.

23. Martinek M, Stevenson WG, Inada K, et al. QRS characteristics fail to reliably identify ventricular tachycardias that require epicardial ablation in ischemic heart disease. J Cardiovasc Electrophysiol 2012;23(2):188–93. https://doi.org/10.1111/j.1540-8167.2011.02179.x.

24. Vallès E, Bazan V, Marchlinski FE. ECG criteria to identify epicardial ventricular tachycardia in nonischemic cardiomyopathy. Circ Arrhythm Electrophysiol 2010;3(1):63–71. https://doi.org/10.1161/CIRCEP.109.859942.

25. de Mello RP, Szarf G, Schvartzman PR, et al. Delayed enhancement cardiac magnetic resonance imaging can identify the risk for ventricular tachycardia in Chagas' cardiomyopathy. Arq Bras Cardiol 2012;98(5):421–30.

26. Melendez-Ramirez G, Soto ME, Velasquez Alvarez LC, et al. Comparison of the amount and patterns of late enhancement in Chagas disease according to the presence and type of ventricular tachycardia. J Cardiovasc Electrophysiol 2019;30(9):1517–25. https://doi.org/10.1111/jce.14015.

27. Pisani CF, Romero J, Lara S, et al. Efficacy and safety of combined endocardial/epicardial catheter ablation for ventricular tachycardia in Chagas disease: a randomized controlled study. Heart Rhythm 2020;17(9):1510–8. https://doi.org/10.1016/j.hrthm.2020.02.009.

28. Garcia FC, Bazan V, Zado ES, et al. Epicardial substrate and outcome with epicardial ablation of ventricular tachycardia in arrhythmogenic right ventricular cardiomyopathy/dysplasia. Circulation 2009;120(5):366–75. https://doi.org/10.1161/CIRCULATIONAHA.108.834903.

29. Berruezo A, Fernández-Armenta J, Mont L, et al. Combined endocardial and epicardial catheter ablation in arrhythmogenic right ventricular dysplasia incorporating scar dechanneling technique. Circ Arrhythm Electrophysiol 2012;5(1):111–21. https://doi.org/10.1161/CIRCEP.110.960740.

30. Jiang R, Nishimura T, Beaser AD, et al. Spatial and transmural properties of the reentrant ventricular tachycardia circuit in arrhythmogenic right ventricular cardiomyopathy: simultaneous epicardial and endocardial recordings. Heart Rhythm 2021;18(6):916–25. https://doi.org/10.1016/j.hrthm.2021.01.028.

31. Mathew S, Saguner AM, Schenker N, et al. Catheter ablation of ventricular tachycardia in patients with arrhythmogenic right ventricular cardiomyopathy/dysplasia: a sequential approach. J Am Heart Assoc 2019;8(5):e010365. https://doi.org/10.1161/JAHA.118.010365.

32. Bai R, Di Biase L, Shivkumar K, et al. Ablation of ventricular arrhythmias in arrhythmogenic right ventricular dysplasia/cardiomyopathy: arrhythmia-free survival after endo-epicardial substrate based mapping and ablation. Circ Arrhythmia Electrophysiol 2011;4(4):478–85. https://doi.org/10.1161/CIRCEP.111.963066.

33. SHEN LS, LIU LM, ZHENG LH, et al. Ablation strategies for arrhythmogenic right ventricular cardiomyopathy: a systematic review and meta-analysis. J Geriatr Cardiol 2020;17(11):694–703. https://doi.org/10.11909/j.issn.1671-5411.2020.11.001.

34. Pappone C, Brugada J, Vicedomini G, et al. Electrical substrate elimination in 135 consecutive patients with brugada syndrome. Circ Arrhythmia Electrophysiol 2017;10(5). https://doi.org/10.1161/CIRCEP.117.005053.

35. Nademanee K, Veerakul G, Chandanamattha P, et al. Prevention of ventricular fibrillation episodes in brugada syndrome by catheter ablation over the anterior right ventricular outflow tract epicardium. Circulation 2011;123(12):1270–9.

36. MD KN. Ablation in brugada Syndrome for Prevention of VF - a randomized, multi-center Study of epicardial Ablation in brugada syndrome Patients to prevent arrhythmia recurrence. clinicaltrials.gov. 2020. Available at: https://clinicaltrials.gov/ct2/show/NCT02704416. Accessed January 12, 2022.

37. Dukkipati SR, d'Avila A, Soejima K, et al. Long-term outcomes of combined epicardial and endocardial ablation of monomorphic ventricular tachycardia related to hypertrophic cardiomyopathy. Circ Arrhythmia Electrophysiol 2011;4(2):185–94. https://doi.org/10.1161/CIRCEP.110.957290.

38. Santangeli P, Di Biase L, Lakkireddy D, et al. Radiofrequency catheter ablation of ventricular arrhythmias in patients with hypertrophic cardiomyopathy: safety and feasibility. Heart Rhythm 2010;7(8):1036–42. https://doi.org/10.1016/j.hrthm.2010.05.022.

39. Peretto G, Sala S, Rizzo S, et al. Ventricular arrhythmias in myocarditis: characterization and relationships with myocardial inflammation. J Am Coll Cardiol 2020;75(9):1046–57. https://doi.org/10.1016/j.jacc.2020.01.036.

40. Peretto G, Sala S, Basso C, et al. Inflammation as a predictor of recurrent ventricular tachycardia after ablation in patients with myocarditis. J Am Coll Cardiol 2020;76(14):1644–56. https://doi.org/10.1016/j.jacc.2020.08.012.

41. Papageorgiou N, Providência R, Bronis K, et al. Catheter ablation for ventricular tachycardia in patients with cardiac sarcoidosis: a systematic review. EP Europace 2018;20(4):682–91. https://doi.org/10.1093/europace/eux077.

42. Kaur D, Roukoz H, Shah M, et al. Impact of the inflammation on the outcomes of catheter ablation of drug-refractory ventricular tachycardia in cardiac sarcoidosis. J Cardiovasc Electrophysiol 2020;31(3):612–20. https://doi.org/10.1111/jce.14341.

43. Dinov B, Fiedler L, Schönbauer R, et al. Outcomes in catheter ablation of ventricular tachycardia in dilated nonischemic cardiomyopathy compared with ischemic cardiomyopathy. Circulation 2014;129(7):728–36. https://doi.org/10.1161/CIRCULATIONAHA.113.003063.

44. Vaseghi M, Hu TY, Tung R, et al. Outcomes of catheter ablation of ventricular tachycardia based on etiology in nonischemic heart disease: an international ventricular tachycardia ablation center collaborative study. JACC: Clin Electrophysiol 2018;4(9):1141–50. https://doi.org/10.1016/j.jacep.2018.05.007.

45. Cano O, Hutchinson M, Lin D, et al. Electroanatomic substrate and ablation outcome for suspected epicardial ventricular tachycardia in left ventricular nonischemic cardiomyopathy. J Am Coll Cardiol 2009;54(9):799–808. https://doi.org/10.1016/j.jacc.2009.05.032.

46. McCrohon Ja, Moon Jc c, Prasad Sk, et al. Differentiation of heart failure related to dilated cardiomyopathy and coronary artery disease using gadolinium-enhanced cardiovascular magnetic resonance. Circulation 2003;108(1):54–9. https://doi.org/10.1161/01.CIR.0000078641.19365.4C.

47. Santangeli P, Marchlinski FE, Zado ES, et al. Percutaneous epicardial ablation of ventricular arrhythmias arising from the left ventricular summit. Circ Arrhythmia Electrophysiol 2015;8(2):337–43. https://doi.org/10.1161/CIRCEP.114.002377.

48. Estner HL, Zviman MM, Herzka D, et al. The critical isthmus sites of ischemic ventricular tachycardia are in zones of tissue heterogeneity, visualized by magnetic resonance imaging. Heart Rhythm 2011;8(12):1942–9. https://doi.org/10.1016/j.hrthm.2011.07.027.

49. Bogun FM, Desjardins B, Good E, et al. Delayed-enhanced magnetic resonance imaging in nonischemic cardiomyopathy. J Am Coll Cardiol 2009;53(13):1138–45. https://doi.org/10.1016/j.jacc.2008.11.052.

50. Acosta J, Fernández-Armenta J, Penela D, et al. Infarct transmurality as a criterion for first-line endo-epicardial substrate–guided ventricular tachycardia ablation in ischemic cardiomyopathy. Heart Rhythm 2016;13(1):85–95. https://doi.org/10.1016/j.hrthm.2015.07.010.

51. Piers SRD, Tao Q, de Riva Silva M, et al. CMR-based identification of critical isthmus sites of ischemic and nonischemic ventricular tachycardia. JACC Cardiovasc Imaging 2014;7(8):774–84. https://doi.org/10.1016/j.jcmg.2014.03.013.

52. Piers S, Tao Q, Taxis C. Contrast-enhanced MRI-derived scar patterns and associated ventricular tachycardias in nonischemic cardiomyopathy: implications for the ablation strategy. Circ Arrhythm Electrophysiol 2013;6:875–83.

53. Soto-Iglesias D, Acosta J, Penela D, et al. Image-based criteria to identify the presence of epicardial arrhythmogenic substrate in patients with transmural

myocardial infarction. Heart Rhythm 2018;15(6): 814–21. https://doi.org/10.1016/j.hrthm.2018.02.007.

54. Andreu D, Penela D, Acosta J, et al. Cardiac magnetic resonance–aided scar dechanneling: influence on acute and long-term outcomes. Heart Rhythm 2017;14(8):1121–8. https://doi.org/10.1016/j.hrthm.2017.05.018.

55. Berruezo A, Penela D, Jáuregui B, et al. The role of imaging in catheter ablation of ventricular arrhythmias. Pacing Clin Electrophysiol 2021. https://doi.org/10.1111/pace.14183. Published online February 1.

56. Soto-Iglesias David, Penela Diego, Beatriz Jáuregui, et al. Cardiac magnetic resonance-guided ventricular tachycardia substrate ablation. JACC: Clin Electrophysiol 2020;6(4):436–47. https://doi.org/10.1016/j.jacep.2019.11.004.

57. Komatsu Y, Cochet H, Jadidi A. Regional myocardial wall thinning at multi-detector computed tomography correlates to arrhythmogenic substrate in post-infarction ventricular tachycardia: assessment of structural and electrical substrate. Circ Arrhythm Electrophysiol 2013;6:342–50.

58. Yamashita S, Sacher F, Hooks DA, et al. Myocardial wall thinning predicts transmural substrate in patients with scar-related ventricular tachycardia. Heart Rhythm 2017;14(2):155–63. https://doi.org/10.1016/j.hrthm.2016.11.012.

59. Komatsu Y, Daly M, Sacher F, et al. Endocardial ablation to eliminate epicardial arrhythmia substrate in scar-related ventricular tachycardia. J Am Coll Cardiol 2014;63(14):1416–26. https://doi.org/10.1016/j.jacc.2013.10.087.

60. Esposito A, Palmisano A, Antunes S, et al. Cardiac CT with delayed enhancement in the characterization of ventricular tachycardia structural substrate: relationship between CT-segmented scar and electro-anatomic mapping. JACC: Cardiovasc Imaging 2016;9(7):822–32. https://doi.org/10.1016/j.jcmg.2015.10.024.

61. Bunch TJ, Weiss JP, Crandall BG, et al. Image integration using intracardiac ultrasound and 3D reconstruction for scar mapping and ablation of ventricular tachycardia. J Cardiovasc Electrophysiol 2010;21(6):678–84. https://doi.org/10.1111/j.1540-8167.2009.01680.x.

62. Bala R, Ren JF, Hutchinson MD, et al. Assessing epicardial substrate using intracardiac echocardiography during VT ablation. Circ Arrhythmia Electrophysiol 2011;4(5):667–73. https://doi.org/10.1161/CIRCEP.111.963553.

63. Aryana A, d'Avila A. Epicardial approach for cardiac electrophysiology procedures. J Cardiovasc Electrophysiol 2020;31(1):345–59. https://doi.org/10.1111/jce.14282.

64. Khan M, Hendriks AA, Yap SC, et al. Damage to the left internal mammary artery during anterior

65. Weerasooriya R, Jais P, Sacher F, et al. Utility of the lateral fluoroscopic view for subxiphoid pericardial access. Circ Arrhythmia Electrophysiol 2009;2(4): e15–7. https://doi.org/10.1161/CIRCEP.108.803676.

66. Mathew S, Feickert S, Fink T, et al. Epicardial access for VT ablation: analysis of two different puncture techniques, incidence of adhesions and complication management. Clin Res Cardiol 2021;110(6):810–21. https://doi.org/10.1007/s00392-020-01711-z.

67. Sacher F, Roberts-Thomson K, Maury P, et al. Epicardial ventricular tachycardia ablation: a multicenter safety study. J Am Coll Cardiol 2010;55(21): 2366–72. https://doi.org/10.1016/j.jacc.2009.10.084.

68. Page SP, Duncan ER, Thomas G, et al. Epicardial catheter ablation for ventricular tachycardia in heparinized patients. Europace 2013;15(2):284–9. https://doi.org/10.1093/europace/eus258.

69. Miyamoto K, Killu AM, Kella DK, et al. Feasibility and safety of percutaneous epicardial access for mapping and ablation for ventricular arrhythmias in patients on oral anticoagulants. J Interv Card Electrophysiol 2019;54(1):81–9. https://doi.org/10.1007/s10840-018-0441-0.

70. Nakamura T, Davogustto GE, Schaeffer B, et al. Complications and anticoagulation strategies for percutaneous epicardial ablation procedures. Circ Arrhythmia Electrophysiol 2018;11(11). https://doi.org/10.1161/CIRCEP.118.006714.

71. Jurko A, Minarik M, Cisarikova V, et al. Congenital complete and partial absence of the left pericardium. Wien Med Wochenschr 2013;163(17–18): 426–8. https://doi.org/10.1007/s10354-013-0178-4.

72. Lennon Collins K, Zakharious F, Mandal A, et al. Pericardial cyst: never too late to diagnose. JCM 2018; 7(11):399. https://doi.org/10.3390/jcm7110399.

73. Patel J, Park C, Michaels J, et al. Pericardial cyst: case reports and a literature review. Echocardiography 2004;21(3):269–72. https://doi.org/10.1111/j.0742-2822.2004.03097.x.

74. Subramanian M, Ravilla VV, Yalagudri S, et al. CT-guided percutaneous epicardial access for ventricular tachycardia ablation: a proof-of-concept study. J Cardiovasc Electrophysiol 2021. https://doi.org/10.1111/jce.15210.

75. D'avila A, Neuzil P, Thiagalingam A, et al. Experimental efficacy of pericardial instillation of anti-inflammatory agents during percutaneous epicardial catheter ablation to prevent postprocedure pericarditis. J Cardiovasc Electrophysiol 2007;18(11):1178–83. https://doi.org/10.1111/j.1540-8167.2007.00945.x.

76. Wan SH, Killu AM, Hodge DO, et al. Obesity does not increase complication rate of percutaneous

epicardial access. J Cardiovasc Electrophysiol 2014; 25(11):1174–9. https://doi.org/10.1111/jce.12485.

77. Roberts-Thomson KC, Seiler J, Steven D, et al. Percutaneous access of the epicardial space for mapping ventricular and supraventricular arrhythmias in patients with and without prior cardiac surgery. J Cardiovasc Electrophysiol 2010;21(4): 406–11. https://doi.org/10.1111/j.1540-8167.2009. 01645.x.

78. Tschabrunn CM, Haqqani HM, Cooper JM, et al. Percutaneous epicardial ventricular tachycardia ablation after noncoronary cardiac surgery or pericarditis. Heart Rhythm 2013;10(2):165–9. https:// doi.org/10.1016/j.hrthm.2012.10.012.

79. Soejima K, Couper G, Cooper JM, et al. Subxiphoid surgical approach for epicardial catheter-based mapping and ablation in patients with prior cardiac surgery or difficult pericardial access. Circulation 2004;110(10):1197–201. https://doi.org/10.1161/ 01.CIR.0000140725.42845.90.

80. Li A, Hayase J, Do D, et al. Hybrid surgical vs percutaneous access epicardial ventricular tachycardia ablation. Heart Rhythm 2018;15(4): 512–9. https://doi.org/10.1016/j.hrthm.2017.11. 009.

81. Gunda S, Reddy M, Pillarisetti J, et al. Differences in complication rates between large bore needle and a long micropuncture needle during epicardial access: time to change clinical practice? Circ Arrhythm Electrophysiol 2015;8(4):890–5. https://doi. org/10.1161/CIRCEP.115.002921.

82. Lakkireddy D, Afzal MR, Lee RJ, et al. Short and long-term outcomes of percutaneous left atrial appendage suture ligation: results from a US multicenter evaluation. Heart Rhythm 2016;13(5): 1030–6. https://doi.org/10.1016/j.hrthm.2016.01. 022.

83. Di Biase L, Burkhardt JD, Reddy V, et al. Initial international multicenter human experience with a novel epicardial access needle embedded with a real-time pressure/frequency monitoring to facilitate epicardial access: feasibility and safety. Heart Rhythm 2017;14(7):981–8. https://doi.org/10.1016/ j.hrthm.2017.02.033.

84. Burkland DA, Ganapathy AV, John M, et al. Near-field impedance accurately distinguishes among pericardial, intracavitary, and anterior mediastinal position. J Cardiovasc Electrophysiol 2017;28(12): 1492–9. https://doi.org/10.1111/jce.13325.

85. Nakatsuma K, Yamamoto E, Watanabe S, et al. Ultrathin endoscopy-guided pericardiocentesis: a pilot study in a swine model. J Invasive Cardiol 2016; 28(3):78–80.

86. Juliá J, Bokhari F, Uuetoa H, et al. A new era in epicardial access for the ablation of ventricular arrhythmias. JACC: Clin Electrophysiol 2021;7(1): 85–96. https://doi.org/10.1016/j.jacep.2020.07.027.

87. Koruth JS, d'Avila A. Management of hemopericardium related to percutaneous epicardial access, mapping, and ablation. Heart Rhythm 2011;8(10): 1652–7. https://doi.org/10.1016/j.hrthm.2011.03. 059.

88. Beyls C, Hermida A, Duchateau J, et al. Management of acute cardiac tamponade by direct autologous blood transfusion in interventional electrophysiology. J Cardiovasc Electrophysiol 2019;30(8):1287–93. https://doi.org/10.1111/jce. 14050.

89. Koruth JS, Aryana A, Dukkipati SR, et al. Unusual complications of percutaneous epicardial access and epicardial mapping and ablation of cardiac arrhythmias. Circ Arrhythm Electrophysiol 2011;4(6): 882–8. https://doi.org/10.1161/CIRCEP.111.965731.

90. D'Avila A, Gutierrez P, Scanavacca M, et al. Effects of radiofrequency pulses delivered in the vicinity of the coronary arteries: implications for nonsurgical transthoracic epicardial catheter ablation to treat ventricular tachycardia. Pacing Clin Electrophysiol 2002;25(10):1488–95. https://doi.org/10.1046/j. 1460-9592.2002.01488.x.

91. Viles-Gonzalez JF, de Castro Miranda R, Scanavacca M, et al. Acute and chronic effects of epicardial radiofrequency applications delivered on epicardial coronary arteries. Circ Arrhythm Electrophysiol 2011;4(4):526–31. https://doi.org/10. 1161/CIRCEP.110.961508.

92. Fan R, Cano O, Ho SY, et al. Characterization of the phrenic nerve course within the epicardial substrate of patients with nonischemic cardiomyopathy and ventricular tachycardia. Heart Rhythm 2009;6(1):59–64. https://doi.org/10.1016/j.hrthm. 2008.09.033.

93. Kumar S, Barbhaiya CR, Baldinger SH, et al. Epicardial phrenic nerve displacement during catheter ablation of atrial and ventricular arrhythmias: procedural experience and outcomes. Circ Arrhythmia Electrophysiol 2015;8(4):896–904. https://doi.org/10.1161/CIRCEP.115.002818.

94. Di Biase L, Burkhardt JD, Pelargonio G, et al. Prevention of phrenic nerve injury during epicardial ablation: comparison of methods for separating the phrenic nerve from the epicardial surface. Heart Rhythm 2009;6(7):957–61. https://doi.org/ 10.1016/j.hrthm.2009.03.022.

95. Yamada T, McElderry HT, Platonov M, et al. Aspirated air in the pericardial space during epicardial catheterization may elevate the defibrillation threshold. Int J Cardiol 2009;135(1):e34–5. https:// doi.org/10.1016/j.ijcard.2008.03.074.

96. Sroubek J, Anter E. Multielectrode epicardial mapping. In: d'Avila A, Aryana A, Reddy VY, et al, editors. Percutaneous epicardial interventions: a guide for cardiac electrophysiologists. Hopkins, MN: Cardiotext Publishing; 2020. p. 185–9.

97. Abbara S, Desai JC, Cury RC, et al. Mapping epicardial fat with multi-detector computed tomography to facilitate percutaneous transepicardial arrhythmia ablation. Eur J Radiol 2006;57(3):417–22. https://doi.org/10.1016/j.ejrad.2005.12.030.

98. Saba MM, Akella J, Gammie J, et al. The influence of fat thickness on the human epicardial bipolar electrogram characteristics: measurements on patients undergoing open-heart surgery. EP Europace 2009;11(7):949–53. https://doi.org/10.1093/europace/eup156.

99. Tung R, Nakahara S, Ramirez R, et al. Distinguishing epicardial fat from scar: analysis of electrograms using high-density electroanatomic mapping in a novel porcine infarct model. Heart Rhythm 2010;7(3):389–95. https://doi.org/10.1016/j.hrthm.2009.11.023.

100. Sacher F, Wright M, Derval N, et al. Endocardial versus epicardial ventricular radiofrequency ablation: utility of in vivo contact force assessment. Circ Arrhythmia Electrophysiol 2013;6(1):144–50. https://doi.org/10.1161/CIRCEP.111.974501.

101. Aryana A, O'Neill PG, Pujara DK, et al. Impact of irrigation flow rate and intrapericardial fluid on cooled-tip epicardial radiofrequency ablation. Heart Rhythm 2016;13(8):1602–11. https://doi.org/10.1016/j.hrthm.2016.05.008.

102. Yokokawa M, Latchamsetty R, Good E, et al. Ablation of epicardial ventricular arrhythmias from non-epicardial sites. Heart Rhythm 2011;8(10):1525–9. https://doi.org/10.1016/j.hrthm.2011.06.020.

103. Kumar S, Barbhaiya CR, Sobieszczyk P, et al. Role of alternative interventional procedures when endo- and epicardial catheter ablation attempts for ventricular arrhythmias fail. Circ Arrhythm Electrophysiol 2015;8(3):606–15. https://doi.org/10.1161/CIRCEP.114.002522.

104. Obel OA, d'Avila A, Neuzil P, et al. Ablation of left ventricular epicardial outflow tract tachycardia from the distal great cardiac vein. J Am Coll Cardiol 2006;48(9):1813–7. https://doi.org/10.1016/j.jacc.2006.06.006.

105. Baman TS, Ilg KJ, Gupta SK, et al. Mapping and ablation of epicardial idiopathic ventricular arrhythmias from within the coronary venous system. Circ Arrhythmia Electrophysiol 2010;3(3):274–9. https://doi.org/10.1161/CIRCEP.109.910802.

106. Kreidieh B, Rodríguez-Mañero M, Schurmann P, et al. Retrograde coronary venous ethanol infusion for ablation of refractory ventricular tachycardia. Circ Arrhythm Electrophysiol 2016;9(7). https://doi.org/10.1161/CIRCEP.116.004352 e004352.

107. Aziz Z, Moss JD, Jabbarzadeh M, et al. Totally endoscopic robotic epicardial ablation of refractory left ventricular summit arrhythmia: first-in-man. Heart Rhythm 2017;14(1):135–8. https://doi.org/10.1016/j.hrthm.2016.09.005.

108. Nguyen DT, Tzou WS, Sandhu A, et al. Prospective multicenter experience with cooled radiofrequency ablation using high impedance irrigant to target deep myocardial substrate refractory to standard ablation. JACC: Clin Electrophysiol 2018;4(9):1176–85. https://doi.org/10.1016/j.jacep.2018.06.021.

109. Robinson CG, Samson PP, Moore KMS, et al. Phase I/II trial of electrophysiology-guided noninvasive cardiac radioablation for ventricular tachycardia. Circulation 2019;139(3):313–21. https://doi.org/10.1161/CIRCULATIONAHA.118.038261.

# Catheter Ablation of Ventricular Tachycardia in Arrhythmogenic Right Ventricular Cardiomyopathy

Alessio Gasperetti, MD, Harikrishna Tandri, MD*

## KEYWORDS

- Arrhythmogenic right ventricular dysplasia/ cardiomyopathy • Ventricular tachycardia
- Catheter ablation • Epicardial ablation • Ventricular tachycardia recurrence

## KEY POINTS

- Ventricular tachycardias (VT) are common in patients with ARVC.
- VT ablation has been shown effective in reducing the burden of VT in patients with ARVC.
- Due to a frequent epicardial substrate, VT ablation strategies in ARVC should employ a epicardial component.

## INTRODUCTION

Arrhythmogenic right ventricular cardiomyopathy (ARVC) is an inherited desmosomal myopathy[1] characterized by progressive fibrofatty replacement of the myocardium, right ventricular (RV) enlargement, and malignant ventricular arrhythmias (VAs). Several pathogenic desomosomal mutations have been reported in the last decade, and genotype-phenotype association has been systematically described, with specific desmosomal genes associated with early left ventricular (LV) involvement.

Ventricular tachycardia (VT) is one of the most common initial presentation in patients with ARVC.[1] Implantable cardioverter defibrillators (ICDs) are a cornerstone of the management of this disease. Most patients with ARVC receive ICD (either transvenous or subcutaneous) for secondary prevention or primary prevention of sudden death, in accordance with current guidelines and risk stratification tools.[2,3] Given the high arrhythmic burden of this disease, ICD therapies including anti-tachycardia pacing and/or ICD shocks are not uncommon during clinical follow up. Significant association exist between physical exercise, Vas, and ARVC.[4,5] Most patients are treated with beta-blockers and many pharmacological approaches are available to treat VAs including sotalol, flecainide, and amiodarone.

### Catheter Ablation of Arrhythmogenic Right Ventricular Cardiomyopathy

VT ablation is an invasive management strategy that has been shown effective in reducing the burden of arrhythmic events in patients with ARVC.[6] It is often offered as an additional therapeutic step for patients whose arrhythmia are not adequately controlled with a pharmacological approach. Currently, the most common reason for VT ablation is an ICD shock resulting from failure of antiarrhythmic drug therapy. Recurrent ATP-terminated VT is also considered for VT ablation, as failure of anti-tachycardia pacing and/or acceleration of VT to ventricular fibrillation occurs with some frequency, necessitating an ICD shock. Moreover, it is well recognized that recurrent ICD

ARVC Program, Division of Cardiology, Johns Hopkins University School of Medicine, 600 Wolfe Street, Baltimore, MD 21287, USA
* Corresponding author.
*E-mail address:* htandri1@jhmi.edu

Card Electrophysiol Clin 14 (2022) 679–683
https://doi.org/10.1016/j.ccep.2022.08.004

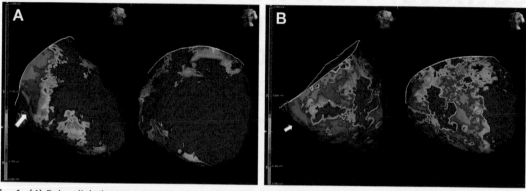

**Fig. 1.** (*A*) Epicardial electroanatomic voltage map RAO (left) and LAO (right) projections in early Plakophilin 2 ARVC showing limited scar in the RV subtricuspid region (*white arrowhead*) with relative sparing of the anterior RV and the apex. (*B*) Epicardial electroanatomic map of an advanced Plakophilin 2 ARVC is shown. In the RAO projection (left) inferior RV scar is seen (*white arrow* head) with involvement of the entire perivalvular and inferior RV wall. In the LAO projection (right), low voltage extends to the RV outflow tract with sparing of the left ventricle. LAO, left anterior oblique; RAO, right anterior oblique.

shocks lead to anxiety and depression, which is very prevalent in patients receiving ICD therapy.

Recently, two randomized controlled trials addressing the role of VT ablation at the time of ICD shock were published. In the PARTITA trial, enrolling a mixed cohort of patients with ischemic and nonischemic cardiomyopathies implanted with ICDs, early VT ablation after first ICD shock was shown to significantly reduce a combined endpoint of death and worsening heart failure hospitalizations.[7] The PAUSE-SCD trial reported similar results in cohort of patients with cardiomyopathy, 35% of them were diagnosed with ARVC.[8] These findings addressed a severely under investigated topic in cardiac electrophysiology and provided strong evidence supporting for considering VT ablation after the first ICD shock in patients with ARVC.

## Approach to Ventricular Tachycardia Ablation in Arrhythmogenic Right Ventricular Cardiomyopathy

Patient selection and accurate planning are critical to harvest all the benefits associated with VT ablation in patients with ARVC. Patients at the highest risk of defibrillator therapy are those with a high burden of premature ventricular contraction (PVC), nonsustained ventricular tachycardia, inducibility of VT during EP study, and high level of physical activity.[9] Patients experiencing frequent episodes of slow VTs, below the detection rate of transvenous ICDs and, more commonly, subcutaneous ICDs represent another cohort of patients that could benefit from VT ablation.

Preprocedural imaging is an important aspect of planning VT ablation. Several studies have

demonstrated the importance of preablation imaging for defining the putative sites of VAs.[10,11] This is particularly important for procedures in ARVC. Classic forms of ARVC often affect the basal subtricuspid region of the lateral and inferior wall of the RV, with areas of scarring and reentry VT circuits commonly localizing in that area[12,13] (**Fig. 1**). Presence of basal aneurysm or abnormal dilatation in the basal region often gives a clue to the anatomic site that needs to be mapped for the VT. It is, however, not uncommon to see other mimics of ARVC, such as sarcoidosis or chronic myocarditis, to present with similar abnormalities both in the LV and the interventricular septum.[14–16] Preprocedural imaging can therefore also be useful for reconfirming the diagnosis, as the underlying cardiac disease influences the approach required for VT ablation (ie, likelihood of epicardial substrate).

Another important aspect of VT ablation in ARVC is streamlining the procedural workflow and clearly definining of the right ablation target. VT induction for clear morphology annotation is generally performed at the beginning of the procedure. In our experience, in early ARVC, VT inducibility is dependent on level of sedation. It is not uncommon to encounter patients that are noninducible after general anesthesia, even when they initially presented with multiple episodes of sustained monomorphic VT. It is routine practice at our center to perform noninvasive programmed stimulation prior to intubation with mild sedation to define the target VT, based on the cycle lengths of treated VT on ICD electrograms and also based on far field morphology. The next step is to adequately identify the arrhythmic substrate sustaining the observed VT. Although there has been enormous interest in substrate-based ablation and excellent results are reported,[17] it is always

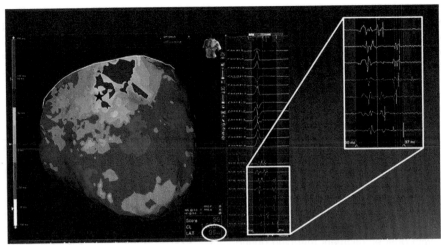

**Fig. 2.** Epicardial substrate. Isochronal late activation map in ARVC showing distinct late potentials and delayed activation with isochronal crowding in the RV basal anterior wall (star).

good practice to define the specific substrate. The substrate for VT ablation in ARVC is epicardial in the majority of cases (**Fig. 2**).[6,18] As such, epicardial access is required in most cases and it is a good practice to plan and consent patients for both endocardial and epicardial procedures.

### Epicardial Access

Epicardial access and ablation is best done at centers that have experience in these procedures to minimize complications and optimize success rates. At our center, epicardial access is obtained in all patients, even for patients presenting for the first procedure. Epicardial VT ablation of ARVC is performed under general anesthesia at our center. Use of dedicated pericardial access micropuncture needle significantly reduces risk of complications. For mapping and ablation of the RV, we recommend an anterior epicardial access and the use of a deflectable sheath (Agilis sheath, Abbott Labs). Anterior approach avoids complications related to

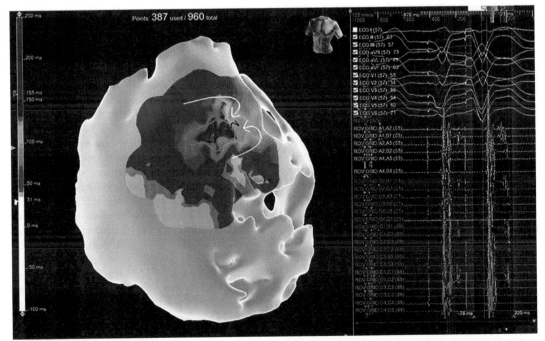

**Fig. 3.** DeEP mapping in ARVC. Decremental evoked potential mapping in the epicardium delineates the VT circuit demonstrating the region of conduction block with impulse propagating around the scar (*curved arrows*) and entering from the opposite direction.

hepatic injury, bowel perforation, and coronary injury.[19] A limited endocardial only approach is generally discouraged, but it may be an option in patients with VT morphology suggestive of RV outflow tract, as epicardial mapping in these areas is hampered by the presence of excessive fat and ablation in the same region risks coronary injury. Serial dilations are often required over a stiff wire to avoid damage to the tip of the deflectable sheath. Once within the RV, a detailed voltage map along with a sinus activation map is performed to identify areas of conduction slowing and late potentials. It is fairly common to see late potentials well beyond the QRS close to the tricuspid annulus even in early ARVC, even in the absence of wall motion abnormalities. Pace mapping to identify potential exit sites along with brief entrainment mapping during VT to identify critical mid-diastolic sites, ensures successful ablation of the targeted VT. It is important to carefully annotate the atrioventricular groove and the interventricular groove to avoid ablation in these regions. Once critical sites are identified, ablation is performed using irrigated radiofrequency energy (30–35 W) with frequent aspirations of the pericardial space every 4 minutes. Recently, decrement evoked potential (DeEP) mapping has been proposed as a way to unmask regions of conduction slowing and late activation and we have found this method to be extremely useful in predicting sites of unidirectional block and likely sites of reentry (**Fig. 3**). Once the critical circuits are identified and ablated in the epicardium, and the patient is not inducible, further ablation of the substrate can be performed, if the substrate is limited. This, however, is often not the case in patients with moderate or advanced ARVC with extensive epicardial substrate, wherein complete elimination of late potentials is not possible and is often not required for long-term VT free survival. Use of intrapericardial steroids at the end of the procedure seems to reduce the risk of pericarditis although there are no systematic studies of its use in patients with ARVC. With current methods of high-density mapping and targeted VT ablation 2 years VT free survival was approximately 80% in this population.[6]

## SUMMARY

In summary, invasive management of ARVC with VT ablation is an effective strategy in reducing arrhythmic burden for those patients. Preprocedural imaging should be implemented routinely, to identify myocardial scarring and increase access safety. Given the epicardial localization of the arrhythmic substrate, epicardial access should routinely be obtained. Programmed VT stimulation and epicardial high-density DeEP mapping could be leveraged to identify the critical area of arrhythmic substrate sustaining the clinical VT. Through substrate homogenization, observed long-term outcomes after VT ablation in ARVC are positive.

## CLINICS CARE POINTS

- Arrhythmic subtrate of patients with ARVC is most often localized epicardially.
- VT ablation, including an epicardial component, is helpful in reducing the arrhythmic burden and the number of implantable cardioverter defibrillator shocks in patients with ARVC.
- While helpful in reudcing the arrhythmic burden, there is no evidence that VT ablation could replace ICD implantation for sudden cardiac death in patients with ARVC.

## REFERENCES

1. Corrado D, Link MS, Calkins H. Arrhythmogenic right ventricular cardiomyopathy. Jarcho JA. N Engl J Med 2017;376:61–72.
2. Corrado D, Wichter T, Link MS, et al. Treatment of arrhythmogenic right ventricular cardiomyopathy/dysplasia: an international task force consensus statement. Circulation 2015;132:441–53.
3. Cadrin-Tourigny J, Bosman LP, Nozza A, et al. A new prediction model for ventricular arrhythmias in arrhythmogenic right ventricular cardiomyopathy. Eur Heart J 2019. Available at: https://academic.oup.com/eurheartj/advance-article/doi/10.1093/eurheartj/ehz103/5419784.
4. James CA, Bhonsale A, Tichnell C, et al. Exercise increases age-related penetrance and arrhythmic risk in arrhythmogenic right ventricular dysplasia/cardiomyopathy–associated desmosomal mutation carriers. J Am Coll Cardiol 2013;62:1290–7.
5. Gasperetti A, Russo AD, Busana M, et al. Novel risk calculator performance in athletes with arrhythmogenic right ventricular cardiomyopathy. Heart Rhythm 2020;17(8):1251–9. https://doi.org/10.1016/j.hrthm.2020.03.007.
6. Daimee UA, Assis FR, Murray B, et al. Clinical outcomes of catheter ablation of ventricular tachycardia in patients with arrhythmogenic right ventricular cardiomyopathy: insights from the Johns Hopkins ARVC Program. Heart Rhythm 2021;18:1369–76.
7. Della Bella P, Baratto F, Vergara P, et al. Does timing of ventricular tachycardia ablation affect prognosis in patients with an implantable cardioverter

defibrillator? results from the multicenter randomized partita trial. Circulation 2022;145:1829–38.

8. Tung R, Xue Y, Chen M, et al. First-line catheter ablation of monomorphic ventricular tachycardia in cardiomyopathy concurrent with defibrillator implantation: the PAUSE-SCD randomized trial. Circulation 2022;145:1839–49.

9. Bhonsale A, James CA, Tichnell C, et al. Incidence and predictors of implantable cardioverter-defibrillator therapy in patients with arrhythmogenic right ventricular dysplasia/cardiomyopathy undergoing implantable cardioverter-defibrillator implantation for primary prevention. J Am Coll Cardiol 2011;58:1485–96.

10. Mukherjee RK, Whitaker J, Williams SE, et al. Magnetic resonance imaging guidance for the optimization of ventricular tachycardia ablation. EP Europace 2018;20:1721–32.

11. Esposito A, Palmisano A, Antunes S, et al. Cardiac CT with delayed enhancement in the characterization of ventricular tachycardia structural substrate. JACC: Cardiovasc Imaging 2016;9:822–32.

12. Te Riele ASJM, James CA, Philips B, et al. Mutation-positive arrhythmogenic right ventricular dysplasia/cardiomyopathy: the triangle of dysplasia displaced: ARVD/C: the triangle of dysplasia displaced. J Cardiovasc Electrophysiol 2013;24:1311–20.

13. Jiang R, Nishimura T, Beaser AD, et al. Spatial and transmural properties of the reentrant ventricular tachycardia circuit in arrhythmogenic right ventricular cardiomyopathy: simultaneous epicardial and endocardial recordings. Heart Rhythm 2021;18:916–25.

14. Gasperetti A, Rossi VA, Chiodini A, et al. Differentiating hereditary arrhythmogenic right ventricular cardiomyopathy from cardiac sarcoidosis fulfilling 2010 ARVC Task Force Criteria. Heart Rhythm 2020;18(2):231–8.

15. Philips B, Madhavan S, James CA, et al. Arrhythmogenic right ventricular dysplasia/cardiomyopathy and cardiac sarcoidosis: distinguishing features when the diagnosis is unclear. Circ Arrhythm Electrophysiol 2014;7:230–6.

16. Pieroni M, Dello Russo A, Marzo F, et al. High prevalence of myocarditis mimicking arrhythmogenic right ventricular cardiomyopathy. J Am Coll Cardiol 2009;53:681–9.

17. Gökoğlan Y, Mohanty S, Gianni C, et al. Scar homogenization versus limited-substrate ablation in patients with nonischemic cardiomyopathy and ventricular tachycardia. J Am Coll Cardiol 2016;68:1990–8.

18. Mathew S, Saguner AM, Schenker N, et al. Catheter ablation of ventricular tachycardia in patients with arrhythmogenic right ventricular cardiomyopathy/dysplasia: a sequential approach. J Acad Hosp Adm 2019;8:e010365.

19. Subramanian M, Ravilla VV, Yalagudri S, et al. CT-guided percutaneous epicardial access for ventricular tachycardia ablation: a proof-of-concept study. Cardiovasc Electrophysiol 2021;32:2665–72.

# Advances in Ventricular Arrhythmia Ablation for Brugada Syndrome

Ronpichai Chokesuwattanaskul, MD[a], Koonlawee Nademanee, MD[a,b,c],*

## KEVYWORDS

• Brugada syndrome • Catheter ablation • Sudden cardiac death • Ventricular arrhythmia

## KEY POINTS

• Arrhythmogenic substrates of BrS are characterized by markedly fractionated prolonged duration of the electrograms harboring over the RVOT/RV epicardium.
• Marked epicardium and interstitial fibrosis are the pathology underlying these abnormal epicardial electrograms.
• Ablations at these substrate sites normalize the ECG pattern and prevent recurrent VF recurrence.
• Catheter ablation of BrS substrates is a promising therapeutic modality for symptomatic BrS patients.

 Video content accompanies this article at http://www.cardiacep.theclinics.com.

## INTRODUCTION

Three decades have passed since the Brugada syndrome (BrS) clinical entity was introduced in the early 1990s.[1] During the first 2 decades, treatment of patients with BrS was challenging because there were limited treatment options, and an implantable cardioverter-defibrillator (ICD) was the only choice for high-risk patients with BrS, that is, those who had aborted sudden cardiac death or had previous ventricular fibrillation (VF) episodes.[2–4] However, even though ICDs are effective at reverting VF episodes to sinus rhythm, they do not prevent VF occurrence.[3,5] Thus, when some patients with BrS experience frequent recurrences of VF episodes with appropriate ICD discharges, electrophysiologists face the formidable task of suppressing such VF episodes. No antiarrhythmic drug has been effective at preventing VF recurrences in BrS except quinidine, which is

not available in many countries.[6] In addition, quinidine is sometimes ineffective in severely symptomatic BrS. Thus, it was imperative to find an alternate solution for such patients with BrS. Fortunately, over the last decade, advances have been made about our understanding of the arrhythmogenic substrate in BrS. Remarkably, radiofrequency (RF) ablations at these substrate sites can normalize the Brugada electrocardiogram (ECG) pattern and prevent recurrent VF episodes.[7,8] In this article, we focus on these advances and how to treat patients with BrS with catheter ablation.

### Brugada Syndrome Substrate

Between 2009 and 2010, we studied 9 patients with severely symptomatic BrS with recurrent VF episodes.[7] We performed electroanatomic mapping of the right ventricle (RV)—both endocardially

[a] Department of Medicine, Center of Excellence in Arrhythmia Research Chulalongkorn University, 1873 Rama IV Road, Pathumwan, Bangkok 10330 Thailand; [b] Bumrungrad Hospital, Bangkok and Pacific Rim Electrophysiology Research Institute, Bangkok, Thailand; [c] Las Vegas, NV, USA
* Corresponding author. King Chulalongkorn Memorial Hospital, Bangkok, Thailand.
E-mail address: wee@pacificrimep.com

Card Electrophysiol Clin 14 (2022) 685–692
https://doi.org/10.1016/j.ccep.2022.08.006

and epicardially—and epicardial mapping of the left ventricle (LV) during sinus rhythm. All had abnormal electrograms (EGMs) characterized by low voltage (<1 mV), prolonged duration (>120 msec), and fractionated late potentials (beyond QRS complex) clustering in the anterior aspect of the right ventricular outflow tract (RVOT) epicardium: **Fig. 1** demonstrates one such example from a patient with BrS with recurrent VF episodes. It shows multiple fractionated late potential EGMs recorded from both proximal and distal pair electrodes of the NaviStar-ThermoCool catheter (Biosense Webster, Diamond Bar, CA, USA). These signature EGMs with late activation identify ideal ablation sites. Interestingly, the unipolar electrogram recorded from the distal electrode also exhibit local coved ST morphology electrogram similar to that of Brugada curved type, known to be associated with local activation failure.[9] Ablation at these sites rendered ventricular tachycardia (VT)/VF noninducible and normalization of the Brugada ECG pattern. In this study, all patients had VT-/VF-free survival, off medications (except on amiodarone), and almost 90% of the patients had Brugada ECG pattern normalized.[7]

These abnormal fractionated late potentials initially puzzled us as these types of EGMs are usually associated with fibrosis,[10] but none of the 9 patients had overt structural abnormalities based on cardiac imaging (either cardiac MRI or computed tomography [CT] imaging). We then conducted a collaborative study that demonstrated epicardial and interstitial fibrosis and reduced gap junction expressions in the RVOT of sudden cardiac death victims with BrS family history and negative routine autopsy.[11] In addition, there was a significant increase in the collagen content in all ventricular walls in sudden death victims diagnosed with BrS (as compared with age- and sex-matched controls). In the same study, we also performed open thoracotomy for direct mapping and ablations in 6 patients with symptomatic BrS with frequent ICD discharges (4 patients from our center in Thailand and 2 from Prof. Nogami's laboratory at Tsukuba University). The indication for thoracotomy was lead extraction (n = 4) for infection or to permit epicardial access for ablation after a failed endocardial ablation attempt (n = 2). Tissue biopsies from the substrate sites that harbored abnormal fragmented and delayed conduction revealed epicardial and

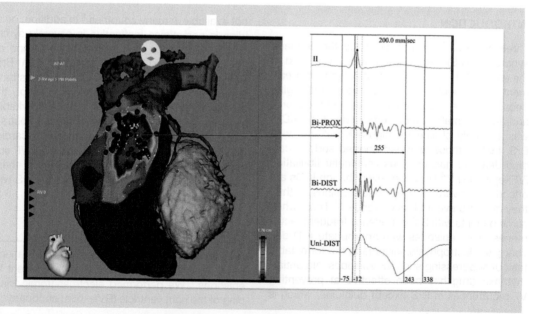

**Fig. 1.** A composite picture of CARTO-Merge maps shows cardiac computed tomography of the right ventricle (RV), left ventricle (LV), aorta, pulmonary artery, and coronary arteries that are merged with the electroanatomic maps of the RV outflow tract epicardium. The double annotation map displays the magnitude of prolonged electrogram duration; the purple area indicates very prolonged duration of the electrogram (>150 msec). The sample electrograms recorded from this area are shown (*right*). The bipolar electrogram recorded from the distal pair electrodes (Bi-DIST) and the proximal pair (Bi-PROX) of the NaviStar-ThermoCool catheter at the purple area of the map is low voltage and fractionated with the electrogram width of 225 msec from the proximal pair. The unipolar electrogram recorded from the distal electrode is also shown, along with the ECG Lead II. The red dots represent ablation points. Uni-DIST, unipolar distal.

interstitial fibrosis (**Fig. 2**). Interestingly, all had normal cardiac imaging including CT/MRI as well as a normal-appearing heart on direct visualization during thoracotomy. Similar findings were also reported by Coronel and colleagues who did biopsy and mapping studies on the explanted heart of a patient with BrS with SCN5A mutation and heart failure from VF storm, necessitating a heart transplantation.[12] The explanted heart showed found evidence of interstitial fibrosis causing conduction delay. Thus, one can unequivocally conclude that the interstitial fibrosis and reduced gap junction expression in the epicardium of the RVOT are the key structural abnormalities creating the arrhythmogenic substrate for BrS.

## Sodium Channel Blockade and Brugada Syndrome Substrates

It is well known that sodium channel blockers (eg, ajmaline, procainamide, flecainide) can unmask the typical coved type of ST elevation (STE) in the right precordial leads of patients with BrS.[3,4,13] But it had been unclear as to how these drugs unmask the Brugada pattern and adversely

affect the BrS substrate. We studied 32 patients with BrS (age $40 \pm 12$ years) with frequent VF and performed electroanatomical mapping and ECG imaging mapping before and after ajmaline administration. In 4 patients, epicardial mapping was performed using open thoracotomy with targeted biopsies.[14] We found that ajmaline, by reducing $I_{Na}$, markedly delays impulse conduction in these RVOT substrate sites with underlying fibrosis, thereby increasing the areas of the late activation and in turn increasing STE over the right precordial ECG leads. **Fig. 3** shows an example of how ajmaline unmasked the arrhythmogenic substrate over the anterior RVOT epicardium in a patient who underwent epicardial mapping during a thoracotomy. Ajmaline (30 mg intravenously) caused changes in bipolar and unipolar EGMs of areas 3, 8, and 13 from relatively normal EGMs to markedly abnormal fractionated EGMs, coinciding with an appearance of STE in the unipolar EGMs in these areas. In particular, the unipolar EGMs after ajmaline infusion have a monophasic morphology (resembling an action potential), especially in panels B, E, and G; this is a sign of absence of local activation (similar to that

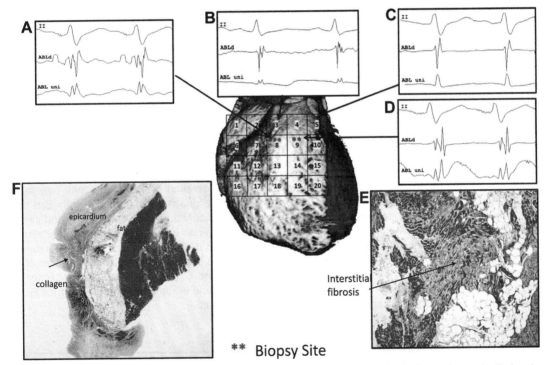

**Fig. 2.** Computed tomography scan of the heart (*center*) of a patient with Brugada syndrome (BrS) showing anatomic grid over the anterior RV outflow tract. ECG Lead II and a distal bipolar (0.4 mV/cm voltage scale at 30–300 Hz filter settings) and unipolar (5 mV/cm voltage scale at 0.05–300 Hz filter settings) electrogram at labeled sites given in surrounding panels. Abnormal fractionated electrograms are in the panel A and D recorded from the biopsy sites (sites 8 and 9) and normal electrograms in the panel B and C. Epicardial biopsy and histology at these sites shows both thickened epicardial and interstitial fibrosis by H&E stain in the panel E and thickened collagen content at this site (*blue*) by Masson trichrome stain at this site (*F*).

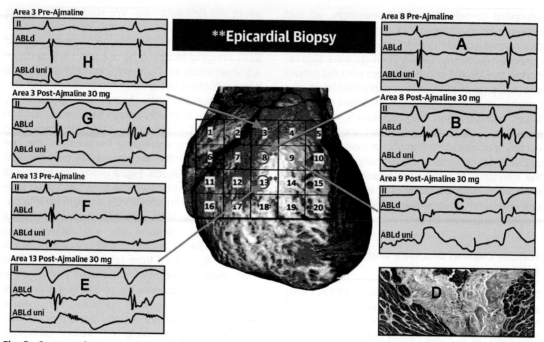

**Fig. 3.** Computed tomography scan of the heart (*center*) from a patient with BrS undergoing open thoracotomy mapping and ablation showing RV anatomic grid. ECG Lead II and a distal bipolar (0.4 mV/cm voltage scale at the filter 30–300 Hz) and unipolar electrogram (5 mV/cm voltage scale at the filter 0.05–300 Hz) are displayed in insets of the surrounding panels. Clockwise from the right are panels A and B, which display electrograms from site 8 at baseline and after ajmaline, respectively; panel C shows electrograms recorded from site 9 after ajmaline; panel D is histology of the biopsy specimen (Masson trichrome stain) from site 8 showing epicardial fibrosis; panels E and F and panels G and H display electrograms recorded from sites 13 and 3 after ajmaline and at baseline, respectively.

recorded from a monophasic action potential catheter).[15] This phenomenon is present at sites 3, 8, and 13. Biopsies at sites 8 and 13 and their histology demonstrate marked epicardial fibrosis (panel D). Furthermore, ajmaline unmasks the substrate by creating excitation failure, manifesting as the genesis of monophasic EGMs or as late monophasic components of unipolar EGMs in fibrotic tissue. The drug, therefore, compromises impulse conduction in the BrS substrates and can uncover the fibrotic sites by producing fractionated EGMs, conduction block, or excitation failure that create the milieu for current-to-load mismatch phenomenon, culminating in VF genesis and the signature Brugada ECG pattern.[14] It is estimated that ajmaline administration approximately increases the size of the target area for ablation by 2-fold. Thus, it is imperative to use sodium channel blockers, ajmaline, procainamide, or pilsicainide, to guide successful catheter ablation of BrS substrates for better long-term outcomes.

## Catheter Ablation of Brugada Substrates

After our initial observations of substrate ablation in the RVOT, several individual case reports as

well as collaborative studies have confirmed our findings that abnormal fractionated late potentials are ubiquitous in the RVOT epicardium/anterior RV of patients with BrS, and substrate ablation in this region has been increasing used to treat symptomatic BrS worldwide.[16–20]

With increasing experience in performing mapping and ablation of BrS substrates, we found that about one-third of patients with BrS also have significant substrate on RV body and inferior epicardium and infrequently, in the LV epicardium as well.[8,20] Thus, one must be very deliberate and meticulous in performing detailed mapping of the substrate, to obtain excellent ablation outcomes. Our workflow in mapping and ablating for BrS is described later.

## Mapping

Gaining epicardial access is crucial to perform high-density mapping of the BrS arrhythmogenic substrate, and knowledge of cardiac anatomy and expertise in safe pericardial puncture is necessary.[21] We are comfortable with technique described by Sosa and colleagues[22] and believe that epicardial access can be achieved with very minimal risk for patients. After advancing the needle into pericardial space, manual contrast injection confirms the needle tip position in the pericardial space. A stiff wire is then inserted to wrap around the heart borders, and fluoroscopic images are used to ascertain that the wire crosses the midline in LAO view. After successful epicardial access, endocardial and epicardial electroanatomic mapping of the RV as well as epicardial mapping of the LV can then be performed with a high-density mapping catheter. In our laboratory, a multipole-electrode catheter with small interelectrode distance such as the PentaRay, a circular mapping catheter (Lasso) or a decapolar catheter (DecaNav, Biosense Webster, Diamond Bar, CA, USA) are used for high-resolution and high-density mapping. Image integration tools such as CARTO Merge and CARTOUNIVU for radiographic/fluoroscopic/angiographic image integration with the electroanatomic mapping system are very helpful to create detailed epicardial and endocardial maps. Such maps can be displayed based on either voltage or duration of local potentials. An example of the map is shown in **Fig. 4**, which was obtained from a patient with BrS with multiple ICD therapies for recurrent VF episodes. The ablation target areas were tagged based on EGM characteristics of abnormal low-voltage fractionated signals (panel A), using the double annotation map that shows that the patient has prolonged ventricular EGMs (>150 msec), as displayed in purple in this area. These abnormal EGMs were not found at the endocardial site of the same area of the RVOT (panel B). Panel C shows epicardial EGMs recorded from various sites of the epicardium in both LV and RV. Panel D demonstrates the effect of the ablation on the ECG pattern; the patient had a typical type 1 Brugada ECG pattern in V1 and V2, which normalized during the ablation.

As mentioned earlier, mapping of the RV epicardium after the administration of sodium channel blocker is essential. The signal of interest is defined by multiple components, greater than 20 ms isoelectric segments between peaks of individual components, and equal to or greater than 70 ms duration (long duration), or presence of late potential beyond the end of QRS complex.

We do not routinely perform coronary angiograms during epicardial mapping and ablation, as adequate coronary anatomy is obtained through detailed endocardial and epicardial mapping and by recognizing the location of annulus and RV septum. However, careful observation for ST segment deviation during RF application is important to avoid inadvertent coronary injury in patients with BrS with anatomic variation of coronary anomaly.

### Ablation Protocol and Endpoint

An irrigated tip catheter with contact force greater than or equal to 5 g is required for RF application. RF power is titrated from 30 to 50 W to achieve greater than or equal to 10 $\Omega$ impedance reduction from baseline. Rapid disappearance of EGMs and a decline in recorded signal amplitude ascertain sufficient acute elimination effect on the target area (Supplemental Video 1). Our endpoint is complete elimination of all substrate sites, after sodium channel blockade.

### Efficacy and Safety of Catheter Ablation for Brugada Syndrome

Brugada substrate ablation now has been accepted as an important effective treatment modality and is being used in several centers worldwide. However, long-term outcomes are still needed. Therefore, we have created a worldwide Brugada Ablation of VF Substrate Ongoing Multicenter (BRAVO) registry study of catheter ablation (ClinicalTrials.gov #NCT04420078) for treatment of patients with symptomatic BrS and presented the interim results at the 39th Annual Heart Rhythm Scientific Sessions in 2019 (full manuscript is under review). BRAVO results confirm our initial observation that BrS substrate ablation is safe and effective and provide excellent long-term outcomes (over 95% patients had no VF recurrences). The only major complication is pericardial bleeding (~1%), with no procedural deaths recorded in the registry. The main predictor of VF recurrence necessitating repeat ablation is continuing presence of Brugada ECG pattern and a combined BrS and early repolarization (ER).

### Combined Syndrome of Brugada and Early Repolarization Syndrome

A combined Brugada and ER ECG pattern either in the inferior leads (II, III, and atrial VF) or lateral leads (V4–V6) or both inferior and lateral leads—the so-called J Wave syndrome—is not uncommon, especially in Southeast Asia.[23,24] Several studies in the past decade show that these overlapping features of BrS and ER syndrome (ERS) increased the risk of recurrent VT/VF much higher than that posed by BrS alone.[25–27] Catheter ablation in the combined BrS and ERS cohort is more challenging than for patients with BrS alone, as the VF recurrence rate after the first session of ablation is higher. This is likely because of larger substrate in the combined syndrome than those of BrS alone; besides RVOT substrate sites, patients with

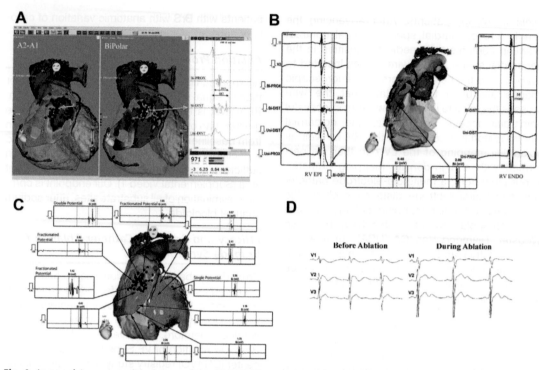

**Fig. 4.** In panel A a composite picture of the CARTO-Merge maps shows the cardiac computed tomography that is merged with the electroanatomic maps of the right ventricular outflow tract (RVOT) epicardium. The double annotation map (A2-A1), shown on the left, illustrates the scale of abnormal prolonged duration of the ventricular electrograms in the anterior RVOT as displayed in the color-coded area; the purple represents the longest duration (>160 msec) during sinus rhythm. The voltage map, shown in the middle, is the same as the A2-A1 map, but is displayed differently, with the color-coded area of low voltage in red and high voltage in purple. The right inset displays the electrograms recorded from the NaviStar-ThermoCool catheter at the site of the anterior aspect of the RVOT epicardium (*arrow*). Red dots represent ablation points. The voltage map and the representative tracing of the bipolar and unipolar electrograms are recorded from the anterior aspect of the RVOT epicardium. Note that the duration of the electrograms in this area is quite prolonged (>150 msec) and low voltage (<1 mV). The bipolar electrogram recorded from this site shows the electrogram is low voltage (0.84 mV), fractionated, and has prolonged duration (183 msec) and delayed depolarization beyond the end of the lead II-QRS complex (160 msec). Bi-DIST, bipolar distal; Bi-PROX, bipolar proximal; Uni-DIST, unipolar distal. Panel B shows a left lateral view of the RVOT displays the difference in ventricular electrograms between the endocardial and epicardial site of the anterior RVOT. The left and right insets display bipolar and unipolar electrograms recorded from the epicardium and endocardium from the same site of the RVOT, respectively. Uni-PROX, unipolar proximal. Panel C shows comparison of ventricular electrograms recorded from different sites in both the LV and RV of the same patient. The cluster of abnormal electrograms, fractionated electrograms, and double potential is only seen in the anterior aspect of the RV epicardium, not anywhere else in the RV or LV. In panel D the right precordial leads (V1–V3) from the same patient show normalization of the Brugada ECG pattern during the ablation. See text for detail. (*From* Nademanee K, Veerakul G, Chandanamattha P, et al. Prevention of ventricular fibrillation episodes in Brugada syndrome by catheter ablation over the anterior right ventricular outflow tract epicardium. Circulation. 2011;123(12):1270-1279. doi:10.1161/CIRCULATIONAHA.110.972612; with permission.)

combined BrS/ERS commonly have arrhythmogenic substrate located in the RV inferior wall and RV inferolateral areas close to the tricuspid annulus.[21]

## FUTURE DIRECTIONS

We believe that catheter ablation is clearly the only and most effective treatment modality for VF prevention in BrS. Recently, several patients who have been free of VF for several years and did not want an ICD anymore requested that the device be taken out or did not want a replacement device at the end of the current ICD's battery life. Similarly, new patients with symptomatic Brugada who sought ablation treatment did not want an ICD implanted after the ablation.

We believe that it would be premature to recommend catheter ablation alone without an ICD for patients with symptomatic BrS, especially those who survived sudden cardiac death. One must be mindful that BrS is part of J-wave syndrome that includes ERS, and often the 2 syndromes coexist. This combined BrS and ERS has a higher rate of VF recurrence after ablation, and thus many of those with J-wave syndrome will continue to need ICD implantation.

In patients with symptomatic BrS without overlapping BrS/ERS syndrome, we hypothesize that patients can be managed after substrate ablation without an ICD, if normalization of the right precordial ECG in higher intercostal lead position can be achieved after sodium channel blocker challenge. To address this hypothesis, we are carrying out a randomized clinical trial, Brugada Syndrome Ablation for the prevention of VF Episodes (BRAVE study, ClinicalTrials.gov NCT02704416). Once this trial is completed, it is very likely that we will have an answer as to whether we can treat patients with symptomatic BrS without an ICD.

## CLINICS CARE POINTS

- In the past, treatment of symptomatic BrS had been limited to only ICD and quinidine.
- Catheter ablation for treatment of symptomatic BrS is highly safe and effective.
- Catheter ablation of BrS substrates emerges as an alternating therapeutic treatment for prevention of VF recurrence in BrS patients.
- Catheter ablation of BrS substrates is indicated in BrS patients with VF recurrences necessitating ICD discharges.

## CONFLICT OF INTEREST

Dr R. Chokesuwattanaskul has no conflict of interest. Dr K. Nademanee has royalty income and consultant honoraria from Biosense Webster, Inc. and research grants from Biosense Webster, Inc and Medtronic Inc.

## DISCLOSURE

This work is partially supported by The National Research Council of Thailand and Grant-in-Aid from Bumrungrad Hospital, Bangkok, Thailand and Medtronic Inc.

## SUPPLEMENTARY DATA

Supplementary data related to this article can be found online at https://doi.org/10.1016/j.ccep.2022.08.006.

## REFERENCES

1. Brugada P, Brugada J. Right bundle branch block, persistent ST segment elevation and sudden cardiac death: a distinct clinical and electrocardiographic syndrome: a multicenter report. J Am Coll Cardiol 1992;20:1391–6.
2. Nademanee K, Veerakul G, Nimmannit S, et al. Arrhythmogenic marker for the sudden unexplained death syndrome in Thai men. Circulation 1997;96: 2595–600.
3. Veerakul G, Nademanee K. Brugada syndrome: two decades of progress. Circ J 2012;76:2713–22.
4. Antzelevitch C, Brugada P, Borggrefe M, et al. Brugada syndrome: report of the second consensus conference: endorsed by the heart rhythm society and the European heart rhythm association. Circulation 2005;111:659–70.
5. Nademanee K, Veerakul G, Mower M, et al. Defibrillator vs. Beta-blockers for Unexplained Death in Thailand (DEBUT). A randomized clinical trial. Circulation 2003;107:2221–6.
6. Viskin S, Wilde AA, Guevara-Valdivia ME, et al. Quinidine, a life-saving medication for Brugada syndrome, is inaccessible in many countries. J Am Coll Cardiol 2013;61(23):2383–7.
7. Nademanee K, Veerakul G, Chandanamattha P, et al. Prevention of ventricular fibrillation episodes in Brugada syndrome by catheter ablation over the anterior right ventricular outflow tract epicardium. Circulation 2011;123(12):1270–9.
8. Nademanee K, Hocini M, Haissaguerre M. Epicardial substrate ablation for Brugada syndrome. Heart Rhythm 2017;14(3):457–61.
9. Haissaguerre M, Cheniti G, Nademanee K, et al. Dependence of epicardial T-wave on local activation voltage in Brugada syndrome. Heart Rhythm 2022; S1547-5271(22):02053–7.
10. de Bakker JM, Wittkampf FH. The pathophysiologic basis of fractionated and complex electrograms and the impact of recording techniques on their detection and interpretation. Circ Arrhythm Electrophysiol 2010;3:204–13.
11. Nademanee K, Raju H, de Noronha SV, et al. Fibrosis, connexin-43, and conduction abnormalities in the Brugada syndrome. J Am Coll Cardiol 2015; 66(18):1976–86.
12. Coronel R, Casini S, Koopmann TT, et al. Right ventricular fibrosis and conduction delay in a patient with clinical signs of Brugada syndrome: a combined electrophysiological, genetic, histopathologic,

and computational study. Circulation 2005;112(18): 2769–77.

13. Wilde AA, Antzelevitch C, Borggrefe M, et al. Proposed diagnostic criteria for the Brugada syndrome: consensus report. Circulation 2002; 106(19):2514–9.

14. Nademanee K, Veerakul G, Nogami A, et al. Mechanism of the effects of sodium channel blockade on the arrhythmogenic substrate of Brugada syndrome. Heart Rhythm 2022;19:407–16.

15. Coronel R, de Bakker JM, Wins-Schopman FL, et al. Monophasic action potentials and activation recovery intervals as measure of ventricular action potential duration. Experimental evidence to resolve some controversies. Heart Rhythm 2006;3:1043–50.

16. Pappone C, Brugada J, Vicedomini G, et al. Electrical substrate elimination in 135 consecutive patients with Brugada syndrome. Circ Arrhythm Electrophysiol 2017;10(5):e005053.

17. Chung FP, Raharjo SB, Lin YJ, et al. A novel method to enhance phenotype, epicardial functional substrates, and ventricular tachyarrhythmias in Brugada syndrome. Heart Rhythm 2017;14:508–17.

18. Fernandes GC, Fernandes A, Cardoso R, et al. Ablation strategies for the management of symptomatic Brugada syndrome: a systematic review. Heart Rhythm 2018;15:1140–7.

19. Zhang P, Tung R, Zhang Z, et al. Characterization of the epicardial substrate for catheter ablation of Brugada syndrome. Heart Rhythm 2016;13:2151–8.

20. Chokesuwattanaskul R, Nademanee K. Role of catheter ablation for ventricular arrhythmias in Brugada syndrome. Curr Cardiol Rep 2021;23(5):54.

21. Romero J, Shivkumar K, Di Biase L, et al. Mastering the art of epicardial access in cardiac electrophysiology. Heart Rhythm 2019;16(11):1738–49.

22. Sosa E, Scanavacca M, d'Avila A, et al. A new technique to perform epicardial mapping in the electrophysiology laboratory. J Cardiovasc Electrophysiol 1996;7(6):531–6.

23. Nademanee K, Haïssaguerre M, Hocini, et al. Mapping and ablation of ventricular fibrillation associated with early repolarization syndrome. Circulation 2019;140:1477–90.

24. Nademanee K, Veerakul G. Overlapping risks of early repolarization and Brugada syndrome. JACC 2014;63:2139–40.

25. Tokioka K, Kusano KF, Morita H, et al. Electrocardiographic pa- rameters and fatal arrhythmic events in patients with Brugada syn- drome: combination of depolarization and repolarization abnormalities. J Am Coll Cardiol 2014;63:2131–8.

26. Sarkozy A, Chierchia GB, Paparella G, et al. Inferior and lateral electrocardiographic repolarization abnormalities in Brugada syndrome. Circ Arrhythm Electrophysiol 2009;2:144–50.

27. Letsas KP, Sacher F, Probst V, et al. Prevalence of early repolarization pattern in inferolateral leads in patients with Brugada syndrome. Heart Rhythm 2008;5:1685–9.

# Catheter Ablation for Ventricular Arrhythmias in Hypertrophic Cardiomyopathy

Muthiah Subramanian, MD, DM[a], Auras R. Atreya, MD, MPH, FACC, FHRS[a,b],
Sachin D. Yalagudri, MD, DM[a], P. Vijay Shekar, MD, DM[a],
Daljeet Kaur Saggu, MD, DM[a], Calambur Narasimhan, MD, DM[a,*]

## KEYWORDS

- Ventricular arrhythmias • Hypertrophic cardiomyopathy • Epicardial ablation • Apical aneurysm
- Ventricular tachycardia

## KEY POINTS

- In patients with hypertrophic cardiomyopathy, the substrate for ventricular arrhythmias can be present in the endocardium, midmyocardium, and/or epicardium.
- Areas with late gadolinium enhancement can be used to target arrhythmic substrate.
- A combination of endocardial and epicardial mapping and ablation leads to reasonable long-term clinical outcomes.
- Bipolar ablation, surgical apical aneurysmectomy, and stereotactic radioablation are options in patients with refractory ventricular arrhythmias with difficult to ablate substrate.

## INTRODUCTION

Although the advent of implantable cardioverter-defibrillators (ICDs) and earlier detection of disease has reduced mortality (<1%) in contemporary cohorts, sudden cardiac death remains a common cause of mortality in patients with hypertrophic cardiomyopathy (HCM).[1] Ventricular ectopics occur in most patients with HCM, with up to one-quarter of patients having greater than 30 ventricular ectopics per hour.[2] The prevalence of nonsustained ventricular tachycardia (NSVT) seems to be dependent on age and left ventricular thickness.[3,4] In large, nontertiary patient populations, the frequency of NSVTs is estimated to be between 20% and 30% on 24-hour and 48-hour ambulatory electrocardiographic (ECG) monitoring.[4] Sustained ventricular tachycardia (VT) or ventricular fibrillation (VF) account for more than 50% of HCM related deaths.[4] An ICD-based study in patients with HCM revealed that the cause of ICD therapy was monomorphic VT, VF, and polymorphic VT in 86%, 9%, and 5% of patients, respectively.[5]

## MECHANISMS OF VENTRICULAR ARRHYTHMIAS

The high risk of ventricular arrhythmias (VA) in patients with HCM can be attributed to an interplay of many factors. Underlying ventricular fibrosis, myocyte disarray, calcium hypersensitivity, along with triggering factors such as physical exertion and microvascular ischemia contribute to the proarrhythmic state in HCM.[6] The widespread fibrosis seen in HCM is strongly implicated as the main arrhythmic substrate, and the fibrotic scar burden increases over time. Myocardial fibrosis does not quantitatively correlate with the degree of ventricular hypertrophy because it occurs due to a combination of energy depletion, microvascular ischemia, and hypertrophy.[7] The typical patchy fibrosis that occurs in HCM can even occur in very early stages of the disease, when hypertrophy is not apparent.

a Electrophysiology Section, AIG Hospitals Institute of Cardiac Sciences and Research, Mindspace Road, Gachibowli, Hyderabad 500032, India; b Division of Cardiovascular Medicine, Electrophysiology Section, University of Arkansas for Medical Sciences, Little Rock, AR, USA
* Corresponding author. 1, Mindspace Road, Gachibowli, Hyderabad, 500032, India
E-mail address: calambur1@gmail.com

Card Electrophysiol Clin 14 (2022) 693–699
https://doi.org/10.1016/j.ccep.2022.08.005

Myocyte disarray can also potentiate arrhythmogenesis by disrupting cell-to-cell alignment, creating conduction delays and unidirectional block, which can initiate and sustain VAs.[8]

One of the hallmark intracellular abnormalities that are present in patients with HCM is an increase in myofilament calcium sensitivity. This increased cytosolic calcium sensitivity can cause delayed after depolarizations.[9] Increased cytosolic calcium can result in changes in the duration of action potentials and cause dispersion of conduction velocities.[10] These can potentially lead to VAs even in the absence of fibrosis. Myocyte hypertrophy causes electrical remodeling and is associated with a down regulation of potassium channels, accentuating the proarrhythmic dispersion of cardiac repolarization.[11] As a result of the above pathogenic processes, the predominant VA mechanism in HCM is re-entry. The presence of patchy fibrosis in HCM can lead to a macro-reentrant mechanism, similar to postinfarction VT. Nonuniform anisotropic conduction due to myocyte disarray can lead to source-sink mismatches and create a substrate for functional re-entry.[12]

Monomorphic VT has been known to occur in patients with apical aneurysms and in those with dilated phase HCM. Apical aneurysms have been identified as a predictor of worse prognosis, and increased risk of VAs in HCM, largely due to the scarred rim of the aneurysms, which serves as substrate for re-entry.[13] These aneurysms may explain the significantly higher rate of VAs in patients with apical HCM compared with septal HCM.[14] In a case series of 15 patients with HCM and apical aneurysm, VT was related to the apical aneurysms in all patients.[15]

## ENDOCARDIAL VERSUS EPICARDIAL SUBSTRATE

Scattered fibrosis within the left ventricle (LV) can manifest as either an endocardial, epicardial, or a combination of both substrates. A high prevalence of midmyocardial and epicardial fibrotic areas have been demonstrated in patients with HCM.[16] Detailed endocardial ventricular surface mapping of patients with HCM revealed a significantly higher unipolar voltage in HCM compared with healthy persons or ischemic cardiomyopathy patients.[17] This suggests that an epicardial substrate may be more common in patients with HCM. Intramural and epicardial circuits have been demonstrated in patients with HCM with recurrent VAs. *Santangeli and colleagues* found that epicardial ablation was necessary to treat VT in close to 60% of cases.[18] Understanding the location and extent of the substrate can help not only in guiding the ablation strategy but also in overall clinical prognostication.

## SELECTION OF PATIENTS FOR CATHETER ABLATION

Indications for catheter ablation for VAs in patients with HCM is not clearly defined and needs to be tailored for each patient. Most patients have antiarrhythmic drug refractory monomorphic VT with multiple ICD shocks. In a subset of patients, especially those with apical aneurysms and sustained VT, it may be worthwhile to consider catheter ablation before ICD implantation to reduce the arrhythmic burden. Adequate management of LV outflow obstruction and obstructive sleep apnea can reduce VAs and potentially affect the progression of fibrosis.[19,20] Patients with end-stage HCM and VT present a clinical challenge because they are prone to hemodynamic collapse. VT ablation with the aid of mechanical circulatory support can be tried in a subset of these advanced patients with HCM. Most of the patients with advanced disease will require left ventricular assist devices and/or cardiac transplantation.

## UTILITY OF PREOPERATIVE IMAGING BEFORE ABLATION

In patients with HCM, multimodality imaging can help in identification of the arrhythmogenic substrate and the anatomic components of the VT circuit. Cardiac magnetic resonance imaging (CMR) can be used to identify specific patterns of scar in patients with HCM.[16] Areas with late gadolinium enhancement (LGE) have been used to target arrhythmogenic substrates during ablation. **Fig. 1** illustrates the spectrum and distribution of LGE in patients with HCM. The pattern of myocardial fibrosis in HCM is significantly different from those observed in coronary artery disease and dilated cardiomyopathy. Patients with HCM have a high prevalence of midmyocardial and epicardial fibrotic areas. As the disease evolves to end-stage HCM, patients can develop wall thinning, ventricular cavity enlargement, aneurysm formation, and a transmural scar.[21]

Advances in CMR imaging have increased our understanding of the myocardial architecture and their prognostic value in predicting future VAs in HCM. Native T1 mapping and extracellular volume fraction are quantitative methods that reflect focal and diffuse interstitial fibrosis in HCM. Global native T1 mapping has been shown to provide incremental prognostic value in predicting VAs and major cardiac event risk.[22] Myocardial disarray is

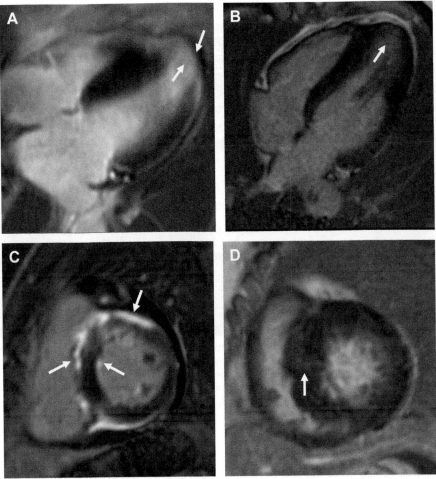

**Fig. 1.** Spectrum of LGE in HCM. Patterns of LGE (*white arrows*) in patients with HCM before ablation of ventricular arrhythmias are shown in Panel A–D. Apical aneurysm showing transmural LGE (*A*) and apical pouching with only endocardial LGE (*B*) are observed in midventricular obstruction hypertrophic cardiomyopathy (*A*). A patient with end-stage HCM (LVEF 33%) had extensive epicardial LGE and myocardial wall thinning (*arrow*) (*C*). Patchy endocardial LGE was present in another patient with recurrent monomorphic VT and normal LV ejection fraction (*D*). HCM, hypertrophic cardiomyopathy; LGE, late gadolinium enhancement; LV, left ventricle; LVEF, left ventricular ejection fraction; VT, ventricular tachycardia.

a microstructural abnormality that can be detected by mapping the preferential diffusion of water along cardiac muscle fibers. Diffusion tensor CMR quantification of fractional anisotropy has been recently shown to be an independent risk factor of VAs in HCM.[23] Therefore, it is possible both fibrosis and disarray contribute to VAs in some patients.

## OUTCOMES OF ABLATION IN HYPERTROPHIC CARDIOMYOPATHY

Overall, there are limited data on the outcomes of patients with HCM who undergo VT ablation. *Santangeli and colleagues* demonstrated modest efficacy in 22 patients with HCM and drug refractory VT.[18] Most patients in this series had developed burnt out disease with an left ventricular ejection fraction (LVEF) less than 35%. Of the 18 patients with hemodynamically stable VT, the exit site of VT was often from the junction of LV and right ventricle (RV) either at the level of the basal or apical LV segments. Epicardial radiofrequency ablation was needed in most patients (13/22 = 59.1%). After a mean follow-up of 20 ± 9 months, 6 patients developed one or more episodes of sustained VT. **Fig. 2** illustrates successful ablation of monomorphic VT in a patient with minimal endocardial substrate and a large scar burden in the epicardium.

Given the ventricular wall thickness in HCM, traditional endocardial mapping and ablation

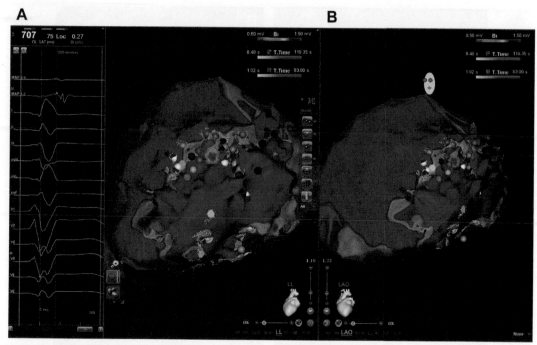

**Fig. 2.** Epicardial VT ablation in HCM. A young man with recurrent monomorphic VT initially underwent endocardial ablation. There were only few areas with fractionated late potentials in the LV endocardium. 3D epicardial bipolar voltage map (0.5–1.5 mV border zone) showed dense scar in the lateral wall of the LV (*A* and *B*, left lateral and left anterior oblique view, respectively). Substrate modification of the areas with fractionated late potentials within the epicardium led to noninducibility of VT. HCM, hypertrophic cardiomyopathy; LV, left ventricle; VT, ventricular tachycardia.

may be of limited value. *Dukkipati and colleagues* showed that a combined epicardial and endocardial mapping and ablation is feasible and effective in a select group of patients with HCM and refractory monomorphic VT.[24] Electrophysiologically identified epicardial scar was present in 80% of the study patients compared with 60% with endocardial scar. Only 1 patient had endocardial scar without concomitant epicardial involvement. Approximately 78% of patients were free of ICD shocks over a follow-up of 37 ± 17 months. An apical scar was present in 70% of patients and an apical aneurysm was observed in 30% in this cohort.

Patients with HCM and an apical aneurysm have a higher rate of sudden death and progressive heart failure. In a multicenter study, *Igarashi and colleagues* found endocardial radiofrequency ablation was effective in suppressing monomorphic VT.[15] Although epicardial or intramural origin of VT was suspected in 7 patients, endocardial ablation suppressed VT at or within the low voltage area. Of the cohort of 15 patients, epicardial ablation was needed in 1 patient. VT recurrence was observed in 2 patients during the 12 month follow-up period. In patients with an apical

aneurysm and an epicardial VT exit site, endocardial ablation may still be effective in the area of the thinned out aneurysmal wall. However, manipulating the ablation catheter within the apical aneurysm through a narrow aneurysmal neck can be challenging, leading to ablation failure. **Fig. 3** shows successful ablation of VT from an apical aneurysm in a patient with a midcavity obstruction.

Few patients with HCM display evidence of His-Purkinje conduction disease, including bundle branch block during the course of the disease. Underlying conduction disease along with cardiac myocyte disarray can lead to bundle branch reentry in HCM. Sustained bundle-branch reentry has been reported as the mechanism of VT in some patients with HCM.[25] **Fig. 4** shows a patient with end-stage HCM who had a counterclockwise bundle branch re-entrant VT (BBRVT) that was rendered noninducible by radiofrequency ablation of the right bundle branch.

## STRATEGIES TO IMPROVE ABLATION OUTCOMES

Because it can be difficult to create transmural lesions in patients with thickened ventricular walls,

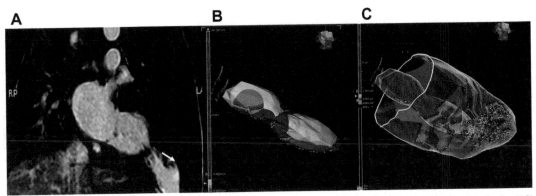

**Fig. 3.** Monomorphic VT in a patient with HCM and apical aneurysm. In a patient with midcavity obstructive HCM and monomorphic VT exiting from the apical aneurysm, preablation CMR revealed LGE in the apical aneurysm (*white arrow, panel A*). 3D electroanatomical mapping revealed endocardial scar in the apical aneurysm (*panel B*). However, due to the narrow neck, entry into the apical aneurysm was difficult. Substrate-guided late potential mapping and ablation in the epicardial surface of the aneurysm (*Panel C*) made the VT noninducible. CMR, cardiac magnetic resonance imaging; HCM, hypertrophic cardiomyopathy; LGE, late gadolinium enhancement; VT, ventricular tachycardia.

some strategies include higher power, longer duration lesions, and the use of low-ionic irrigant (half-normal saline) for ablation. In addition, simultaneous unipolar or bipolar ablation is a viable option in some patients with HCM. *Igarashi and colleagues* demonstrated successful bipolar ablation in 3 patients with HCM.[26] In two of these patients with an LV free wall ablation target site, bipolar ablation was delivered between an LV

endocardial and epicardial catheter. In the other patient with a deep septal intramural substrate, ablation was delivered from RV and LV endocardium simultaneously. Bipolar ablation seems to be effective for VTs using a deep intramural VT circuit. It is also plausible that a needle radiofrequency ablation catheter would be able to deliver deep intramural lesions but this remains to be studied clinically in patients with HCM.

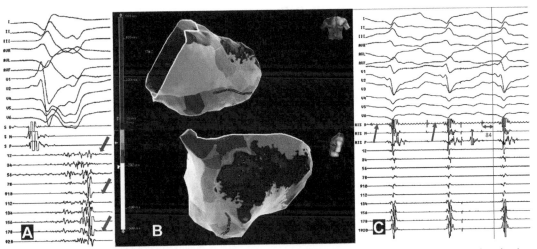

**Fig. 4.** Recurrent BBRVT in HCM. A patient with end-stage HCM (LVEF 30%) had extensive endocardial and epicardial scar. *Panel A* shows late potentials recorded on a decapolar catheter within the epicardium (*red arrows*). *Panel B* shows a late potential 3D electroanatomical map (Ensite Precision, NAVX, Abbott) with most delayed potentials shown in purple (along the left lateral aspect of the epicardial map). Panel C shows the positive HV interval (HV = 84 milliseconds) wide complex tachycardia with proximal to distal his bundle activation (*red arrow*) in the same patient. The counterclockwise BBRVT was terminated with ablation of the distal right bundle. BBRVT, bundle branch re-entrant ventricular tachycardia; HCM, hypertrophic cardiomyopathy; LVEF, left ventricular ejection fraction.

Another option to consider in failed ablations is stereotactic radioablation. *Park and colleagues* performed radioablation to control VT and VF storm in a patient in whom catheter ablation was unsuccessful.[27] A total of 24 Gray was administered, divided into 3 fractions around the apical aneurysm. Immediately after the initiation of radioablation, the daily burden of total VAs and treated VT/VF episodes began to decrease rapidly. During the follow up of 6 months, ICD shocks were no longer required. Surgical apical aneurysmectomy could be another choice for patients with apical aneurysm-related VT.[28] The resection of the aneurysms is a reliable treatment of refractory malignant arrhythmias.

## SUMMARY

In patients with HCM and VAs, patient selection and utilization of preablation CMR can improve the outcomes of ablation therapy. Although available data suggest a recurrence rate of 20% to 30%, optimization of endocardial and epicardial ablation techniques can potentially lead to better outcomes in this challenging cohort. With the advent of newer modalities such as image integration, bipolar ablation, radioablation, the success rate of catheter ablation is likely to improve in this subset of patients.

## DISCLOSURES

Dr C. Narasimhan and Dr D. K Saggu receive support for fellowship program from Medtronic. Dr D. K. Saggu receives honoraria from Boston Scientific. Dr A.R. Atreya receives honoraria or consultancy fees from Abbott, Connected Care and Abiomed. Dr S.D. Yalagudri receives honoraria or consultancy fees from Boston Scientific, Medtronic and Johnson & Johnson. All other authors have no conflicts of interest to disclose relevant to the content of this article.

## REFERENCES

1. Maron BJ, Rowin EJ, Casey SA, et al. Hypertrophic cardiomyopathy in Adulthood associated with low Cardiovascular mortality with contemporary management strategies. J Am Coll Cardiol 2015;65: 1915–28.
2. Adabag AS, Maron BJ. Implications of arrhythmias and prevention of sudden death in hypertrophic cardiomyopathy. Ann Noninvasive Electrocardiol 2007; 12:171–80.
3. Adabag AS, Casey SA, Kuskowski MA, et al. Spectrum and prognostic significance of arrhythmias on ambulatory Holter electrocardiogram in hypertrophic cardiomyopathy. J Am Coll Cardiol 2005;45: 697–704.
4. Monserrat L, Elliott PM, Gimeno JR, et al. Non-sustained ventricular tachycardia in hypertrophic cardiomyopathy: an independent marker of sudden death risk in young patients. J Am Coll Cardiol 2003;42:873–9.
5. O'Mahony C, Lambiase PD, Rahman SM, et al. The relation of ventricular arrhythmia electrophysiological characteristics to cardiac phenotype and circadian patterns in hypertrophic cardiomyopathy. Europace 2012;14:724–33.
6. Hutchings D, Sankaranarayanan R, Venetucci L. Ventricular arrhythmias complicating hypertrophic cardiomyopathy. Br J Hosp Med (Lond) 2012;73: 502–8.
7. Vakrou S, Abraham MR. Hypertrophic cardiomyopathy: a heart in need of an energy bar? Front Physiol 2014;5:309.
8. Michels M. Appropriate implantable cardioverter defibrillator therapy in hypertrophic cardiomyopathy: what happens on Sunday afternoons in May? Europace 2012;14:621–2.
9. Santini L, Coppini R, Cerbai E. Ion channel Impairment and myofilament Ca(2+) Sensitization: two Parallel mechanisms Underlying arrhythmogenesis in hypertrophic cardiomyopathy. Cells 2021;10.
10. Watkins H, McKenna WJ, Thierfelder L, et al. Mutations in the genes for cardiac troponin T and alpha-tropomyosin in hypertrophic cardiomyopathy. N Engl J Med 1995;332:1058–64.
11. Coppini R, Ferrantini C, Mugelli A, et al. Altered Ca(2+) and Na(+) Homeostasis in Human hypertrophic cardiomyopathy: Implications for arrhythmogenesis. Front Physiol 2018;9:1391.
12. Kotadia I, Whitaker J, Roney C, et al. Anisotropic cardiac conduction. Arrhythm Electrophysiol Rev 2020;9:202–10.
13. Maron MS, Finley JJ, Bos JM, et al. Prevalence, clinical significance, and natural history of left ventricular apical aneurysms in hypertrophic cardiomyopathy. Circulation 2008;118:1541–9.
14. Steinberg C, Nadeau-Routhier C, Andre P, et al. Ventricular arrhythmia in septal and apical hypertrophic cardiomyopathy: the French-Canadian Experience. Front Cardiovasc Med 2020;7:548564.
15. Igarashi M, Nogami A, Kurosaki K, et al. Radiofrequency catheter ablation of ventricular tachycardia in patients with hypertrophic cardiomyopathy and apical aneurysm. JACC Clin Electrophysiol 2018;4: 339–50.
16. Amano Y, Kitamura M, Takano H, et al. Cardiac MR imaging of hypertrophic cardiomyopathy: techniques, findings, and clinical relevance. Magn Reson Med Sci 2018;17:120–31.
17. Perez-Alday EA, Haq KT, German DM, et al. Mechanisms of Arrhythmogenicity in hypertrophic

cardiomyopathy: Insight from non-invasive Electro-cardiographic imaging. Front Physiol 2020;11:344.

18. Santangeli P, Di Biase L, Lakkireddy D, et al. Radio-frequency catheter ablation of ventricular arrhythmias in patients with hypertrophic cardiomyopathy: safety and feasibility. Heart Rhythm 2010;7:1036–42.

19. Vriesendorp PA, Liebregts M, Steggerda RC, et al. Long-term outcomes after medical and invasive treatment in patients with hypertrophic cardiomyopathy. JACC Heart Fail 2014;2:630–6.

20. Wang SCH, Ji K, Zhu C, et al. Relationship between obstructive sleep apnea and late gadolinium enhancement and their Effect on cardiac arrhythmias in patients with hypertrophic obstructive cardiomyopathy. Nat Sci Sleep 2021;447–56.

21. Soler R, Mendez C, Rodriguez E, et al. Phenotypes of hypertrophic cardiomyopathy. An illustrative review of MRI findings. Insights Imaging 2018;9:1007–20.

22. Qin L, Min J, Chen C, et al. Incremental values of T1 mapping in the prediction of sudden cardiac death risk in hypertrophic cardiomyopathy: a Comparison with two Guidelines. Front Cardiovasc Med 2021;8:661673.

23. Ariga R, Tunnicliffe EM, Manohar SG, et al. Identification of myocardial disarray in patients with hypertrophic cardiomyopathy and ventricular arrhythmias. J Am Coll Cardiol 2019;73:2493–502.

24. Dukkipati SR, d'Avila A, Soejima K, et al. Long-term outcomes of combined epicardial and endocardial ablation of monomorphic ventricular tachycardia related to hypertrophic cardiomyopathy. Circ Arrhythm Electrophysiol 2011;4:185–94.

25. Mittal S, Coyne RF, Herling IM, et al. Sustained bundle branch reentry in a patient with hypertrophic cardiomyopathy and nondilated left ventricle. J Interv Card Electrophysiol 1997;1:73–7.

26. Igarashi M, Nogami A, Fukamizu S, et al. Acute and long-term results of bipolar radiofrequency catheter ablation of refractory ventricular arrhythmias of deep intramural origin. Heart Rhythm 2020;17:1500–7.

27. Park JS, Choi Y. Stereotactic cardiac radiation to control ventricular tachycardia and fibrillation storm in a patient with apical hypertrophic cardiomyopathy at Burnout stage: case Report. J Korean Med Sci 2020;35:e200.

28. Spina R, Granger E, Walker B, et al. Ventricular tachycardia in hypertrophic cardiomyopathy with apical aneurysm successfully treated with left ventricular aneurysmectomy and cryoablation. Eur Heart J 2013;34:3631.

# Ventricular Tachycardia in Granulomatous Myocarditis: Role of Catheter Ablation

Daljeet Kaur Saggu, MD, DM[a], Sachin D. Yalagudri, MD, DM[a],
Muthiah Subramanian, MD, DM[a], Auras R. Atreya, MD, MPH, FACC, FHRS[a,b],
Calambur Narasimhan, MD, DM[a,*]

**KEYWORDS**

- Ventricular tachycardia • Catheter ablation • Granuloma • Sarcoidosis • Tuberculosis
- Inflammatory myocarditis

**KEY POINTS**

- Outcome of catheter ablation (CA) in granulomatous myocarditis (GM) is better when performed after underlying inflammation is adequately treated.
- Immunosuppressive therapy (antitubercular therapy in cardiac tuberculosis) and antiarrhythmic drugs should be the mainstay of treatment during the inflammatory phase of the disease. CA may be considered among highly resistant cases during this phase of the disease.
- Results of CA in the scar phase of the disease (PET-computed tomography uptake absent) are excellent and should be considered as first-line therapy.
- In the non-inflammatory (scar) phase, epicardial ventricular tachycardicircuits are common in patients with GM and upfront or early epicardial access may be useful in suspected cases.

## INTRODUCTION

Ventricular tachycardia (VT) is a common clinical presentation of granulomatous myocarditis (GM). Cardiac sarcoidosis (CS) and cardiac tuberculosis (CTB) are the usual underlying causes of granulomatous disease and early diagnosis can be challenging for a variety of reasons.[1–13] The granulomatous inflammation and resultant fibrosis in these conditions creates anatomic and functional substrate for re-entrant VT by creating zones of slow conduction in areas of scar.[1,5,14] Delayed diagnosis has serious implications, resulting in a significant increase in morbidity and mortality.[15–18] A high index of suspicion, early diagnosis, and treatment with disease-specific/modifying drugs are key for improving clinical outcomes. Imaging modalities such as PET and cardiac MRI (CMRI) in patients with unexplained ventricular arrhythmias (VA), especially when there are coexistent conduction system abnormalities, fractionated QRS on baseline ECG and or ventricular dysfunction will help early diagnosis (**Fig. 1**).

## SPECTRUM OF DISEASE

VAs in GM can present as frequent premature ventricular complex (PVCs), monomorphic VT, pleomorphic VT, bidirectional VT, Purkinje-related VT, epicardial VT, polymorphic VT, and ventricular fibrillation (VF) (**Fig. 2**).[1,4,5,19–25] Managing VAs in GM can be difficult because of the inability to diagnose and characterize the underlying disease.[26] Ongoing inflammation, scar-related re-entry, or a combination of both may result in VAs.[5,15,26,27]

[a] Electrophysiology Section, AIG Hospitals Institute of Cardiac Sciences and Research, Hyderabad, India;
[b] Division of Cardiovascular Medicine, Electrophysiology Section, University of Arkansas for Medical Sciences, Little Rock, AR, USA
* Corresponding author. 1, Mindspace Road, Gachibowli, Hyderabad 500032, India.
E-mail address: calambur1@gmail.com

Card Electrophysiol Clin 14 (2022) 701–707
https://doi.org/10.1016/j.ccep.2022.08.001

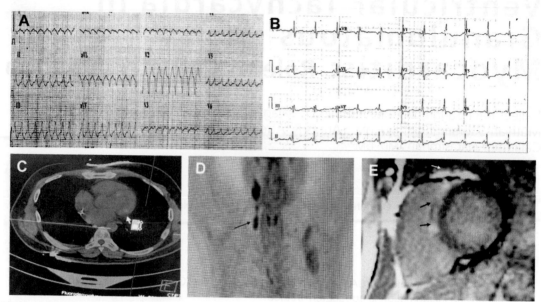

**Fig. 1.** A 37-year-old man presented with (*A*) VT of RVOT morphology with (*B*) underlying sinus rhythm ECG showing RBBB along with fractionated distal QRS in lead III, avF, V2, and V3. His echocardiogram was reported as normal. Cardiac PET-CT with FDG (*C, D*) showing diffuse uptake in left ventricular myocardium along with interventricular septum. FDG uptake is seen in right supraclavicular lymph node (*black arrow* in *D*). Cardiac MRI with LGE (*E*) showing delayed uptake suggestive of scar in the right side of interventricular septum (*black arrows*) along with epicardial scar (*white arrow*). In this case, lymph node biopsy confirmed the diagnosis of cardiac sarcoidosis. FDG, fluorodeoxy glucose; LGE, late gadolinium enhancement; CT, computed tomography; RBBB, right bundle branch block; RVOT, right ventricular outflow tract; VT, ventricular tachycardia.

A practical framework for the management of VA in GM can be formulated based on the disease activity in the myocardium:[26]

1. *Ventricular arrhythmia in inflammatory phase (Stage A).* Patients with VAs and increased myocardial 18-fluoro deoxyglucose (18FDG) uptake on PET and computed tomography (PET-CT) scan in CS and acute phase of disease in CTB.

2. *Ventricular arrhythmia due to myocardial scar (stage B).* Patients with GM presenting with VT and no abnormal myocardial FDG uptake. CMRI with late gadolinium enhancement (LGE) may indicate a scar in the myocardium (burnt-out phase).

3. *Ventricular arrhythmia due to disease reactivation (stage C).* Patients who were treated for VAs due to CS in the past and presented with VAs again along with evidence of reactivation (increased myocardial FDG uptake on PET-CT scan) after being stable for at least 6 months of therapy.

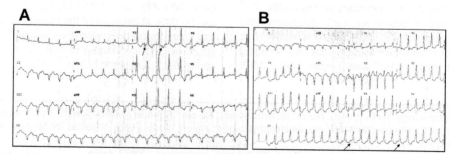

**Fig. 2.** 12-lead ECG of a case of cardiac sarcoidosis showing. (*A*) Narrow QRS (QRS duration = 80 ms) Purkinje fiber-related ventricular tachycardia (VT). (*B*) Wide QRS VT with pattern break in V2 suggestive of epicardial VT in the same patient. Black arrows show evidence of V-A dissociation.

Waxing and waning of inflammation leading to variability in arrhythmic burden are not uncommon in CS. Reactivation of disease activity can occur months to years after the quiescent phase leading to the recurrence of VAs. Scar-related VT (in the burnt-out phase) can occur at any time during the course of CS and CTB.

## TREATMENT MODALITIES

A stepwise approach for the management of VT/VA in GM includes the following (**Fig. 3**):

1) Implantation of implantable cardioverter defibrillator (ICD) for secondary prevention of sudden cardiac arrest (SCA) is indicated in all patients of GM, irrespective of stage of disease.[28] Antiarrhythmic drugs (AADs) are indicated to suppress the VA as required.
2) Steroids followed by steroid-sparing immunosuppressants for CS in stage A and stage C.[26]
3) Antitubercular therapy (ATT) for CTB and a combination of steroids and ATT in patients with CS and latent TB. Low-dose steroids along with ATT can be considered in CTB during the intensive phase (initial 2 months) of therapy. This is to prevent an immune reactivation or reconstitution following ATT, which paradoxically worsens the preexisting infectious process and can present as a VT storm and heart failure.

Therapy with disease-specific agents not only decreases the disease burden but in conjunction with AADs, reduces VT burden in more than 50% of patients in the active or recrudescent phase of the disease (stages A and C).[19,24,29–31] Thus, timely treatment of underlying inflammation, can improve clinical outcomes in this disease. On the contrary, immunosuppressant therapy should be avoided in patients presenting in stage B with scar-related VT.

## ROLE OF CATHETER ABLATION IN PATIENTS WITH GRANULOMATOUS MYOCARDITIS

Catheter ablation (CA) of VT in GM has an adjunctive role along with abovementioned therapies. Outcome of CA depends on the stage (inflammation vs. scar) and extent of disease, with better results in patients with more localized involvement[32] as compared with extensive myocardial involvement.[23] Epicardial scar may be more extensive, and not corresponding to endocardial scar in GM. [23,33] In our series of CA for VT in CS, 60% required epicardial access.[33] Thus, it is better to obtain epicardial access upfront or be prepared for one during the CA procedure. It is not uncommon to induce nonclinical and multiple morphologies of VTs in the electrophysiology (EP) laboratory (**Fig. 4**). [26,33] Induction of nonclinical multiple morphology VTs is more common in stage A and stage C disease with ongoing inflammation. Number of clinical VTs and VT induced in the EP laboratory decreases once underlying inflammation is treated.

In the patients undergoing CA, it is very important to define the underlying substrate; this complements information obtained from preprocedural imaging. During substrate mapping, it is better to *create a unipolar map along with bipolar voltage maps*, preferably with a multipolar catheter. High-definition mapping with closely spaced electrodes is likely to help to define the substrate (endo, epicardial, and/or intramural circuits) more accurately. Tagging the *Purkinje potentials during substrate mapping* would be of added advantage, as some of the VTs may be Purkinje system-related circuits.[24,34] It is better to avoid neuromuscular blockade with paralytic agents during GA as phrenic nerve location needs to be delineated while mapping the epicardium.

The reasons for failure to abolish VTs are deep intramural/intraseptal circuits, extensive scarring with multiple re-entry circuits giving rise to multiple morphology VTs, epicardial site of origin adjacent to phrenic nerve or a major epicardial coronary artery, or due to VT from parahisian region precluding safe ablation.[23] All these factors increase the technical challenges of VT ablation, necessitating simultaneous unipolar or bipolar

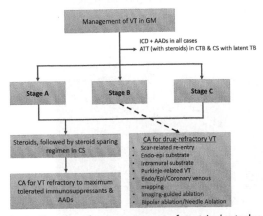

**Fig. 3.** Flowchart for management of ventricular tachycardia in granulomatous myocarditis. AAD, antirhythmic drugs; ATT, antitubercular therapy; CTB, cardiac tuberculosis; CS, cardiac sarcoidosis; GM, granulomatous myocarditis; ICD, implantable cardioverter defibrillator; TB, tuberculosis; VT, ventricular tachycardia; Stage A: inflammatory phase; Stage B: scar phase; Stage C: reactivation of inflammation in cardiac sarcoidosis; CA, catheter ablation. See text for details.

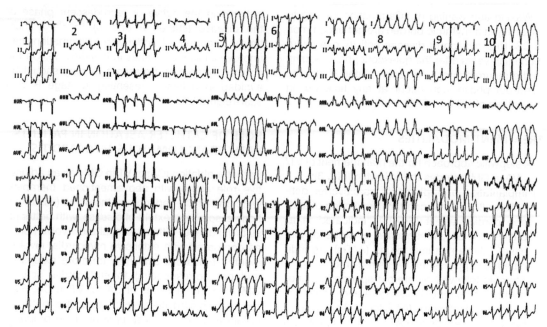

**Fig. 4.** Showing 10 different morphologies of ventricular tachycardia induced in the electrophysiology laboratory in a case of cardiac sarcoidosis.

ablation for intramural circuits, (**Fig. 5**) phrenic nerve protection (balloon inflation in the pericardium) for VT circuits near the phrenic nerve, (**Fig. 6**) coronary venous mapping, and surgical ablation for multiple epicardial VT circuits. CA of VT for these cases are better performed in tertiary care centers experienced in complex high-risk VT ablation.

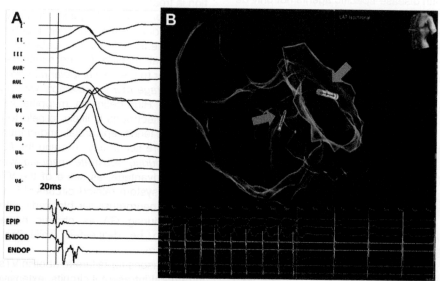

**Fig. 5.** Catheter ablation of VT in cardiac sarcoidosis. (*A*) 12-lead surface ECG and intracardiac electrogram during VT mapping showing high frequency early signal (−20 ms) during epicardial mapping (RFA was unsuccessful at this site), endocardial signal at the diagonally opposite site showing low frequency early signal. (*B*) Three-dimensional NAVX/Ensite electroanatomic map in LAO showing successful ablation with endocardial (blue *arrow*) to epicardial bipolar lesion (yellow *arrow*), suggestive of deep intramural VT circuit. Lower panel shows termination of VT during RFA. CS, coronary sinus signal; EPID, epicardial distal; EPIP: epicardial proximal; ENDOD: endocardial distal; ENDOP, endocardial proximal; LAO, left anterior oblique; RFA, radiofrequency ablation; RAO, right anterior oblique; VT, ventricular tachycardia.

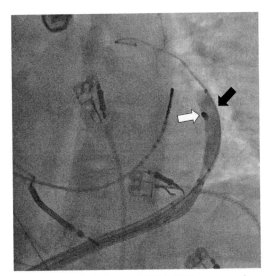

**Fig. 6.** Fluoroscopic image in LAO 25° in a case of cardiac sarcoidosis with epicardial VT showing: a use of noncompliant 10 mm × 40 mm peripheral balloon (*black arrow*) to separate phrenic nerve (on parietal pericardium) from the site of epicardial ablation (*white arrow* showing ablation catheter). VT, ventricular tachycardia.

## IMPACT OF INFLAMMATION ON CATHETER ABLATION

GM is characterized by myocardial inflammation and interstitial fibrosis which can lead to conduction slowing and macro-reentrant arrhythmias.[14,16,22,23,35–38] Thus, re-entrant substrate is present in both the active and scar phase. Induction of re-entrant VTs has also been shown during the active phase of disease,[5] which may be due to dispersion of ventricular activation and recovery processes. VT can be initiated with programmed ventricular extra stimulation further proving the re-entrant mechanism. As expected, induction of multiple morphologies in the EP lab is associated with a decreased success rate.[33] It is imperative to understand if there is evidence of myocardial inflammation before attempting VT ablation. Reviewing CMRI and 18-FDG PET-CT data is useful as they provide complementary information.

Outcome of CA for VT is better when performed during the scar phase (stage B) of the disease. Recurrence of VT after CA is more often observed among patients with ongoing inflammation. Late recurrence of VT (>6 months) is common with proven reactivation of inflammation on PET CT scan in patients with CS (stage C).[33] CA for VA is better considered for patients with drug-refractory VT or electrical storm not responding to AADs, preferably after the inflammation is adequately treated.[26,33] Patients with acute inflammation are better managed with disease-specific treatment along with intensification of AADs until the acute phase subsides.

## RESPONSE TO THERAPY

Response to therapy can be monitored by the clinical response: measured by decrease in number of VT episodes and improvement in heart failure symptoms. The resolution of myocardial inflammation on the follow-up PET-CT scan and improvement in the left ventricular ejection fraction are good indicators for treatment response. Close clinical follow up is important as remissions and relapses are common in CS. In CS patients with inadequate clinical response, serial FDG-PET scans help to identify steroid resistance.[39] Specialized rheumatologist/immunologist consultation will help in managing these patients better in the long term.

## DISCLOSURE

Dr C. Narasimhan and Dr D.K. Saggu receive fellowship programmatic support Medtronic. Dr D.K. Saggu receives honoraria from Boston Scientific. Dr S.D. Yalagudri receives honoraria or consultancy fees from Boston Scientific, Medtronic and Johnson & Johnson. Dr A.R. Atreya receives honoraria or consultancy fees from Abbott, Connected Care and Abiomed. All other authors have no conflicts of interest to disclose relevant to the content of this article.

## REFERENCES

1. Duke C, Rosenthal E. Sudden death caused by cardiac sarcoidosis in childhood. J Cardiovasc electrophysiol 2002;13(9):939–42.
2. Thachil A, Christopher J, Sastry BK, et al. Monomorphic ventricular tachycardia and mediastinaladenopathy due to granulomatous infiltration in patients with preserved ventricular function. J Am Coll Cardiol 2011;58(1):48–55.
3. Matsui Y, Iwai K, Tachibana T, et al. Clinicopathological study of fatal myocardial sarcoidosis. Ann N Y Acad Sci 1976;278:455–69.
4. Winters SL, Cohen M, Greenberg S, et al. Sustained ventricular tachycardia associated with sarcoidosis: assessment of the underlying cardiac anatomy and the prospective utility of programmed ventricular stimulation, drug therapy and an implantable antitachycardia device. J Am Coll cCardiol 1991;18:937–43.
5. Furushima H, Chinushi M, Sugiura H, et al. Ventricular tachyarrhythmia associated with cardiac sarcoidosis: its mechanisms and outcome. ClinCardiol 2004;27:217–22.
6. Sharma SK, Mohan A.. Tuberculosis: from an incurable scourge to a curable disease—journey over a millennium. Indian J Med Res 2013;137:455–93.

7. Roberts WC, McAllister HA, Ferrans VJ. Sarcoidosis of the heart. A clinicopathologic study of 35 necropsy patients (group 1) and review of 78 previously described necropsy patients (group 11). Am J Med 1977;63:86–108.

8. Veinot JP, Johnston B. Cardiac sarcoidosis–an occult cause of sudden death: a case report and literature review. J Forensic Sci 1998;43(3):715–7.

9. Wallis PJ, Branfoot AC, Emerson PA. Sudden death due to myocardial tuberculosis. Thorax 1984;39(2): 155–6.

10. Rose AG. Cardiac tuberculosis. A study of 19 patients. Arch Pathol Lab Med 1987;111:422–6.

11. Schnitzer R. Myocardial tuberculosis with paroxysmal ventricular tachycardia. Br Heart J 1947; 9(3):213–9.

12. Agarwal R, Malhotra P, Awasthi A, et al. Tuberculous dilated cardiomyopathy: an under-recognized entity? BMC Infect Dis 2005;5:29.

13. Gulati GS, Kothari SS. Diffuse infiltrative cardiac tuberculosis. Ann Pediatr 2011;4:87–9.

14. Koplan BA, Soejima K, Baughman K, et al. Refractory ventricular tachycardia secondary to cardiac sarcoid: electrophysiologic characteristics, mapping, and ablation. Heart Rhythm 2006;3:924–9.

15. Banba K, Kusano KF, Nakamura K, et al. Relationship between arrhythmogenesis and disease activity in cardiac sarcoidosis. Heart Rhythm 2007;4(10): 1292–9.

16. Soejima K, Yada H. The work-up and management of patients with apparent or subclinical cardiac sarcoidosis: with emphasis on the associated heart rhythm abnormalities. J Cardiovasc electrophysiol 2009;20(5):578–83.

17. Terasaki F, Ishizaka N. Deterioration of cardiac function during the progression of cardiac sarcoidosis: diagnosis and treatment. Intern Med 2014;53(15): 1595–605.

18. Padala SK, Peaslee S, Sidhu MS, et al. Impact of early initiation of corticosteroid therapy on cardiac function and rhythm in patients with cardiac sarcoidosis. Int J Cardiol 2017;227:565–70.

19. Bargout R, Kelly RF. Sarcoid heart disease: clinical course and treatment. Int J Cardiol 2004;97:173–82.

20. Uusimaa P, Ylitalo K, Anttonen O, et al. Ventricular tachyarrhythmia as a primary presentation of sarcoidosis. Europace 2008;10(6):760–6.

21. Kirchhof P, Eckardt L, Haverkamp, et al. IntracardiacTuberculoma causing "idiopathic" ventricular tachycardia in a patient without Detectable heart disease. J Cardiovasc Electrophysiol 2001;12:118.

22. Latcu DG, Duparc A, Chabbert V, et al. Systemic sarcoidosis revealed by ventricular tachycardia: electrocardiography and MRI correspondence. Pacing Clin Electrophysiol 2007;30(12):1566–70.

23. Kumar S, Barbhaiya C, Nagashima K, et al. Ventricular tachycardia in cardiac sarcoidosis: characterization of ventricular substrate and outcomes of catheter ablation. Circ Arrhythm Electrophysiol 2015;8(1):87–93.

24. Naruse Y, Sekiguchi Y, Nogami A, et al. Systematic treatment approach to ventricular tachycardia in cardiac sarcoidosis. Circ Arrhythm Electrophysiol 2014; 7(3):407–13.

25. Panda S, Kaur D, Lalukota K, et al. Pleomorphism during ventricular tachycardia: a Distinguishing Feature between cardiac sarcoidosis and idiopathic VT. Pacing Clin Electrophysiol 2015;38(6):694–9.

26. Yalagudri S, Zin Thu N, Devidutta S, et al. Tailored approach for management of ventricular tachycardia in cardiac sarcoidosis. J Cardiovasc Electrophysiol 2017. https://doi.org/10.1111/jce.13228.

27. Blankstein R, Osborne M, Naya M, et al. Cardiac positron emission tomography enhances prognostic assessments of patients with suspected cardiac sarcoidosis. J Am Coll Cardiol 2014;63:329–36.

28. Birnie DH, Sauer WH, Bogun F, et al. HRS expert consensus statement on the diagnosis and management of arrhythmias associated with cardiac sarcoidosis. Heart Rhythm 2014;11:1305–23.

29. Yodogawa K, Seino Y, Ohara T, et al. Effect of corticosteroid therapy on ventricular arrhythmias in patients with cardiac sarcoidosis. Ann Noninvasive Electrocardiol 2011;16(2):140–7.

30. Tung R, Bauer B, Schelbert H, et al. Incidence of abnormal positron emission tomography in patients with unexplained cardiomyopathy and ventricular arrhythmias: the potential role of occult inflammation in arrhythmogenesis. Heart Rhythm 2015;12(12): 2488–98.

31. Walsh MJ. Systemic sarcoidosis with refractory ventricular tachycardia and heart failure. Br Heart J 1978;40:931–3.

32. Jefic D, Joel B, Good E, et al. Role of radiofrequency catheter ablation of ventricular tachycardia in cardiac sarcoidosis: report from a multicenter registry. Heart Rhythm 2009;6(2):189–95.

33. Kaur D, Roukoz H, Shah M, et al. Impact of the inflammation on the outcomes of catheter ablation of drug-refractory ventricular tachycardia in cardiac sarcoidosis [published online ahead of print, 2020 Jan 9]. J Cardiovasc Electrophysiol 2020. https://doi.org/10.1111/jce.14341.

34. Shirai Yasuhiro, Goya Masahiko, Tao Susumu, et al. Delayed Purkinje potential during sinus rhythm in cardiac sarcoidosis with multiple focal Purkinje ventricular tachycardias: ablation target or bystander? Heart Rhythm Case Rep 2022. https://doi.org/10.1016/j.hrcr.2022.05.005.

35. Noda T, Suyama K, Shimizu W, et al. Ventricular tachycardia with figure eight pattern originating from the right ventricle in a patient with cardiac sarcoidosis. Pacing Clin Electrophysiol 2004;27: 561–2.

36. Santucci PA, Morton JB, PickenMM, et al. Electranatomic mapping of the right ventricle in a patient with a giant epsilon wave, ventricular tachycardia and cardiac sarcoidosis. J Cardivasc electrophysiol 2004;15:1091–4.

37. Dechering DG, Kochhauser S, Wasmer K, et al. Electrophysiological characteristics of ventricular tachyarrhythmias in cardiac sarcoidosis versus arrhythmogenicrightventricular cardiomyopathy. Heart Rhythm 2013;10:158–64.

38. Sekiguchi M, Hiroe M, Take M, et al. Clinical and histopathological profile of sarcoidosis of the heart and acute idiopathic myocarditis. Concepts through a study employing endomyocardial biopsy.II. Myocarditis. Jpncirc J 1980;44: 264–73.

39. Shelke AB, Aurangabadkar HU, Bradfield JS, et al. Serial FDG-PET scans help to identify steroid resistance in cardiac sarcoidosis. Int J Cardiol 2017; 228:717–22.

# Ventricular Tachycardia Ablation in Adult Congenital Heart Disease

Justin Wallet, MD[a,b,c], Yoshitaka Kimura, MD, PhD[a,b,c],
Katja Zeppenfeld, MD, PhD[a,b,c],*

## KEYWORDS

- Congenital heart disease • Tetralogy of Fallot • Ventricular tachycardia
- Electroanatomical mapping • Catheter ablation • Surgical ablation

## KEY POINTS

- The prevalence of adults with congenital heart disease (CHD) and the clinical relevance of late ventricular tachycardia (VT) is increasing.
- Slow conducting anatomical isthmuses (SCAI) are the dominant substrate for monomorphic VT in repaired tetralogy of Fallot and have been described in other CHD.
- SCAI is a well-defined target and can be identified and transected during stable rhythm, offering curative and possibly preventive treatment in carefully selected patients.
- To improve outcome, it is paramount to confirm block across linear ablation line with differential pacing as an additional endpoint of ablation in patients with SCAI-dependent monomorphic VT.
- Surgical or percutaneous pulmonary valve replacement may cover parts of SCAI, making it inaccessible to catheter ablation and supporting ablation before or concomitant with revalving.

## INTRODUCTION

The relevance of congenital heart disease (CHD) is growing. Approximately 0.8% of all infants born alive are affected.[1] Over the last decades, improvement in medical care has led to a significant increase in life expectancy of patients with CHD.[2] Advances in surgical repair performed at a young age have reduced mortality during childhood in particular in patients with moderate and severe forms, including tetralogy of Fallot (TOF), its morphological spectrum, and the transposition of the great arteries (d-TGA) complex.[2] Survivors can live productive lives often without restrictions.[3] However, with increasing age, new problems arise. Late ventricular arrhythmias (VA) are an important sequela. The prevalence of VA in unselected patients with CHD is approximately 5%, but higher in those who require ventricular incisions and patch closure during intracardiac repair.[4] In particular, in adults with repaired TOF (rTOF), the ventricular tachycardia (VT) burden is considerable, and with 14.2% prevalence, it is the dominant arrhythmia subtype.[4,5] Of note, VA in CHD is not necessarily related to cardiac function.[4–6] Patients may present with palpitations or syncope, but resuscitated cardiac arrest or sudden cardiac death may be the first arrhythmic manifestation.[7] Implantable cardioverter-defibrillator (ICD) can effectively terminate VA. However, they do not prevent VA, are not without complications, and additional treatment is often required.[8] The feasibility of catheter and surgical ablation of VT has already been reported in the early 1980s. However, an improved understanding of the underlying substrate has profoundly changed the approach to patients with CHD and VT.[6,9,10]

In this review, we provide an overview of VT substrates in patients with CHD, in the context of the

[a] Department of Cardiology, Heart Lung Center, Leiden University Medical Center, Postbus 9600, Leiden 2300 RC, the Netherlands; [b] Center for Congenital Heart Disease Amsterdam-Leiden (CAHAL), the Netherlands; [c] Willem Einthoven Center of Arrhythmia Research and Management
* Corresponding author.
*E-mail address:* k.zeppenfeld@lumc.nl

Card Electrophysiol Clin 14 (2022) 709–727
https://doi.org/10.1016/j.ccep.2022.06.008
1877-9182/22/© 2022 Elsevier Inc. All rights reserved.

surgical era. Catheter and surgical ablation strategies, endpoints of ablation, reasons for ablation failure, and potential solutions are summarized. Evolving indications for mapping and ablation are also discussed.

## PREPROCEDURAL EVALUATION

Preprocedural assessment of hemodynamics and identification of residual or new lesions, which may require surgical or percutaneous intervention, is important, for example, pulmonary valve regurgitation or significant residual ventricular septal defect (VSD) (**Fig. 1**). If surgical repair is indicated, intraoperative ablation, in close collaboration between an electrophysiologist and congenital cardiac surgeon may be favored over catheter ablation. Imaging, including late gadolinium enhancement cardiac magnetic resonance (LGE-CMR), can raise suspicion for cardiac pathology not related to the CHD or unexpected scar location and related VT substrates, such as right ventricular (RV) basal aneurysm.[11]

## EVOLVING MAPPING AND ABLATION TECHNIQUES

Early ablation procedures were based on activation and entrainment mapping (**Table 1**), guided by fluoroscopy. Studies reported an excellent reproducibility of VT-induction during programmed electrical stimulation (PES) [median 100%, interquartile range (IQR) 86–100%]. However, hemodynamic tolerance during VT was essential for mapping. Hemodynamic instability during the typically fast VTs was reported in up to 50%–60% of patients, leading to ablation failure in early reports.[12–15] In 2007, Kriebel and colleagues[16] used noncontact mapping to facilitate swift mapping in patients with compromised hemodynamics during VT as one potential solution. An alternative approach relies on three-dimensional (3D) electroanatomical mapping (EAM) during stable sinus rhythm (SR), allowing for the identification of VT substrates, without the need for mapping during VT (**Box 1**).[6,9,10]

## PATIENT POPULATION

The vast majority of catheter ablation data in CHD are derived from patients with rTOF (246/338, 73%), with limited data from repaired d-TGA (n = 11, 3%), VSD closure (n = 18, 5%), or Ebstein's anomaly (EA) (n = 31, 9%) (see **Table 1**), and only one surgical ablation study reports on other etiologies than the rTOF morphological spectrum (**Table 2**).

The relevance of rTOF patients for the clinical electrophysiologist is also reflected by ICD studies; rTOF was the dominant subgroup among all CHD patients implanted with ICDs for primary or secondary prevention, followed by patients with d-TGA.[8]

Based on pooled data from published series, the reported acute procedural success, usually defined as VT noninducibility after ablation, was 228/298 (77%). After procedural success, VT recurred in 32/180 (18%) during follow-up, ranging between 13 months and 6.7 years. These data support the feasibility of catheter ablation with promising outcomes if performed in experienced centers. As rTOF is the most frequent CHD subtype among patients considered for ablation, we specifically focus on rTOF.

## TETRALOGY OF FALLOT

TOF is the most common cyanotic heart defect with an incidence of 0.42 per 1000 live births.[1] The morphological key feature is the antero-cephalad deviation of the outlet (or conal) septum, a muscular structure, separating the subaortic from the subpulmonary outlet. The deviation causes a malalignment with the remainder of the ventricular septum resulting in a subaortic, and in most cases perimembranous *VSD*. Rarely there is a muscular rim between the VSD and the tricuspid annulus, which is important to recognize. The degree of *aortic override* can vary (>50% overriding is considered double-outlet right ventricle). Another important feature is the *obstruction of the right ventricular outflow tract* (RVOT), often because of subpulmonary stenosis, determined by septum deviation and hypertrophy of the septoparietal trabeculations. The subpulmonary obstruction often coexists with pulmonary valve stenosis, or in extreme cases pulmonary atresia. *RV hypertrophy* is regarded as a hemodynamic consequence of the earlier discussed features.[17]

Surgical approaches to TOF have changed over time. The details are important for an interventional electrophysiologist (**Fig. 2**). Although the intracardiac repair was already successfully performed in 1954 by Lillehei, the high perioperative mortality in subsequent series led to a "two-stage repair.[3] A palliative shunt operation to augment pulmonary blood flow was followed by intracardiac repair in childhood. For resection of the subpulmonary stenosis and VSD closure, large transverse or longitudinal RV incisions were made (see **Fig. 2**A). To enlarge a coexisting narrow pulmonary annulus, the longitudinal incisions were often extended through the annulus followed by the insertion of large transannular patches. Because of the

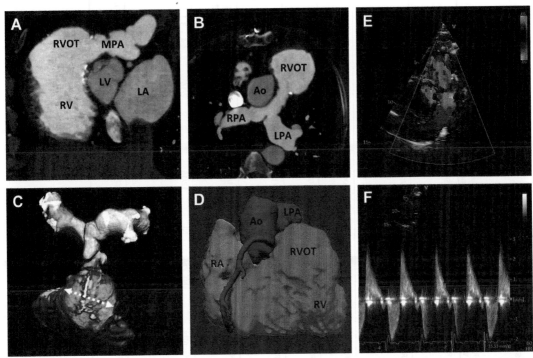

**Fig. 1.** Preprocedural evaluation. (*A–D*) Example of a cardiac CT of an rTOF patient with severe RVOT dilatation/aneurysm (5 × 4 cm) in combination with MPA stenosis. The two images below (*C, D*) are 3D reconstructions. This malformation could necessitate surgical or percutaneous relief of pulmonary obstruction and/or RVOT plication. (*E, F*) Example of a cardiac echocardiogram of an rTOF patient with severe pulmonary regurgitation. Electrophysiological evaluation may be important before PVR. Ao, aorta; LA, left atrium; LV, left ventricle; RPA/LPA/MPA, right, left, and main pulmonary artery; RV(OT), right ventricle (outflow tract). (*Courtesy of* Dr. P. Kies, LUMC, Leiden, the Netherlands.)

adverse hemodynamic consequences of the pulmonary regurgitation and large RV incision, a combined transatrial-transpulmonary approach has been introduced (see **Fig. 2**B). This operation is nowadays performed early in life. Patch augmentation of the RVOT is avoided or limited to the pulmonary annulus.[18]

## VENTRICULAR TACHYCARDIA SUBSTRATE AND MAPPING STRATEGIES IN REPAIRED TETRALOGY OF FALLOT

ICD interrogation demonstrated that 81.5% of all appropriate shocks in primary and secondary prevention were delivered for monomorphic VT, which were fast with a median rate of 213 bpm.[12] Early mapping studies have already identified macroreentry as the important underlying mechanism for monomorphic VT, typically related to the RVOT.[19] Zeppenfeld and colleagues[9] could demonstrate in 2007 that anatomical isthmuses (AI) bordered by unexcitable boundaries were harboring the critical part of these macroreentrant circuits. The boundaries comprised prior surgical incisions, patches, and valve tissue. Activation,

entrainment mapping, and VT termination of briefly induced VTs by radiofrequency catheter ablation (RFCA) confirmed the link between AI and VT. In rTOF, four distinct AIs have been identified by EAM, namely between (1) RV incision/RVOT patch and a tricuspid annulus; (2) non-transannular RV incision/RVOT patch and the pulmonary annulus; (3) pulmonary annulus and VSD patch; and (4) VSD patch and tricuspid annulus (see **Fig. 2**).[6,9,10,20,21] In postmortem studies the prevalence of AI 1, 2, 3, and 4 were 88–99%, 25–42%, 94–99%, and 6–13%, respectively.[20,21] In particular, AI4 is rare because in the majority this area is part of the fibrous mitral-tricuspid continuity.

Of importance, not all AIs are arrhythmogenic and (potentially) related to VT. In 2017, Kapel and colleagues[6] systematically measured the width, length, and conduction velocities (CV) of AIs as determined by EAM during SR in 74 rTOF patients who underwent mapping either for VT treatment, risk stratification, or before revalving (see **Box 1**, **Fig. 3**D). In contrast to AI in patients without VT, the AIs in patients with clinical and/or inducible VT (n = 28) were narrower (20 ± 8 vs.

**Table 1**
Overview of studies on catheter ablation of ventricular tachycardia in congenital heart disease

| Author, Year | Inclusion Period (Y) | Congenital Heart Defect (n) | Patients (n) | Age at Intracardiac Repair (Median, Y) | Age at Ablation (Median/Mean, Y) | Clinical VA | Inducible sVT (n of pts) | Median VTCL (Induced VT) | Presumed VT Mechanism | Mapping and Ablation Methods | Endpoint | Complete Success | CB | Recurrence of VA after Abl Success | Follow-up Period |
|---|---|---|---|---|---|---|---|---|---|---|---|---|---|---|---|
| Gonska et al,[36] 1996 | a | rTOF 9, VSD 4, PS 2, d-TGA + VSD 1 | 16 | 5(IQR 3–16) | 41 (IQR 20–43) | SVT 8, nsVTS 8 | 11/16 | 325 (IQR 304–369)[b] | Reentry 12, undetermined 4 | ENT, AM, PM | NI of sVT or nsVT | 15/16 | a | 1/15 | 13M (IQR 8–24) |
| Hebe et al,[37] 2000 | < 1999 | rTOF 8, VSD 3, RVOTO 1, PA 1, dTGA + DORV + VSD 1 | 14 | a | 24 ± 11[c] | a | 14/14 | a | Reentry | ENT, AM, LL | Unclear | 8/14 | Unclear | 2/14[i] | Unclear |
| Morwood et al,[13] 2004 | 1990–2003 | rTOF 8, VSD 3, EA 1, SV 1, AoS 1 | 14 | a | 22 ± 14 | a | a | a | Reentry | ENT, AM, PM | NI | 10/20 | CB in newer cases | 4/10 | 3.8 ± 2.0Y |
| Furushima et al,[38] 2006 | a | rTOF 4, DORV 3 | 7 | 3(IQR 3–9) | 24 (IQR 18–29) | SVT | 7/7 | 360 (IQR 310–393) | Reentry | ENT, AM, PM, LL | NI | 4/7 | a | 0/4 | 55M (IQR 51–75) |
| Kriebel et al,[16] 2007 | a | rTOF | 10 | a | 34 (IQR 17–39) | SVT 6, nsVT 4 | 10/10 | 265 (IQR235–302) | Reentry 11, focal 2[d] | AM (NC), LL | NI | 8/10 | CB | 2/8 | Mean 35M (range 3–52) |
| Zeppenfeld et al,[9] 2007 | 1998–2007 | rTOF 9, d-TGA + VSD 1, AVSD 1 | 11 | 10 (IQR 9–13) | 46 (IQR 36–50) | sVT 10, nsVT 1 | 11/11 | 255 (IQR236–300) | Reentry | ENT, AM, PM, SSM, LL | NI | 11/11 | CB (not routinely) | 1/11 | 30.4 ± 29.3 M (range 4–103) |
| Tokuda et al,[39] 2012 | 1999–2010 | rTOF 8, VSD 3, d-TGA 1, DORV 1, PS 1, other 2 | 16 | a | 45 ± 15 | a | a | a,e | Reentry | ENT, PM, SSM, LL | NI | 12/16 | a | 2/16[i] | 4.4 ± 3.3 Y[f] |
| Schneider et al,[25] 2012 | a | rTOF 5, rTOF + PA 2 | 7 | a | 33 median (range 14–49) | SVT | 7/7 | 300 (IQR 240–310) | Reentry | AM (NC), SSM, LL | NI | 5/7 | CB | 1/5 | Mean 56.3 M |

| Study | Years | Diagnosis | N | | | VT type | | Cycle length | Mechanism | Mapping | | | CB | | Follow-up |
|---|---|---|---|---|---|---|---|---|---|---|---|---|---|---|---|
| Kapel et al,[10] 2015 | 2001–2012 | rTOF 28, d-TGA + PS 1, d-TGA + VSD 1, VSD + PS 1, VSD + bAV 1, PS 1, AVSD1 | 34 | 10 (IQR 5–19) | 48 (IQR 38–59) | SVT 27, sVT suspected 7 | 34/34 | 295 (IQR 242–346) | Reentry | ENT, AM, PM, SSM, LL | NI + CB | 25/34 | CB is endpoint | 1/25 | 46 ± 28M |
| Van Zyl et al,[23] 2016 | 2004–2015 | rTOF 10, d-TGA 4, VSD 2, PA 1, EA 2, AoS 1, TA 1 | 21 | 6 (IQR 5–13) | 45 ± 3 | SVT 10, nsVT 11 | 18/21 | 300 (IQR 265–390) | Reentry 14, focal 7 | ENT, AM, SSM, LL | NI | 17/21 | CB when possible | 3/17[g] | 33±7M |
| Kapel et al,[6] 2017 | 2005–2013 | rTOF | 74 | 6 (IQR 2 –12) | 40 ± 16 | SVT 13, vt risk factors 61 | 28/74[h] | 252 (IQR 231–312) | Reentry, focal 1 | ENT, AM, PM, SSM, LL | NI + CB | 19/28[i] | CB is endpoint | 0/19 | 50 ± 22M |
| Laredo et al,[14] 2017 | 1990–2012 | rTOF | 34 | 5.4 (range 3M-23Y) | 31 ± 10 | SVT 33, nsVT 1 | 33/34 | 294 (mean) | Reentry 13, incomplete data 21 | ENT, AM, PM, SSM, some DCA | NI | 28/34 | [a] | 13/34[i] | 9.5 ± 5.2Y |
| Moore et al,[35] 2018 | 1995–2017 | EA | 24 | [a,j] | 17 (IQR 11–37) | sVT + PVC | [a] | 305 (IQR 268–400) | Reentry 10 focal 15 | ENT, AM, PM, SSM | NI | 23/24 | [a] | 1/23 | Median 3.4 Y |
| Yang et al,[15] 2019 | 2000–2017 | rTOF 29, DORV 2, d-TGA 1, VSD 1, EA4, AoS 2, PS 1, bAV 4, TA 1, LV aneurysm 1, Shone' complex 1, aortic root dilatation 1 | 48 | 5 (range 2M-65Y) | 41 ± 13 | sVT | 42/48 | 299 (IQR 259–330) | Reentry 62, focal 11, His-Purkinje system reentry 4[d] | ENT, AM, PM, SSM, LL | NI | 36/48 | CB when possible | 17/36 | 53M (IQR 15–85) |

(continued on next page)

**Table 1**
*(continued)*

| Author, Year | Inclusion Period (Y) | Congenital Heart Defect (n) | Patients (n) | Age at Intracardiac Repair (Median, Y) Mean, Y) | Age at Ablation (Median/Mean, Y) | Clinical VA | Inducible sVT (n of pts) | Median VTCL (Induced VT) | Presumed VT Mechanism | Mapping and Ablation Methods | Endpoint | Complete Success | CB | Recurrence of VA after Abl Success | Follow-up Period |
|---|---|---|---|---|---|---|---|---|---|---|---|---|---|---|---|
| Kawada[47] et al, 2021 | 2000–2018 | rTOF | 8 | 9 (IQR 5–11) | 43 (IQR 28–56)[k] | sVT 6, VF 2 | 6/8 | 270 [IQR 210–285] | Reentry | ENT, AM, PM, SSM, LL | NI | 7/8 | CB when possible | 1/7 | 81M (IQR 29–131) |

Studies were included if *n* > 5 Data are displayed as number (*n*), median with IQR/range or mean ± standard deviation/range.

*Abbreviations:* abl, ablation; AM, activation mapping; AoS, aortic stenosis; AVSD, atrioventricular septal defect; bAV, bicuspid aortic valve; DCA, direct-current ablation; DORV, double outlet right ventricle; ENT, entrainment mapping; LL, Linear ablation lesions; LV, left ventricle; M, months; NC, noncontact; NI, noninducibility of VT; NICMP, nonischemic cardiomyopathy; nsVT, nonsustained VT; PA, pulmonary atresia; PM, pace mapping; PS, pulmonary stenosis; pts, patients; PVC, premature ventricular contraction; SSM, substrate mapping; SV, single ventricle; sVT, sustained VT; TA, truncus arteriosus; VF, ventricular fibrillation; VT, cycle length; Y, years.

<sup>a</sup> Indicates unknown.

a Indicates unknown.
b VTCL clinical VT.
c Includes 1 with NICMP
d Of all induced VTs.
e 14 pts fastest VTCL <400 ms.
f Total NICMP group.
g No recurrence in pts with CB.
h All pts with clinical sVT were inducible.
i Unknown n were surgically ablated.
j 12/24 with TV surgery.
k Age at ICD implantation.
l Recurrence of VA in all (also unsuccessfully) ablated patients.

*Data from* Refs.[36–39]

**Box 1**
**Workflow for catheter mapping and ablation of VT in patients with rTOF and SCAI**

Electrophysiological evaluation includes PES for VT induction and EAM. The first step in our laboratory is VT induction to obtain the 12-lead VT QRS morphology (template for pace-mapping). Our standard PES protocol includes up to four drive-cycle lengths (600 millisecond, 500 millisecond, 400 millisecond, and 350 millisecond) from the RV apex and at least one RVOT site close to the AI with up to four extrastimuli and isoproterenol infusion, if VT is not inducible at baseline.

Accurate delineation of areas with low voltages, identification of unexcitable tissue (UET) by high-output pacing (eg, scars, valves, patch material), and determination of regions with slow conduction provide a real-time and detailed 3D electroanatomical reconstruction of the potential VT substrate.

Bipolar voltage (BV) < 1.5 mV is usually defined as low voltage, although BV< 1.76 mV has also been suggested as a cut-off.[24] High-output pacing without capture (10 mA/2 millisecond) in these low voltage areas identifies UET (ie, prosthetic materials or valve). In 3D maps, normal voltage areas, UET, and the valve annuli are displayed, together with important structures such as the bundle of His (see **Fig. 3B**). AI are areas that are bordered by UET. AI can be electroanatomically normal, defined as normal BV continuously recorded throughout the AI connecting to areas with normal voltages and a CV through the AI during SR and/or RV pacing within the normal range.

To assess the CV through an AI, the AI length is evaluated by measuring the distance between the first normal bipolar electrogram at each side of the AI, and the conduction time through the AI is determined by measuring the difference in local activation times (LAT) between those points. The CV is calculated by dividing the AI length by the conduction time (see **Fig. 3D**). An SCAI is defined by a CV of less than 0.5 m/s. Of note, in patients with narrow QRS, activation wavefronts during SR may collide at AI3. In these cases, pacing in the vicinity of the AI and measuring LAT on the other side of the AI is required (see **Fig. 3E**). Pacing at VT cycle length within or at the border of an AI may result in a pace-match of the VT supporting the fact that the AI under evaluation is related to the VT.

After identification of an SCAI, a linear RF ablation line is applied, connecting the unexcitable boundaries at the narrowest and easiest accessible part (see **Fig. 3F**). Contact-force catheters and deflectable sheaths are preferable. After each application, pacing with 10 mA at 2 ms pulse width from the distal electrodes of the mapping catheter is performed to confirm appropriate lesion formation. Conduction block along the ablation line can be assumed by the presence of double potentials along the line and the change in activation sequence during intrinsic or paced rhythm after ablation and is further supported by the results of differential pacing from both sides of the AI, similar to proving CB after cavotricuspid isthmus ablation (see **Fig. 3F**). Finally, the entire PES protocol is repeated.

28 ± 11 mm), longer (22 ± 7 vs. 16±7 mm), and had lower CV (0.36 ± 0.34 vs. 0.78 ± 0.24 m/s). An electroanatomically determined CV of <0.5 m/s could identify a slow conducting AI (SCAI) related to VT with high accuracy.

It is important to emphasize the difference between AI and SCAI; AI is present in almost all rTOF patients, whereas SCAI could only be found in 38% of patients who underwent mapping.[6] Of note, an SCAI was the confirmed VT substrate for 93% of patients with induced and/or spontaneous VTs.[6] This strong link between SCAI and VT allows for a systematic mapping and ablation approach during stable rhythm.

## THE IMPACT OF THE SURGICAL ERA ON ELECTROANATOMICAL VENTRICULAR TACHYCARDIA SUBSTRATES

The differences in surgical techniques for TOF impact AI dimensions. A study of postmortem hearts showed that with the modern transatrial-

transpulmonary approach AI2 is abandoned and AI1 contains thicker myocardium (6 ± 2 vs. 5±2 mm), which may be less prone to develop slow conduction over time.[20] Avoidance of large RV incisions and the use of smaller transannular patches increases the distance between the tricuspid annulus and the transannular patch, formally AI1, however, with large dimensions. Different surgical approaches do not alter the presence and dimensions of AI3 and AI4.[20] Consequently, in the majority of contemporary patients with rTOF, AI3, if slow conducting, is the most important remaining potential VT substrate.

## SUBSTRATE ABLATION AND ENDPOINTS

A suggested workflow for substrate mapping and ablation in rTOF is provided in **Box 1** and **Fig. 3**. Endpoints of ablation and the definition of procedural success have evolved over time. Early studies have used VT termination during and noninducibility after ablation as criteria for success.

**Table 2**
Overview of studies on surgical ablation of ventricular tachycardia in congenital heart disease

| Author, Year | Inclusion Period (Y) | Congenital Heart Defect (n) | Patients (n) | Concomitant with (n) | Age at Intracardiac Repair (Median, Y) | Age at Ablation (Median/ Mean, Y) | Clinical VA | Inducible sVT (n of pts) | Presumed VT Mechanism | Mapping Protocol | Mapping and Ablation Methods | Targeted Lesion | Empirical Ablation | Endpoint | Complete Success | Recurrence of VA | Follow-Up Period |
|---|---|---|---|---|---|---|---|---|---|---|---|---|---|---|---|---|---|
| Harrison et al,[40] 1997 | 1990–1994 | rTOF | 18 sVT, 14 periop mapping, 10 ablated | PVR 11, RVOT aneurysm resection 1, MVR 1, cryoablation alone 1 | 9±7[a] | 28±9[a] | Unclear | 14/14 preop 10/14 periop (mean VTCL 261 ms) | Reentry | Preop PES, periop AM | AM, cryo | Site of earliest (AI3, IS-parietal band, or IS-RV free wall) | No | Unclear | 10/10 | 2/10 | 4.0 ± 3.5Y |
| Therrien[41] 2001 | ... | rTOF | 9 | PVR | ... | ... | sVT 9 | ... | Reentry | Preiop AM | AM, cryo | Areas of slow conduction | No | Unclear | 9/9 | 0/9 | 4.7Y (mean) |
| Ashburn et al,[42] 2003 | 1984–2001 | rTOF 35, undefined 8 | 43, 33 ablated | ... | ... | 31 (range 18M-56Y) | sVT 43 | 33/43 periop | Reentry | Preop PES, periop AM | AM, cryo | Site of earliest activation (94% AI3) | No | Unclear | 33/33 | 5/33 | Freedom from VT 88% at 1Y, 80% at 3Y |
| Karamlou et al,[43] 2006 | 1969–2005 | rTOF | 44 with sVT, 31 ablated | Predominantly PVR | ... | ... | sVT 44 | 15/... | Reentry | Preop PES, periop AM | AM, cryo | Site of earliest activation | ... | Unclear | 31/31 | 3/31 | 5.4Y (median)[b] |
| Giamberti et al,[44] 2008 | 2002–2006 | rTOF | 6 | PVR | ... | ... | sVT 6 | ... | ... | Preop EP study | RF | Unclear | Unclear | Unclear | 6/6 | 0/6 | 34M (mean, range 6-52M)[b] |
| Mavroudis et al,[45] 2008 | 1987–2007 | rTOF 6, d-TGA + VSD + LVOTO 2, Uhl anomaly 1, absent PV 1, VSD 2 | 12 | PVR 8, RVOTO resection 1, VSD repair 2, TV annuloplasty 1 | ... | ... | sVT 12 | ... | ... | Unclear | Cryo[c] | Unclear | ... | Postop NI | 10/12 | 1/10 | Unclear |
| Sabate Rotes et al,[46] 2015 | 1988–2010 | rTOF | 22 | PVR | ... | 42 (IQR 31–47)[d] | sVT 4 | 10/12 preop | Reentry | Preop PES, on indication | No mapping, cryo | LL of AI3, AI2, AI1 | Yes[e] | ... | 22/22 | 1/22 | 6.7Y (median)[k] |
| Sandhu et al,[29] 2018 | 2006–2017 | rTOF | 70 pre-PVR PES, 31 ablated | PVR | 4Y | 33 (IQR 24–44)[d] | ... | 34/70 | Reentry | Preop PES, in all and postop PES in pts when ablated | No mapping, cryo | LL of AI3, AI2, and circumferential in RVOT | Yes | Postop NI | 17/31 | 2/53[f] | 6.1 ± 3.2Y |

| Caldaroni et al,[30] 2019 | Nevvazhay et al,[28] 2020 | Kawada[47] et al 2021 |
|---|---|---|
| 2004–2013 | 2013–2019 | 2000–2008 |
| rTOF | rTOF 6, PA + VSD 1 | rTOF |
| 37 pre-PVR PES/EAM, 20 ablated | 27 pre-PVR PES/EAM, 7 ablated | 12 |
| PVR | PVR | PVR |
| 7Y (range 0.1–26Y) | 1.1Y (IQR 1.0–5Y) | 6 (IQR 3–9) |
| 28Y after first repair (median, range 16–39) | 24Y (IQR 17–48) | 45 (IQR 33–55)[i] |
| VA 11 (sVT 6, VF 1, rest unclear) | … | sVT 9, VF 3 |
| 20/37 preop | … | Unclear |
| Reentry | Reentry | Reentry |
| Preop PES, on indication | Preop PES/EAM, periop BL | 4 preop, 4 periop, 4 empirical |
| RF | SSM, cryo | SSM, cryo |
| LL of most frequently AI1 and AI3 | LL of AI3 | LL of AI3 (in 8), AI3+AI4 (in 3), AI1-AI4 (in 1) |
| Yes | No | Yes |
| Postop NI 6M after ablation | BL[i] | … |
| 16/19[g] | 7/7 | 12/12 |
| 2/19[h] | No follow-up data | 2/12 |
| 6.5Y (median, range 6M-10Y) | No follow-up data | 81M (IQR 29–131) |

Studies were included if n > 5 Data are displayed as number (n), median with IQR/range, or mean ± standard deviation/range.

*Abbreviations:* IS, infundibular septum; EP, electrophysiological; periop, perioperative; postop, postoperative; Preop, preoperative; PV, pulmonary valve; rest as in **Table 1.**

a For total 18 sVt.

b Total group VA/atrial.

c Combined with endo or epicardial resection.

d Age at PVR.

e (near)syncope or nonsustained VTs were also indicated for ablation, without preoperative PES.

f n = 53 with negative pre or postop PEs.

g 1 pt died in hospital.

h Both with recurrence were NI during re-PES at 6M.

i BL confirmed by periop differential pacing.

j Age at ICD implantation.

k $of total group of PVR pts, n = 200.

*Data from Refs.*[40–46]

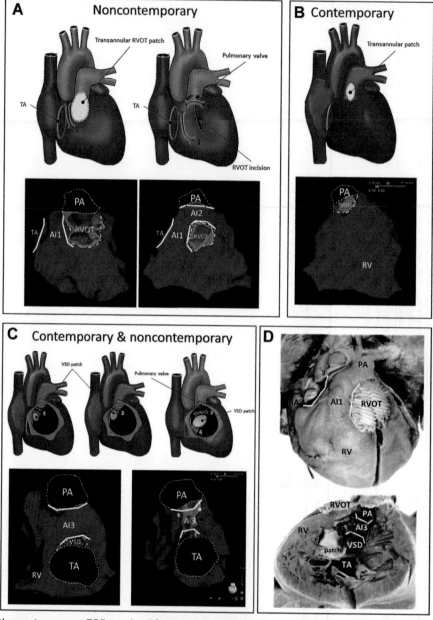

**Fig. 2.** (*A*) Noncontemporary TOF repair with RV incision, with (*left*) or without (*right*) large transannular/RVOT patch. The upper schematics show AI1 and AI2 (see text for AI boundaries). The lower two figures show corresponding bipolar EAM of the RV (anterior view, color-coded according to bar in panel *B*). (*B*) Contemporary TOF repair with transatrial-transpulmonary approach avoids (extensive) RV incision and subsequently AI2. Only a small transannular patch is inserted. Below, the corresponding EAM (anterior view). (*C*) Noncontemporary and contemporary repair both include VSD closure, as boundary of AI3. Two most left schematics show a perimembranous VSD of various sizes, corresponding to variations in AI3 width. AI4 is rare, and present in those with a muscular VSD (*right*). Lower figures show posterior view of bipolar RV EAM. Left figure shows AI3 with normal electroanatomical properties (bipolar voltage >1.5 mV), and the right lower bipolar voltages (<1.5 mV), which could indicate a VT substrate. (*D*) Anatomical rTOF specimens showing AI1 and AI3 (VSD patch removed to the side). TA, tricuspid annulus. (Schematics adapted from Zeppenfeld K, Wijnmaalen AP. Clinical Aspects and Ablation of Ventricular Arrhythmias in Tetralogy of Fallot. Card Electrophysiol Clin. Jun 2017;9(2):285-294; with permission.)

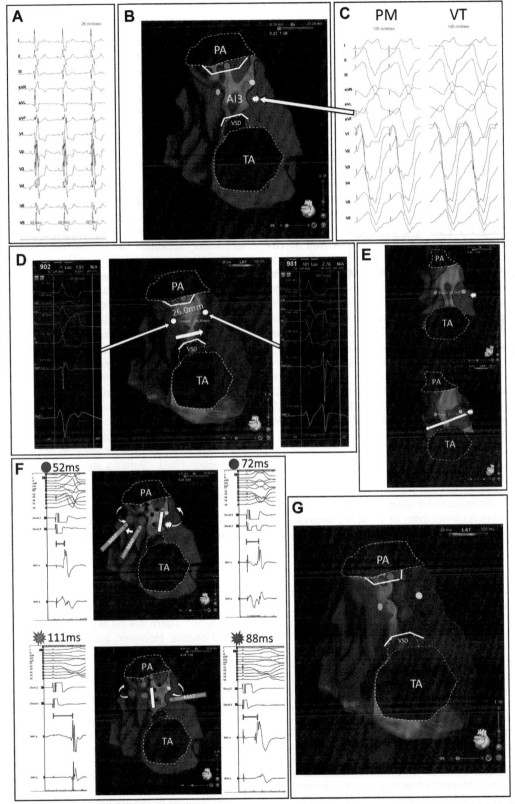

**Fig. 3.** Workflow for substrate mapping and ablation in rTOF. (*A*) SR ECG with right bundle branch block (QRS width 196 millisecond). (*B*) Posterior view of bipolar voltage map of the RV with AI3 (voltages color-coded according to bar). Gray dots indicate UET/scar. (*C*) PM at RV-free wall (symbol indicates pacing location in panel *B*) matches the induced clinical VT (PASO 0.983, VT cycle length 286 millisecond) and is consistent with a VT exit site, which corresponds to a counterclockwise wavefront propagation (if viewed from anterior) through AI3

Although the inducibility of VT in patients referred for ablation is usually high, in 1 series of 252 rTOF patients, 17% of patients with clinical VT were not inducible, supporting the limitation of noninducibility as a sole endpoint.[22] Following the identification of a VT-related SCAI, a linear radiofrequency (RF) ablation line can be applied connecting the unexcitable boundaries of the AI during SR (**Fig. 4**). Facilitated by the 3D mapping systems completeness of the line and bidirectional conduction block (CB) across the ablation line can be tested by differential pacing, thereby providing an established endpoint of ablation (see **Fig. 3**F).

Among recent studies that have introduced confirmation of CB across the ablation line as an essential part of the procedure (see **Box 1**, **Table 1**), long-term freedom of VT recurrence is excellent. After successful SCAI ablation with the endpoint CB, Zeppenfeld and colleagues identified only one VA event, which was ventricular fibrillation (VF) in an rTOF patient with end-stage heart failure.[6,9,10] Similarly, van Zyl and colleagues reported no recurrence of VT after CB verification.[23] In a study by Yang and colleagues, persistent inducibility of the clinical VT after ablation occurred frequently in patients without CB (2/3).[15] These data support the importance of CB across SCAI as the endpoint of ablation of AI-related VTs.

## ABLATION FAILURE AND POTENTIAL SOLUTIONS

Reported reasons for ablation failure in earlier series were noninducibility of VT at the beginning of the procedure, hemodynamic instability during VT, and anatomical limitations. Inducibility and hemodynamic tolerance of VT is no longer a requirement for successful ablation of AI-related VT (substrate ablation), however, anatomical limitations remain.

Withholding of RF delivery at high-risk locations to avoid anticipated complications can explain ablation failure. For example, the proximity of the bundle of His to AI4 may result in complete heart block if AI4 is targeted by RFCA.[10,16,25] The ostia of the coronary arteries, which may be located in an unusual position because of the clockwise rotated overriding aorta in rTOF, and aberrant coronary arteries need to be considered, in particular, if RFCA is intended from the aortic root.[17,23] RFCA may not be effective because of hypertrophied RV myocardium and the desired endpoint of CB may not be reached.[6,10,15] Important additional anatomical obstacles for ablation are prosthetic materials overlying AIs. In particular, valved conduits can make AI3 inaccessible to right-sided catheter ablation (**Fig. 5**).[6,10] In some cases, a left-sided approach from the left ventricular outflow tract or aortic cusps may be helpful but is not without risks.[26] To increase lesion depth and improve efficacy, bail-out strategies have been applied in patients with nonischemic cardiomyopathies, such as bipolar ablation, retractable needle ablation, and the use of half-normal saline for irrigation.[27] However, safety is of concern in the vulnerable CHD patient population. Variable wall thicknesses of the RV and the proximity of structures at risk (eg, coronary arteries, valves, and conduction system) need to be considered. Elegant solutions include strategies that target the (potential) VT substrate before it becomes inaccessible to catheter or surgical ablation (see the section titled, "Surgical ablation").[28–30]

## COMPLICATIONS

In general, RFCA in adult patients with CHD is considered safe. Complications do occur, mainly related to the vascular access sites, including inguinal hematoma, retroperitoneal hemorrhage, and pseudoaneurysm.[10,14,15] Reported severe complications are rare; however, in two patients a low cardiac output during ablation required intervention.[10,14] There are no reports on procedure-related deaths. However, available reports come

during VT. (*D*) The EAM is displayed as an activation map during SR. LAT is color-coded according to bar. The CV was 0.25 m/s, indicating SCAI, calculated by dividing distance between AI3 entrance and exit sites (*white dots*, 26.0 mm) by LAT between these points (LAT101-LAT-1 = 102 milliseconds). (*E*) In patients with narrow QRS and rapid RV conduction collision of wavefronts during SR typically occurs in AI3 (not shown) excluding CV measurement. In these cases, pacing from one site of AI3 (here RV free wall) and measuring CV through AI3 utilizing the paced wavefront can unmask an SCAI (here CV 0.44 m/s). (*F*) After ablation (*red dots*) differential pacing confirms bidirectional block across the ablation line. Upper panel: pacing is first performed at the free wall site of AI (symbol). Latest activation is recorded at the septal side of AI3 (blue dot, stimulus to electrogram 72 milliseconds), while the LAT remote from the line was shorter (*red dot*, 52 milliseconds). Lower panel: Pacing from the septal side close to AI3 (blue symbol, 111 milliseconds) leads to a longer stimulus to electrogram interval than pacing remote from AI3 (*red symbol*, 88 milliseconds). These findings are consistent with bidirectional block. (*G*) Activation map during SR after ablation. Note the change of activation with collision of wavefronts at AI3 (compare with panel *D*). MAP, mapping catheter; PM, pace map; UET, unexcitable tissue.

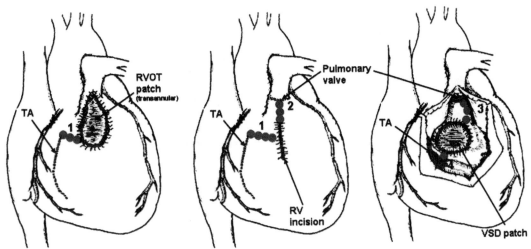

**Fig. 4.** Overview of AI in rTOF with the subsequent ablation lines (*red dots*) connecting the unexcitable boundaries of the isthmus with the aim of achieving bidirectional conduction block (CB). (*Adapted from* Zeppenfeld K, Schalij MJ, Bartelings MM, et al. Catheter ablation of ventricular tachycardia after repair of congenital heart disease: electroanatomic identification of the critical right ventricular isthmus. Circulation. Nov 13 2007;116(20):2241-52; with permission.)

from experienced centers and operators, and more complications may occur in less experienced centers.

## OTHER VENTRICULAR TACHYCARDIA SUBSTRATES IN REPAIRED TETRALOGY OF FALLOT

Apart from SCAI as the dominant substrate for monomorphic VT in rTOF, other substrates for VT have been reported. Ventricular scars in non-outflow tract regions (eg, large free wall scar), in proximity to unexcitable valve annuli, can form AIs related to VTs (**Fig. 6**).[6,10] Furthermore, focal VTs in rTOF have been described in 7 (3.0%), and the bundle of His–Purkinje system-related VT in 2 (0.8%), of a total of 236 rTOF cases (see **Table 1**). Details of the exact location and potential mechanism of focal VTs are often not available, but sources have been reported in the RVOT, aortic sinus, and RV free wall.[15] Successful ablation of a VT originating from an RV basal aneurysm has been case-reported.[11] These data emphasize the importance of detailed substrate mapping, not restricted to the RVOT and VT induction, because VTs may arise from unexpected scars or focal substrates. Accordingly, noninducibility following substrate ablation remains an important additional procedural endpoint.

## SURGICAL ABLATION

Despite the modern surgical approach, transannular patches are still required in a significant number of rTOF patients to enlarge the pulmonary annulus. Subsequent pulmonary valve regurgitation and RV dilatation require revalving later in life. Most of these patients undergo surgical pulmonary valve replacement (PVR), using valved conduits. In 1 series of 1181 rTOF patients, 30% required open surgical procedures, which was PVR in the majority, during a median follow-up of 20 years after the initial repair.[31] Risk of PVR was independent of the surgical era.[31] If during initial intracardiac repair RV-pulmonary artery conduits had been used (54/1181, 5%), the rate of consecutive conduit replacement during follow-up was even higher (41%). Pulmonary regurgitation and RV dilatation have been associated with the occurrence of VTs, however, PVR alone does not remove the anatomical substrate and does not eliminate VT.[32] Therefore, concomitant VT ablation during indicated reoperation has been introduced (see **Table 2**). Similar to catheter mapping, earlier studies have used intraoperative VT induction and epicardial and endocardial activation mapping to determine the critical re-entry circuit and the appropriate site of ablation, which was most commonly the RVOT. With the identification of VT-related AIs in rTOF, a surgical substrate-based ablation approach (AI1, AI2, and AI3) can be performed, without the need for intraoperative VT induction. Different protocols for preoperative work-up and surgical ablations have been reported. Sandhu and colleagues[29] have performed preoperative PES in 70 patients, followed by empirical intraoperative substrate ablation in

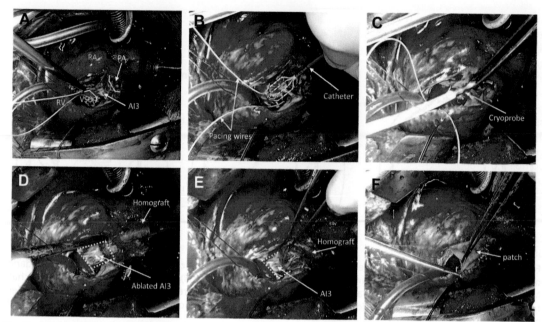

**Fig. 5.** Cryoablation of AI3 concomitant with surgical PVR. (*A*) The RV is incised showing the septal RVOT. Temporary bipolar pacing wires inserted on either side of AI3. (*B*) Multielectrode catheter is utilized to measure CV before and after cryoablation. (*C*) Cryoablation of AI3. (*D*) Ablated part of AI3 is visible. (*E*) Homograft clearly covers parts of AI3, rendering it potentially inaccessible to later catheter ablation. (*F*) Xenopericardial patch for RVOT reconstruction. (*Courtesy of* Dr. T. Nevvazhay, LUMC, Leiden, the Netherlands.)

inducible patients, including AI3, AI2, and a circumferential lesion directly below the pulmonary valve using cryoenergy, if VT was inducible. Caldaroni and colleagues[30] have performed preoperative PES in 37 patients considered at high risk for VT, followed by empirical ablation of AI1 and AI3 in inducible patients before revalving using unipolar RF. Noninducibility after surgical

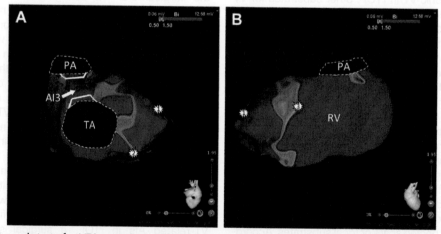

**Fig. 6.** Other substrate for VT in a patient with rTOF. Two bipolar voltage maps are shown, with a posteroinferior view (*A*), and modified lateral view (*B*), color-coded according to bar. EAM identified unexcitable scar continuously through AI3 (*gray dots*, panel *A*) and differential pacing on both sides of AI3 showed that AI3 was already blocked, and therefore no VT substrate. In the basal lateral RV a large confluent low-voltage area was revealed, showing abnormal fragmented electrograms and late potentials during SR. Three different VTs were induced, and PM showed excellent pace-matches for these VTs in or at the border of this area (pacing symbols with number), indicating VT exit sites. Ablation targeted abnormal electrograms (*red dots*). After ablation no VT was inducible.

ablation was achieved in 21% (Sandhu and colleagues) and 10% (Caldaroni and colleagues), respectively. During a mean follow-up of 6.1 years and 6.5 years, respectively, VT occurred in 5/70 and 2/37 patients (see **Table 2**).[29,30] Of note, in both series preoperative evaluation of AI characteristics (CV) and confirmation of CB across the surgical ablation line was not performed, which requires beating heart surgery. In 2020, Nevvazhay and colleagues described a novel approach, combining preoperative PES and substrate mapping to identify SCAI with intraoperative surgical ablation with the endpoint CB (see **Fig. 4**). Only preoperatively identified SCAI was targeted by cryoablation and bidirectional CB across the line could be confirmed after ablation using intraoperative differential pacing in all.[28] Whether this concept of preoperative PES and EAM identification of substrate, followed by intraoperative ablation of SCAI with endpoint CB is superior to empiric AI ablation requires additional data.

## EVOLVING INDICATIONS FOR CATHETER AND SURGICAL ABLATION IN REPAIRED TETRALOGY OF FALLOT

VT ablation is an important treatment option to prevent ICD discharge and symptoms in patients with recurrent VT.[6,22,33] Considering the favorable success and low complication rates RFCA offers an alternative to long-term medical therapy.[33]

In selected rTOF patients with symptomatic monomorphic VT, and preserved biventricular function, catheter or surgical ablation maybe even considered curative, and an alternative to ICD therapy, provided that the appropriate ablation endpoints (noninducibility and CB confirmation) have been reached.[33] This is important, as inappropriate ICD shock rates are reported in 25%, and other complications are reported in 26% of CHD patients with an ICD, during a mean follow-up of 3.7 years.[8] Furthermore, shock-related anxiety, sexual dysfunction, and depression are serious and prevalent issues in ICD recipients.

Prosthetic material, in particular valved conduits covering the most prevalent SCAI3, constitute an important reason for catheter ablation failure (see **Fig. 4**). In line with the current European CHD guidelines, preoperative PES/EAM and transection of VT-related AI before or during surgical or percutaneous PVR is important in rTOF patients with clinical VT.[33] Whether patients without VTs but with SCAI as potential VT substrate benefit from preventive surgical ablation is unclear. Considering the low risk and rapid surgical cryoablation, the potential benefits outweigh the risk, in our opinion. As SCAIs lead to spontaneous VTs at an older age, the gain of this approach for the growing population of adult rTOF patients can be only determined in the long term.[5–7]

## VENTRICULAR TACHYCARDIA SUBSTRATE AND ABLATION STRATEGIES IN OTHER CONGENITAL HEART DISEASE

Ablation of VT in CHD other than rTOF has been reported. Similar to rTOF, isthmus-dependent macroreentrant VT, especially in patients with prior RV incision or insertion of patch material, is one important VA subtype. However, data are limited, and other substrates and mechanisms may be involved. Accordingly, both substrate mapping and VT induction, followed by activation and entrainment mapping to localize critical re-entry circuit isthmus sites or to identify focal sources are important, and noninducibility of VT remains a valid endpoint.

## VENTRICULAR SEPTAL DEFECTS

VSD is the most frequently occurring CHD and is reported in 3.6 per 1000 live births.[1] It is most commonly perimembranous ($\pm$80%), but can also be located in the muscular ($\pm$15%-20%) or outlet septum ($\pm$5%).[33] Most VSDs close spontaneously during childhood, although some require surgical or transcatheter closure. Overall, long-term survival is excellent and monomorphic VTs are rarely encountered considering the high prevalence of VSDs and surgical repair.[8,33] However, catheter ablation of monomorphic VT in patients that have undergone VSD closure has been case-reported (see **Table 1**, 18/338, 5%). One report described a linear RF ablation line targeting AI2 as the critical isthmus, presumably caused by an RV incision for VSD repair.[15] In an RFCA study by Kapel and colleagues two patients with VSD were mentioned, both with concomitant anomalies. The underlying VT mechanism (VT cycle length 424 milliseconds and 400 millisecond) was macroreentrant VT, dependent on AI3 and AI4 in the first, and utilizing a basolateral left ventricular scar in the second patient.[10] In the first patient, RFCA was terminated prematurely to prevent total atrioventricular block because of the proximity of the bundle of His.[10]

## TRANSPOSITION OF THE GREAT ARTERIES

d-TGA is the second most prevalent cyanotic heart disease with an incidence of 0.32 per 1000 live births.[1] Surgical techniques have evolved over time: historically d-TGA patients underwent an atrial switch procedure (ie, Mustard or Senning), which has been replaced by an arterial switch operation which is the standard approach in contemporary patients. Both do not require RV incisions.

However, d-TGA can be associated with additional malformations, defined as complex d-TGA; for example, a VSD accompanies d-TGA in approximately 45% and may require intraventricular repair with a patch closure or the Rastelli operation.[33] ICD interrogation studies in d-TGA patients after atrial switch showed that 49% of appropriate therapy was because of monomorphic VT, the remainder being polymorphic VT (34%) and VF (17%) associated with failure of the systemic RV.[34] In patients with simple d-TGA and no ventricular scars monomorphic VT is uncommon. Focal VTs from the outflow tract region have also been described. In complex d-TGA, monomorphic VT because of macroreentry and subsequent ablation has been case-reported (see **Table 1**, 11/338 with d-TGA (3%), of whom 5 reported as complex). In these patients, patch material, surgical scar, and valve tissue can also form boundaries that can facilitate macroreentry VT via AIs.[10] Catheter manipulation can be challenging because of the anatomic variations, in particular if a retrograde, transaortic approach is required in patients after an arterial switch. Data on ablation outcomes are limited. In one recent study, two patients were successfully ablated without VT recurrence during follow-up.[10]

## EBSTEIN'S ANOMALY

EA is reported in 0.11 per 1000 live births.[1] It is characterized by the anomalous formation of the tricuspid valve (TV) leaflets and displacement toward the RV apex.[33] Because of this downward displacement of the TV, a portion of the morphological RV is atrialized. Monomorphic VT in EA is rare. Moore and colleagues[35] recently combined data of 11 centers between 1995 and 2017; a total of 24 patients with EA underwent VT ablation (see **Table 1**, 31/338, 9% in total). Importantly and in contrast to other CHD, 12 patients had VA without prior surgical TV repair. Substrate location and characteristics differ between patients with and without surgical interventions. Macroreentrant VT was the dominant VT mechanism in patients with prior TV surgery (six macroreentry, four focal, and three PVC). In contrast, in patients without prior repair, focal VTs were more frequently observed (eight focal and four macroreentry). Additionally, in patients after repair, macroreentrant VT substrates were located in the RV-free wall, related to areas of the larger confluent scar.

In patients without repair, the VT substrates were located in the atrialized portion of the RV.[35] Complete ablation success was achieved in 92%, and in only one patient VT recurred during a median follow-up of 3.4 years. There were no procedure-related complications in adults.[35] To date, there are no data supporting preoperative mapping for potential VT substrates in EA patients referred for surgery without documented VT.[33]

## FUTURE DIRECTIONS

Mapping and ablation for VT in patients with CHD are evolving. More data and longer follow-up are needed to (1) further determine the role of ablation as a curative treatment of VT as an alternative to ICD implantation in selected patients with repaired CHD; (2) assess the benefit of intraoperative CB confirmation across surgical ablation lines in terms of VT recurrence; and (3) to evaluate the role of routine EAM and preventive ablation of SCAI in all rTOF patients before PVR. Given that SCAIs are the dominant substrate for VT in rTOF, the future role of LGE-CMR for noninvasively identifying SCAI to select patients for invasive mapping and (preventive) ablation needs to be evaluated.

## SUMMARY

The prevalence of adults with CHD is on the rise as advances in surgical techniques and medical care have significantly improved survival. However, morbidity and mortality due to VA become an important clinical problem in adulthood. Macroreentrant VT constitutes the dominant subtype of VA, especially in CHD patients with ventricular incisions and prosthetic material. The identification of SCAI as the dominant substrate of VT in patients with rTOF (often hemodynamically unstable), has paved the way for substrate-based mapping and ablation, without the need for mapping during VT. The catheter or surgical ablation of SCAI, applying a linear line between the unexcitable boundaries is considered safe, provided that the proximity of vulnerable structures is recognized. SCAI related to VT should be targeted by ablation before they become inaccessible. If recommended endpoints for ablation are reached, namely confirmation of CB along the ablation line and noninducibility of VT, the long-term outcome is excellent. Ablation may be even considered curative in carefully selected patients with a preserved biventricular function. Whether mapping and subsequent ablation of SCAI for risk stratification and prevention of VT are beneficial, requires further studies.

## CLINICS CARE POINTS

- In contemporary patients with repaired tetralogy of Fallot (rTOF), slow-conducting anatomical isthmus (SCAI) 3, between the ventricular septal defect patch and the pulmonary annulus, is the most important remaining substrate for ventricular tachycardia (VT).
- In rTOF patients without a competing ventricular arrhythmia substrate, transection of SCAI with bidirectional conduction block (CB) may be considered as curative treatment for VT.
- The strong link between SCAI and inducible and spontaneous VT supports electroanatomical mapping as a potential tool for risk stratification.
- Surgical ablation with intraoperative confirmation of CB may be the preferred ablation method concomitant with pulmonary valve replacement, if indicated.
- Clinical care of adults with congenital heart disease requires a multidisciplinary team.

## ACKNOWLEDGMENTS

The authors thank Dr. Philippine Kiès and Dr. Timofey Nevvazhay for their aid in providing **Figs. 1** and **4**, respectively. We acknowledge the support from the Netherlands Cardiovascular Research Initiative: An initiative with support of the Dutch Heart Foundation and Hartekind, CVON2019-002 OUTREACH.

## DISCLOSURE

The authors have nothing to disclose.

## REFERENCES

1. Hoffman JI, Kaplan S. The incidence of congenital heart disease. J Am Coll Cardiol 2002;39(12): 1890–900.
2. Khairy P, Ionescu-Ittu R, Mackie AS, et al. Changing mortality in congenital heart disease. J Am Coll Cardiol 2010;56(14):1149–57.
3. Lillehei CW, Varco RL, Cohen M, et al. The first open heart corrections of tetralogy of Fallot. A 26-31 year follow-up of 106 patients. Ann Surg 1986;204(4): 490–502.
4. Engelfriet P, Boersma E, Oechslin E, et al. The spectrum of adult congenital heart disease in Europe: morbidity and mortality in a 5 year follow-up period. The Euro Heart Survey on adult congenital heart disease. Eur Heart J 2005;26(21):2325–33.
5. Khairy P, Aboulhosn J, Gurvitz MZ, et al. Arrhythmia burden in adults with surgically repaired tetralogy of Fallot: a multi-institutional study. Circulation 2010;122(9): 868–75.
6. Kapel GF, Sacher F, Dekkers OM, et al. Arrhythmogenic anatomical isthmuses identified by electroanatomical mapping are the substrate for ventricular tachycardia in repaired Tetralogy of Fallot. Eur Heart J 2017;38(4):268–76.
7. Gatzoulis MA, Balaji S, Webber SA, et al. Risk factors for arrhythmia and sudden cardiac death late after repair of tetralogy of Fallot: a multicentre study. Lancet 2000;356(9234):975–81.
8. Vehmeijer JT, Brouwer TF, Limpens J, et al. Implantable cardioverter-defibrillators in adults with congenital heart disease: a systematic review and meta-analysis. Eur Heart J 2016;37(18):1439–48.
9. Zeppenfeld K, Schalij MJ, Bartelings MM, et al. Catheter ablation of ventricular tachycardia after repair of congenital heart disease: electroanatomic identification of the critical right ventricular isthmus. Circulation 2007;116(20):2241–52.
10. Kapel GF, Reichlin T, Wijnmaalen AP, et al. Re-entry using anatomically determined isthmuses: a curable ventricular tachycardia in repaired congenital heart disease. Circ Arrhythm Electrophysiol 2015;8(1): 102–9.
11. Le Bloa M, Pham M, Mongeon FP, et al. Right ventricular basal aneurysm as a substrate for ventricular tachycardia in tetralogy of fallot. JACC Clin Electrophysiol 2020;6(6):743–4.
12. Khairy P, Harris L, Landzberg MJ, et al. Implantable cardioverter-defibrillators in tetralogy of Fallot. Circulation 2008;117(3):363–70.
13. Morwood JG, Triedman JK, Berul CI, et al. Radiofrequency catheter ablation of ventricular tachycardia in children and young adults with congenital heart disease. Heart Rhythm 2004;1(3):301–8.
14. Laredo M, Frank R, Waintraub X, et al. Ten-year outcomes of monomorphic ventricular tachycardia catheter ablation in repaired tetralogy of Fallot. Arch Cardiovasc Dis 2017;110(5):292–302.
15. Yang J, Brunnquell M, Liang JJ, et al. Long term follow-up after ventricular tachycardia ablation in patients with congenital heart disease. J Cardiovasc Electrophysiol 2019;30(9):1560–8.
16. Kriebel T, Saul JP, Schneider H, et al. Noncontact mapping and radiofrequency catheter ablation of fast and hemodynamically unstable ventricular tachycardia after surgical repair of tetralogy of Fallot. J Am Coll Cardiol 2007;50(22):2162–8.
17. Bashore TM. Adult congenital heart disease: right ventricular outflow tract lesions. Circulation 2007; 115(14):1933–47.
18. Hosseinpour AR, Gonzalez-Calle A, Adsuar-Gomez A, et al. The predicament of surgical correction of tetralogy of fallot. Pediatr Cardiol 2021;42(6):1252–7.

19. Horowitz LN, Vetter VL, Harken AH, et al. Electro-physiologic characteristics of sustained ventricular tachycardia occurring after repair of tetralogy of fallot. Am J Cardiol 1980;46(3):446–52.

20. Kapel GFL, Laranjo S, Blom NA, et al. Impact of surgery on presence and dimensions of anatomical isthmuses in tetralogy of Fallot. Heart 2018; 104(14):1200–7.

21. Moore JP, Seki A, Shannon KM, et al. Characterization of anatomic ventricular tachycardia isthmus pathology after surgical repair of tetralogy of Fallot. Circ Arrhythm Electrophysiol 2013;6(5):905–11.

22. Khairy P, Landzberg MJ, Gatzoulis MA, et al. Value of programmed ventricular stimulation after tetralogy of fallot repair: a multicenter study. Circulation 2004; 109(16):1994–2000.

23. van Zyl M, Kapa S, Padmanabhan D, et al. Mechanism and outcomes of catheter ablation for ventricular tachycardia in adults with repaired congenital heart disease. Heart Rhythm 2016; 13(7):1449–54.

24. Teijeira-Fernandez E, Cochet H, Bourier F, et al. Influence of contact force on voltage mapping: a combined magnetic resonance imaging and electroanatomic mapping study in patients with tetralogy of Fallot. Heart Rhythm 2018;15(8):1198–205.

25. Schneider HE, Schill M, Kriebel T, et al. Value of dynamic substrate mapping to identify the critical diastolic pathway in postoperative ventricular reentrant tachycardias after surgical repair of tetralogy of fallot. J Cardiovasc Electrophysiol 2012; 23(9):930–7.

26. Kapel GF, Reichlin T, Wijnmaalen AP, et al. Left-sided ablation of ventricular tachycardia in adults with repaired tetralogy of Fallot: a case series. Circ Arrhythm Electrophysiol 2014;7(5):889–97.

27. Bhaskaran A, Tung R, Stevenson WG, et al. Catheter ablation of VT in non-ischaemic cardiomyopathies: endocardial, epicardial and intramural approaches. Heart Lung Circ 2019;28(1):84–101.

28. Nevvazhay T, Zeppenfeld K, Brouwer C, et al. Intraoperative cryoablation in late pulmonary valve replacement for tetralogy of Fallot. Interact Cardiovasc Thorac Surg 2020;30(5):780–2.

29. Sandhu A, Ruckdeschel E, Sauer WH, et al. Perioperative electrophysiology study in patients with tetralogy of Fallot undergoing pulmonary valve replacement will identify those at high risk of subsequent ventricular tachycardia. Heart Rhythm 2018; 15(5):679–85.

30. Caldaroni F, Lo Rito M, Chessa M, et al. Surgical ablation of ventricular tachycardia in patients with repaired tetralogy of Fallot. Eur J Cardiothorac Surg 2019;55(5):845–50.

31. Hickey EJ, Veldtman G, Bradley TJ, et al. Late risk of outcomes for adults with repaired tetralogy of Fallot from an inception cohort spanning four decades. Eur J Cardiothorac Surg 2009;35(1):156–64 [discussion: 164].

32. Harrild DM, Berul CI, Cecchin F, et al. Pulmonary valve replacement in tetralogy of Fallot: impact on survival and ventricular tachycardia. Circulation 2009;119(3):445–51.

33. Baumgartner H, De Backer J, Babu-Narayan SV, et al. 2020 ESC guidelines for the management of adult congenital heart disease. Eur Heart J 2021; 42(6):563–645.

34. Khairy P, Harris L, Landzberg MJ, et al. Sudden death and defibrillators in transposition of the great arteries with intra-atrial baffles: a multicenter study. Circ Arrhythm Electrophysiol 2008;1(4):250–7.

35. Moore JP, Shannon KM, Gallotti RG, et al. Catheter ablation of ventricular arrhythmia for Ebstein's anomaly in unoperated and post-surgical patients. JACC Clin Electrophysiol 2018;4(10):1300–7.

36. Gonska BD, Cao K, Raab J, et al. Radiofrequency catheter ablation of right venticular tachycardia late after repair of congenital heart defects. Circulation 1996;94(8):1902–8.

37. Hebe J, Hansen P, Ouyang F, et al. Radiofrequency catheter ablation of tachycardia in patients with congenital heart disease. Pediatr Cardiol 2000; 21(6):557–75.

38. Furushima H, Chinushi M, Sugiura H, et al. Ventricular tachycardia tachycardia late after repair of congenital heart diseases: efficacy of combination therapy with radiofrequency catheter ablation and class III antiarrhythmic agents and long-term outcomes. J Electrocardiol 2006; 39(2):219–24.

39. Tokuda M, Tedrow UB, Kojodjojo P, et al. Catheter ablation of ventricular tachycardia in nonischemic heart disease. Circ Arrhythm Electrophysiol 2012; 5(5):992–1000.

40. Harrison DA, Harris L, Siu SC, et al. Sustained ventricular tachycardia in adult patients late after repair of tetralog of Fallot. J Am Coll Cardiol 1997;30(5):1368–73.

41. Therrien J, Siu SC. Harris, and colleagues Impact of pulmonary valve replacement on arrhythmia propensity late after repair of tetralogy of Fallot. Circulation 2001;103(20):2489–94.

42. Ashburn DA, Harris L, Downar EH, et al. Electrophysiologic surgery in patients with congential heart disease. Semin Thorac Cardiovasc Surg Pediatr Card Surg Annu 2003;6:51–8.

43. Karamlou T, Silber T, Lao R, et al. Outcomes after late reoperation in patients with repaired tetralogy of Fallot: the impact of arrhythmia and arrhythmia surgery. Ann Thorac Surg 2006;81(5):1786–93 [discussion: 1793].

44. Giamberti A, Chessa M, Abella R, et al. Surgical treatment of arrhthmias in adults with congenital heart defects. Int J Cardiol 2008;129(1):37–41.

45. Mavroudis C, Deal BJ, Backer CL, et al. Arrhythmia Surgery in patients with and without congenital heart disease. Ann Thorac Surg 2008;86(3):857–68.

46. Sabate Rotes A, Connolly HM, Warnes CA, et al. Ventricular arrhythmia risk stratification in patients with tetralogy of Fallot at the time of pulmonary valve replacement. Circ Arrhythm Electrophysiol 2015; 8(1):110–6.

47. Kawada S, Chakraborty P, Downar E, et al. The Role of Ablation in Prevention of Recurrent Implantable Cardioverter Defibrillator Shocks in Patients With Tetralogy of Fallot. CJC Open 2021;3(5):619–26.

# Catheter Ablation of Ventricular Fibrillation

Fatima M. Ezzeddine, MD, Ashley M. Darlington, MD, Christopher V. DeSimone, MD, PhD,
Samuel J. Asirvatham, MD*

## KEYWORDS

• Catheter ablation • Autonomic nervous system • Purkinje fibers • Ventricular fibrillation

## KEY POINTS

- Catheter ablation targeting triggers for ventricular fibrillation (VF) can be effective in preventing VF recurrence in some patients.
- The critical substrate residing in the ventricles and His–Purkinje network that are crucial for maintaining VF remain elusive. Rigorous study is needed to identify the substrate of VF to improve targeted therapeutic interventions.
- Autonomic interventions through extracardiac structure neuromodulation including stellate ganglion blockade, sympathectomy, and/or renal sympathetic denervation hold promise as an adjunct to conventional therapies to prevent VF recurrence.

## INTRODUCTION

Consideration of catheter ablation for ventricular fibrillation (VF) has only been possible in recent years with the development of more advanced mapping and ablation tools, along with the identification of common triggers for VF. Much of what has been applied to trigger-based ablation for VF is from a similar conceptual model for paroxysmal atrial fibrillation (AF) ablation where pulmonary veins are the main triggers for initiation of the arrhythmia.[1] Thus, the triggers for VF initiation such as closely coupled premature ventricular complexes (PVCs) from certain regions as the papillary muscles and Purkinje tissue can be mapped and ablated. For persistent AF, non-pulmonary vein substrate is targeted;[2,3] however, there is no valid approach for VF substrate modification given the lack of understanding of the critical substrate required for VF maintenance. Thus, an improved understanding beyond the triggers for VF is critical if we are to move toward improved therapeutic interventions.

To better conceptualize and provide a framework for understanding VF, this rhythm can be described in varying phases: initiation and perpetuation across several phases. These include (1) initiation, (2) transition, (3) maintenance, and (4) evolution (**Fig. 1**).[4] The first phase is *initiation*, which can occur via a PVC, generated by either abnormal automaticity, triggered activity, or reentry through electrically heterogenous ventricular myocardial tissue and/or the specialized His–Purkinje system (HPS).[5] The second phase is *transition* which describes the transformation of the PVC into a sustenance of fibrillatory activity via propagation through an electrically heterogenous substrate in the ventricle and/or HPS. It has been suggested that the transition into fibrillatory activity can occur through initiation of rotor formation, where the activation wave front rotates around a central inert core creating continuous functional reentry.[6,7] The third phase is that of VF *maintenance*, describing the formation of multiple rotor wave fronts or a single "mother rotor" which turns at a high frequency that promotes wave breaks.[8,9] The final phase is that of *evolution*, which describes the process of the sustainment of VF from short to long duration.

Department of Cardiovascular Medicine, Mayo Clinic, 200 First Street Southwest, Rochester, MN, USA
* Corresponding author. Mayo Clinic College of Medicine, 200 First Street Southwest, Rochester, MN 55905.
*E-mail address:* asirvatham.samuel@mayo.edu

Card Electrophysiol Clin 14 (2022) 729–742
https://doi.org/10.1016/j.ccep.2022.06.002
1877-9182/22/© 2022 Elsevier Inc. All rights reserved.

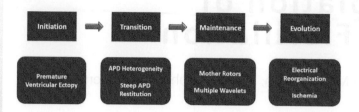

**Fig. 1.** Stages and mechanisms of ventricular fibrillation.

As VF persists, cardiac tissue ischemia ensues, resulting in electrical reorganization and continued sources of sustained VF activity. This not only complicates the rhythm of VF itself, but also complicates our understanding of VF perpetuation. Given the lethal nature of this rhythm, our ability to map it adequately without hypoperfusion or ischemia is limited, and thus we are constrained by a limited amount of mapping, as well as limited time during which these features can be mapped and understood. In addition, given the fast rates of the HPS and ventricular tissue, it is very difficult to decipher at times between ventricular and HPS electrograms given the current fidelity and filtering with the recording/mapping systems we have available. Thus, most of our knowledge is based on animal studies, ex vivo tissue preparations, Langendorff models, as well as computer modeling and simulation.[10–13]

In this review, we summarize the evidence behind catheter ablation of VF focusing on patients with structurally normal hearts. We also highlight and discuss current gaps that exist in our knowledge of VF. Finally, we discuss future directions and research necessary to advance our understanding of VF and expand our approaches to permit effective catheter ablation.

## PREMATURE VENTRICULAR COMPLEX-TRIGGERED VENTRICULAR FIBRILLATION
### Localization of Common Premature Ventricular Complexes

Seminal observations showed a characterizable set of patients with structurally normal hearts in whom VF is initiated by an intervening and reproducible beat rather than a transition directly from normal sinus rhythm.[14–16] In these patients, identifying and ablating the trigger mitigated further risk of recurrent VF albeit with limited success because of the difficulties of mapping infrequent triggers in an unstable myocardium.[15–17] An approach to VF trigger ablation is summarized in **Fig. 2**. Localization of triggering PVCs on the surface electrocardiogram (ECG) and/or cardiac monitoring is critical for planning catheter ablation of VF (**Table 1**). PVC triggers can initiate VF repeatedly and tend to have a similar morphology with a short coupling interval. PVCs or non-sustained polymorphic ventricular tachycardia (PMVT) of similar morphologies may suggest a single anatomic area of origin.[14,17]

Anatomic localization of the trigger is paramount to guiding ablation, which has had some success in treating VF without recurrence.[17,18] In a

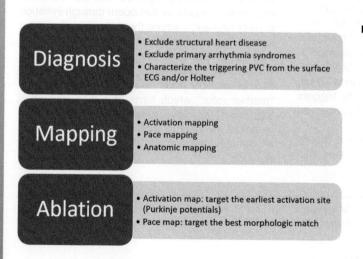

**Fig. 2.** Approach to trigger ablation.

**Table 1**
**Localization of idiopathic premature ventricular complex triggers on electrocardiography and/or cardiac monitoring**

| | Lead V1 | Inferior Leads | Precordial Leads | Additional Notes |
|---|---|---|---|---|
| Left anterior fascicle | RBBB pattern (rsR′) | Inferior, rightward axis | | QRS duration <130 ms |
| Anterolateral papillary muscle | RBBB pattern (R or qR) | Inferior, rightward axis | Transition at leads V3–V5, rS pattern in lead V6 | QRS duration >130 ms |
| Left posterior fascicle | RBBB pattern (rsR′) | Superior, leftward axis | | QRS duration <130 ms |
| Posteromedial papillary muscle | RBBB pattern (R or qR) | Superior, leftward axis | Transition at leads V3–V5, rS pattern in lead V6 | QRS duration >130 ms |
| RV moderator band | LBBB pattern | rS pattern in lead II, negative QRS in lead III | Transition at leads V4–V6 | |
| LVOT | RBBB or LBBB pattern | Inferior axis | Early transition (V1–V2) (lead V3 transition + V2 transition ratio ≥ 0.6) | LCAS/RCAS: Notched QS in lead V1<br>LV summit: V2 transition break |
| RVOT | LBBB pattern | Inferior axis | Late transition (≥V3) (lead V3 transition + V2 transition ratio < 0.6) | Free wall: Inferior notching<br>Septal: Positive lead I, aVR < aVL |

*Abbreviations:* LBBB, left bundle branch block; LCAS, left coronary aortic sinus; LVOT, left ventricular outflow tract; RBBB, right bundle branch block; RCAS, right coronary aortic sinus; RVOT, right ventricular outflow tract.

multicenter study assessing long-term outcomes of trigger ablation in patients with idiopathic VF, 18% of patients had VF recurrence at a median of 4 months during a median follow-up duration of 63 months.[18] Common areas of origin of triggering PVCs include the HPS, the right ventricular outflow tract, the left ventricular outflow tract, papillary muscles of both ventricles, and the right ventricular moderator band.[19–23] When originating from the HPS, PVC complexes are usually of narrow QRS duration and have a RBBB morphology when originating from the left Purkinje network with right or left axis deviation.[17,19] When originating from the right Purkinje network, PVC complexes are of narrow QRS duration with a LBBB morphology.[17,19] It has been shown that the origin of Purkinje ectopics triggering idiopathic VF differs between men and women.[24] Purkinje ectopics arise predominantly from the right ventricle (RV) in men and from the left ventricle (LV) or both ventricles in women.[24] It is unclear as to why this is the cause, but the authors suggest that it may be related to asymmetry in the development and function of the left and right Purkinje networks.

### Mapping Premature Ventricular Complexes: Approach and Common Scenarios of Difficulty

The most successful approach for mapping these PVCs is through activation mapping of the earliest site of activation of the PVC. Ideally, mapping and ablation would be performed during a time of high PVC burden. However, this is not often the case and given the rarity of PVCs during the electrophysiological (EP) study, such challenges can be a major impediment to successful VF ablation. It is often quite difficult to determine the culprit PVC as those that are present and not inducing VF at the time of EP study may not be the desired culprit PVCs of interest to target. However, if spontaneous PVC activity is absent at the time of ablation, attempts can be made to trigger the clinically relevant PVC through noncontact and contact approaches, although each has significant limitations and is likely responsible for only partial success of these procedures.

Triggering PVCs through a noncontact approach can be achieved by intravenous infusion of arrhythmogenic medications, usually those that are adrenergic drivers. Isoproterenol infusion may stimulate arrhythmogenicity through its beta-agonist activity or reveal concealed long QT syndrome, catecholaminergic polymorphic ventricular tachycardia (CPVT), or coronary spasm as underlying causes for VF.[18,21,25] Alternatively, Ajmaline infusion may induce R-on-T ectopy originating from the Purkinje network or reveal Brugada syndrome as the underlying cause for VF through its sodium channel blocking action.[21,26] Unfortunately, up to 25% of patients have no ectopy and thus no ability for elucidation of the trigger for VF using this approach.[21] When PVCs cannot be triggered by medications, it is very difficult to find the trigger source, and this almost certainly causes the efficacy of the procedure rate to diminish. A contact-induced trigger can be attempted via catheter and pacing maneuvers during the EP study but may be of limited clinical value. Introduction of ventricular extra-stimuli (1–3 beats) from the RV or LV is one approach to elicit PVCs, as well as burst pacing from the atrium, RV, or LV.[21,27]

Activation of the His–Purkinje network is noted by the presence of a Purkinje potential, identified as a sharp potential (<10 ms in duration) preceding the QRS complex (<15 ms) on the intracardiac electrogram. Despite this, reliably localizing the origin of the PVC trigger remains difficult given the limitations in mapping the Purkinje network with current intracardiac catheters, as well as current mapping/recording systems. The filtering used by the mapping system can lead to distortion in the signal and obscurement, thus making it difficult to determine which is a HPS electrogram versus a ventricular electrogram, and which is activated first. In addition, Purkinje potentials can be blocked, concealed, or activated retrogradely by inadvertent stimulation of the bundle branches by catheters, inducing interventricular conduction abnormalities that conceal the Purkinje potential.[18,28] The presence of a bundle branch block due to mechanical disruption is an independent predictor for VF recurrence after ablation for this reason.[18]

If spontaneous or triggered PVCs cannot be localized, then pace mapping may indicate the anatomic origin of the triggering PVC. This is performed by delivering low energy stimulation (2–15 mA) to various sites of HPS and/or ventricular myocardium, and then comparing the QRS complexes to the clinically triggering PVC until an identical match is achieved.[28] However, there are several factors that limit the success of pace mapping in these types of regions. First, pace mapping has poorer resolution as similar morphologies can be reproduced over larger areas of myocardium compared with activation mapping.[29] Furthermore, the location identified by pace mapping may also be unreliable if the true site of origin lies deeper within the myocardium that is preferentially conducted to an alternative surface site through preferential fibers.[29] Lastly, pace mapping is not as sensitive for triggers originating from conduction tissue. Delivery of the stimulation simultaneously activates the Purkinje network and the surrounding myocardium, concealing the Purkinje activity and prohibiting reproduction of a PVC originating from the Purkinje network.[28]

When activation mapping and pace mapping are unable to localize the trigger, an anatomic approach can be considered, but only as a last option because of its notably lower success rate, higher rate of complications, and poor outcomes. In this approach, the putative ablation site is not identified by the earliest site of activation or via morphology match with pace-mapping, but rather based on anatomic information elucidated from the morphology of the PVC on the surface ECG. Owing to the less precise nature of this approach, larger areas of ablation can lead to other complications including heterogenous scar formation, which can lead to scar-based VT involving ventricular myocardium and the HPS.

As highlighted above, there are many limitations to accurately localizing the culprit PVC that diminish the success rate and efficacy of VF ablation. One major area for improvement needed to advance procedural outcomes is a more reliable and reproducible approach to induce the culprit PVC, and ultimately permit activation mapping. Catecholamines can be used to simulate stress-induced ectopy or unveil CPVT or long QT syndrome; however, excess catecholamine stimulation can lead to other detrimental physiologic changes including coronary vasoconstriction, increased myocardial oxygen demand, and increased afterload that may lead to ischemic injury.[30,31] Alternatively, mechanical deformation of the myocardium can induce PVCs and VF through mechanical activation of nonselective-cation and potassium channels.[32,33] When activated nonuniformly, as is during mechanical injury, this can create repolarization dispersion of the substrate that is vulnerable to VF when applied during the repolarization period.[34,35] Simulation studies show that sustained recruitment of these channels increases excitability and ectopy, suggesting a novel pharmacologic target for PVC induction that may permit activation mapping.[36]

A key development needed for enhancing our ability to ablate VF would be an innovation involving a novel energy source that is able to selectively ablate either conduction tissue or ventricular tissue, without affecting the other. Such an application could also be administered at "test" doses, similar to cryomapping, which are reversible, will not cause thermal damage, and not induce VF. One possible solution is pulsed-field electroporation, or the application of pulsatile direct current to permeabilize cell membranes. Transient exposure to weaker electrical fields creates permeabilization that is reversible, whereas prolonged exposure results in irreversible permeabilization and cell death.[37,38] This nonthermal energy source has also been shown to successfully ablate conductive tissue with minimal effect to myocardium in a manner that is dose-dependent in a canine model.[39–41]

## VENTRICULAR FIBRILLATION—ROLE OF THE HIS–PURKINJE SYSTEM IN VENTRICULAR FIBRILLATION MAINTENANCE

Maintenance of VF is because of the propagation of a trigger through an electrically heterogeneous substrate. Historically, intramural reentry was thought to be the main factor behind sustained VF.[42] However, a plethora of literature has shed light on the role of the HPS not only in the initiation of VF but also in its maintenance. Early VF mapping studies showed an endocardial to epicardial activation gradient during sustained VF with the activation being more rapid in the endocardium.[43,44] Worley and colleagues[43] showed that this gradient occurred after discontinuing cardiac bypass which indicates a gradient that is setup by ensuing ischemia.

Subsequent studies showed that the Purkinje fibers, which reside in the subendocardium and are more resistant to ischemia than the ventricular myocardium, seemed to be the culprit behind the endocardial to epicardial activation gradient in VF.[45–49] Using three-dimensional electrical mapping of canine hearts, Li and colleagues[46] showed that after 5 min of sustained VF the electrical activation becomes seemingly more organized, starting in the Purkinje fibers of the endocardium and traversing intramurally toward the epicardium. Tabereaux and colleagues[47] found that the Purkinje fibers are highly active 10 min after the onset of VF with antegrade propagation from the Purkinje fibers to the surrounding ventricular myocardium and retrograde propagation from the ventricular myocardium to the Purkinje fibers. Similarly, Lin and colleagues[48] and Wu and colleagues[49] showed a close relationship between repetitive focal endocardial discharges and the maintenance of VF.

An elegant study strongly supporting the role of the HPS in VF maintenance was performed via the use of Lugol's solution creating a chemical ablation of the subendocardial surface and resulted in the inability to sustain VF in animal studies.[48,49] The role of the Purkinje fibers in maintaining VF has been further emphasized in studies focused on mapping long-duration VF (LDVF) which elucidated an organized state driven by endocardial activation as VF progresses to LDVF.[50,51] After defibrillation of LDVF, the earliest post-shock activation was also found to be in the Purkinje network.[52] Within the Purkinje network, Tri and colleagues[53] showed an intramural gradient between the proximal, insulated regions of the HPS and the distal, non-insulated regions of the HPS during VF with the latter being faster, alluding to the notion that the distal conduction system may indeed harbor the critical substrate necessary to sustain VF.

Mechanistically, studies including in vivo animal studies, ex vivo tissue preparations, Langendorff models, as well as computer modeling and simulation, have shown that rotors play a key role in the maintenance of VF.[54] A rotor is defined as a singularity point around which the electrical activity is organized in the form of spiral waves.[55] A rotor forms when a wave front meets an anatomic or functional obstacle resulting in a wave break or wave curling[56] (**Fig. 3**). Rotors can be stationary or drifting depending on the structural and electrophysiological properties of the tissue in which they form.[57] Fibrosis facilitates wave break[58] and inward rectifier potassium currents stabilize rotors.[59,60] Being able to track rotors using dominant frequency mapping and phase mapping was a

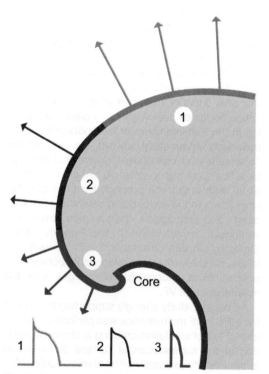

**Fig. 3.** Snapshot of the spiral wave. The rotor or (*) phase singularity is the point where the wave front and the wave tail meet.

step forward in the understanding of rotor dynamics.[57] Krummen and colleagues[61] used phase mapping to map VF episodes in patients undergoing ventricular tachycardia ablation procedures and found that the presence of stable rotors was the distinguishing factor between sustained and self-limiting VF episodes.

Substrate-directed therapies started with using Lugol's solution to chemically ablate the Purkinje system, which resulted in early VF termination and increased the VF induction threshold.[62,63] Furthermore, in studies in isolated swine RVs, VF induction was more difficult after surgical excision of the papillary muscles.[64] Similarly, radiofrequency ablation of the rotors at the LV posteroseptum and posterior papillary muscles reduced VF inducibility in both rabbit and dog hearts.[65] These data, among others, are suggestive of a critical role for the Purkinje system in VF maintenance and pose adequate fodder for further study to elucidate the exact regions that are necessary for this rhythm to continue.

Despite favorable results in the experimental laboratory, many of these findings have failed to translate into clinical research because of their significant risks and impracticality in humans given potential toxicities, surgical interventions, and also the major issue with anesthesia and hemodynamic support necessary to perform such procedures. There have been some limited attempts to translate early proof-of-concept studies though these have been rare. In a clinical proof-of-concept study in a patient with recurrent implantable cardioverter-defibrillator (ICD) shocks because of refractory VF, VF rotor substrate ablation was effective in preventing VF recurrence for at least 2 years post-ablation.[66] In patients with left ventricular assist devices and long-lasting VF, catheter ablation of myocardial scars was shown to reduce the mean dominant frequency and complexity of electrical waves obtained by spectral analysis.[67]

Further research is needed to identify the critical area within the Purkinje network that is responsible for VF maintenance to perform targeted endocardial substrate ablation and avoid extensive damage to the Purkinje network. Tan and colleagues[68] used sequential biventricular endocardial and epicardial mapping in an attempt to understand the spatiotemporal characteristics of VF and identify the critical regions required for VF maintenance. They noted that the regions with the shortest ventricular cycle lengths were in the endocardial aspect of the distal RV during the early stages of VF (0–30 min) followed by a transition to the endocardial aspect of the distal LV during the later stages of VF (30–60 min).[68]

One of the limitations of this study was the lack of consistent and continuous mapping of VF activity in these critical regions. Nonetheless, the dynamic nature of VF was finally appreciated with the first comprehensive report on endocardial and epicardial biventricular mapping with an advancing mapping system and multipolar catheters in an intact large-scale animal model. Much work remains in this area to be done if we are to use the fertile research and translate it into the clinical arena.

## AUTONOMIC MODULATION FOR VENTRICULAR FIBRILLATION

The autonomic nervous system (ANS) plays a key role in the modulation of cardiac arrhythmias. The superior cervical ganglia, the stellate ganglia, and the thoracic ganglia provide cardiac sympathetic innervation via the superior, middle, and inferior cardiac nerves[69] (**Fig. 4**). The vagus nerves provide cardiac parasympathetic innervation via fibers that converge at the level of the third fat pad; the latter is located between the medial superior vena cava and the aorta[70] (see **Fig. 4**). The cardiac ganglia modulate complex autonomic interactions and are mainly located on the posterior surfaces of the atria and along the superior aspect of the ventricles.[71] The ANS has various effects on cardiac arrhythmias. Although some arrhythmias are because of sympathetic overactivity (ventricular arrhythmias in the setting of ischemia, long QT syndrome, and CPVT), others are because of parasympathetic overactivity (Brugada syndrome and AF).[72]

In pediatric patients with idiopathic VF, Frontera and colleagues[73] reported an association between VF and high adrenergic tone. Alternatively, Kasanuki and colleagues[74] described a series of patients in whom idiopathic VF was induced by increased vagal activity. Animal experiments have shown that sympathetic stimulation increases the ventricular action potential duration restitution slope which decreases fibrillation threshold,[75] whereas parasympathetic stimulation has the opposite effects.[76] The effect of sympathetic stimulation becomes more prominent in the setting of ischemia and myocardial infarction which cause regional cellular and tissue remodeling[77] and heterogeneity in sympathetic nervous system innervation.[78]

To explain sudden death in states of increased vagal activity such as during sleep, several investigators studied the role of cholinergic activity in VF initiation and maintenance.[79–81] VF induction and maintenance occurred with a moderate increase in cholinergic activity in the setting of increased adrenergic activity.[81] This was thought to be due to discharge of multiple ectopic pacemakers or to conduction disturbances.[81] Based on these findings, a critical balance between the sympathetic and parasympathetic influences seems to be needed for both VF initiation and maintenance.

### Cardiac Sympathetic Denervation

Cardiac sympathetic denervation aims at interrupting the sympathetic input to the heart. It is commonly performed by left stellate ganglion or bilateral stellate ganglia blockade with the use of an anesthetic agent for temporary block or surgically for permanent block. In a meta-analysis including 38 patients with electrical storm triggered by acute myocardial infarction or QT prolongation, Meng and colleagues[82] showed that stellate ganglion blockade was effective in the management of electrical storm as an adjunct to

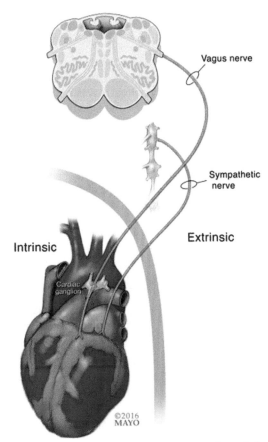

**Fig. 4.** Scheme of the autonomic innervation of the heart. The superior cervical ganglia, the stellate ganglia, and the thoracic ganglia provide cardiac sympathetic innervation, and the vagus nerves provide cardiac parasympathetic innervation.

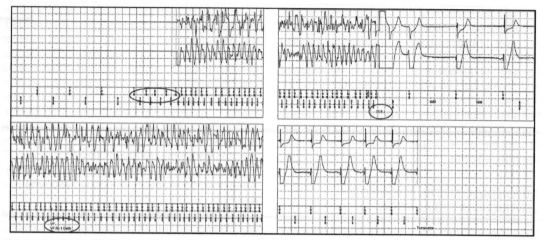

**Fig. 5.** Ventricular fibrillation triggered by premature ventricular ectopy. First circle: premature ventricular contractions; Second circle: ventricular fibrillation detected; Third circle: shock delivery.

conventional therapies. Surgical resection of the lower half of the stellate ganglion has been performed for hopes of a more durable effect. Initially, an open surgical approach was used via a supraclavicular access or thoracotomy.[83] Subsequently, a less invasive approach using video assisted thoracic surgery was adopted.[84] During this procedure, the lower half of the stellate ganglion is removed along with the thoracic ganglia T2 to T4 and its rami communicantes. The upper half of the stellate ganglion is preserved to prevent Horner's syndrome.

### Renal Sympathetic Denervation

Renal sympathetic denervation was first shown to decrease sympathetic stimulation in patients with resistant hypertension.[85,86] It was then used in other diseases or conditions associated with increased adrenergic tone such as heart failure and arrhythmias. Ukena and colleagues[87] first described the use of renal sympathetic denervation for the management of electrical storm. In patients with ICDs and refractory ventricular

arrhythmias, renal sympathetic denervation was associated with a decrease in the burden of ventricular arrhythmias.[88,89]

## CLINICAL CASES

In this section, we present two clinical cases of patients with structurally normal hearts who suffered from VF. We discuss the management strategy and outcomes in each of these cases.

### Case 1

A 16-year-old previously healthy boy had an out-of-hospital cardiac arrest due to VF. ECG, transthoracic echocardiogram, and cardiac magnetic resonance imaging were unremarkable. Genetic testing for inherited channelopathies was negative. The patient underwent single chamber ICD implantation and was discharged on nadolol. Four months later, he had an appropriate ICD shock due to recurrent VF after he had missed a few doses of nadolol. The VF event was triggered by a PVC (**Fig. 5**). Holter monitor and cardiac

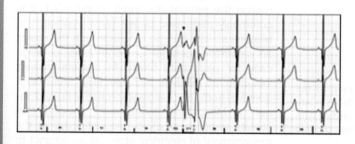

**Fig. 6.** Holter monitoring showing closely coupled premature ventricular contractions (*arrowhead*).

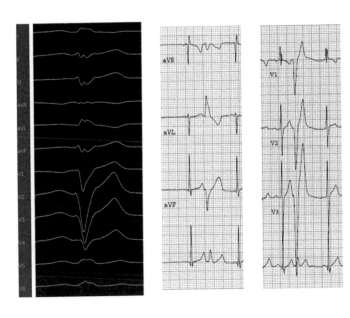

**Fig. 7.** Triggering premature ventricular contraction had a left bundle branch block morphology in lead v1, superior axis, and late transition in the precordial leads concerning for a moderator band focus of ectopy.

exercise stress test showed closely coupled PVCs (**Fig. 6**). In light of these findings, a decision was made to ablate the PVC focus which was suspected to be in the moderator band (**Fig. 7**). The PVC was mapped and ablated at the distal end of the moderator band which is close the junction between the moderator band and the anterior papillary muscle (**Fig. 8**). The earliest ventricular activation was in that area (24 ms before the onset of the QRS complex—**Fig. 9**), and pace mapping showed a 97% morphology match. Furthermore, substrate mapping showed no abnormalities in the RV. At the end of the procedure, there were no spontaneous or inducible PVCs. A year later, the patient continues to do well with no recurrent ventricular arrhythmias off beta blocker therapy.

## Case 2

A 14-year-old previously healthy athlete had an out-of-hospital cardiac arrest and was subsequently diagnosed with CPVT. He underwent single chamber ICD implantation and was started on nadolol 40 mg daily. A few years later, he had appropriate ICD shocks due to VF during a baseball game. No clear discernible trigger could be identified for ablation. The patient was then started on Flecainide 150 mg twice daily. To prevent recurrent ICD shocks, a decision was made to pursue sympathectomy which was done via a left thoracoscopic video-assisted approach. The sympathetic chain was removed just below the ganglion at T4 and extending up to the stellate ganglion which was divided at its midpoint

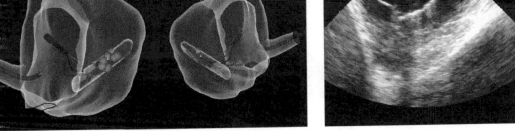

**Fig. 8.** Ablation site at the distal end of the moderator band.

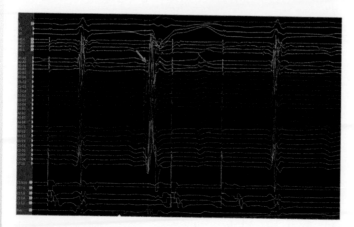

**Fig. 9.** Intracardiac electrograms showing the earliest ventricular activation with a Purkinje potential (*yellow arrow*) noted at the distal end of the moderator band.

(**Fig. 10**). Five years later, the patient continues to do well with no recurrent ventricular arrhythmias.

## SUMMARY

VF is a significant cause of cardiovascular morbidity and mortality. A better mechanistic understanding of the underlying arrhythmogenesis in VF and the use of targeted ablative therapies have enabled us to manage patients with VF more effectively. Catheter ablation targeting triggers including ventricular ectopy and Purkinje potentials has been promising. Autonomic modulation via cardiac and renal sympathetic denervation has also been effective in preventing VF recurrence when used as an adjunct to conventional therapies. Further research is needed to elucidate the substrate needed for VF maintenance and thereby expand the treatment armamentarium for VF.

## CLINICS CARE POINTS

- Adequate localization of the triggering sources of ventricular fibrillation (VF) is critical to the success of trigger-guided ablation.

- The His-Purkinje system (HPS) has been commonly implicated in the initiation of idiopathic VF.

- Substrate modification for VF is limited by current lapses in our understanding of the critical substrate required for VF maintenance.

- Cardiac and renal sympathetic denervation are effective in treating VF storm through interruption of sympathetic input to the heart.

## DISCLOSURE

Dr S.J. Asirvatham receives honoraria or speaker fees from Abiomed, Atricure, Biotronik, Blackwell Futura, Boston Scientific, Medtronic, Medtelligence, Spectranetics, St. Jude, and Zoll. Dr C.V. DeSimone is supported by the Dr Earl Wood, Career Development Benefactor award. Dr C.V. DeSimone and Dr S.J. Asirvatham have several patent submissions regarding novel mapping tools and ablation techniques for ventricular fibrillation. All other authors have no conflicts of interest to disclose relevant to the content of this article.

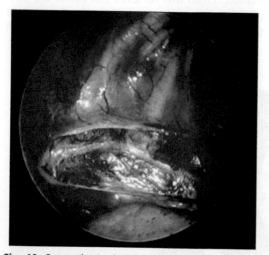

**Fig. 10.** Sympathetic chain at the inferior aspect of the stellate ganglion targeted during sympathetic cardiac denervation.

## REFERENCES

1. Khan R. Identifying and understanding the role of pulmonary vein activity in atrial fibrillation. Cardiovasc Res 2004;64(3):387–94.

2. Willems S, Klemm H, Rostock T, et al. Substrate modification combined with pulmonary vein isolation improves outcome of catheter ablation in patients with persistent atrial fibrillation: a prospective randomized comparison. Eur Heart J 2006;27(23): 2871–8.

3. Roten L, Derval N, Jaïs P. Catheter ablation for persistent atrial fibrillation: elimination of triggers is not sufficient. Circ Arrhythm Electrophysiol 2012; 5(6):1224–32 [discussion: 32].

4. Krummen DE, Ho G, Villongco CT, et al. Ventricular fibrillation: triggers, mechanisms and therapies. Future Cardiol 2016;12(3):373–90.

5. Haissaguerre M, Vigmond E, Stuyvers B, et al. Ventricular arrhythmias and the His-Purkinje system. Nat Rev Cardiol 2016;13(3):155–66.

6. Winfree AT. Spiral waves of chemical activity. Science 1972;175(4022):634–6.

7. Biktasheva IV, Biktashev VN. Wave-particle dualism of spiral waves dynamics. Phys Rev E Stat Nonlin Soft Matter Phys 2003;67(2 Pt 2):026221.

8. Chen J, Mandapati R, Berenfeld O, et al. High-frequency periodic sources underlie ventricular fibrillation in the isolated rabbit heart. Circ Res 2000;86(1): 86–93.

9. Jalife J. Ventricular fibrillation: mechanisms of initiation and maintenance. Annu Rev Physiol 2000;62: 25–50.

10. Gelzer AR, Koller ML, Otani NF, et al. Dynamic mechanism for initiation of ventricular fibrillation in vivo. Circulation 2008;118(11):1123–9.

11. Everett THt, Wilson EE, Foreman S, et al. Mechanisms of ventricular fibrillation in canine models of congestive heart failure and ischemia assessed by in vivo noncontact mapping. Circulation 2005; 112(11):1532–41.

12. Mandapati R, Asano Y, Baxter WT, et al. Quantification of effects of global ischemia on dynamics of ventricular fibrillation in isolated rabbit heart. Circulation 1998;98(16):1688–96.

13. Nanthakumar K, Jalife J, Massé S, et al. Optical mapping of Langendorff-perfused human hearts: establishing a model for the study of ventricular fibrillation in humans. Am J Physiol Heart Circ Physiol 2007;293(1):H875–80.

14. Leenhardt A, Glaser E, Burguera M, et al. Short-coupled variant of torsade de pointes. A new electrocardiographic entity in the spectrum of idiopathic ventricular tachyarrhythmias. Circulation 1994;89(1): 206–15.

15. Saliba W, Abul Karim A, Tchou P, et al. Ventricular fibrillation: ablation of a trigger? J Cardiovasc Electrophysiol 2002;13(12):1296–9.

16. Yap J, Tan VH, Hsu LF, et al. Catheter ablation of ventricular fibrillation storm in a long QT syndrome genotype carrier with normal QT interval. Singapore Med J 2013;54(1):e1–4.

17. Haïssaguerre M, Shoda M, Jaïs P, et al. Mapping and ablation of idiopathic ventricular fibrillation. Circulation 2002;106(8):962–7.

18. Knecht S, Sacher F, Wright M, et al. Long-term follow-up of idiopathic ventricular fibrillation ablation: a multicenter study. J Am Coll Cardiol 2009;54(6): 522–8.

19. Haïssaguerre M, Shah DC, Jaïs P, et al. Role of Purkinje conducting system in triggering of idiopathic ventricular fibrillation. Lancet 2002;359(9307): 677–8.

20. Van Herendael H, Zado ES, Haqqani H, et al. Catheter ablation of ventricular fibrillation: importance of left ventricular outflow tract and papillary muscle triggers. Heart Rhythm 2014;11(4):566–73.

21. Haïssaguerre M, Duchateau J, Dubois R, et al. Idiopathic ventricular fibrillation: role of Purkinje system and microstructural myocardial abnormalities. JACC Clin Electrophysiol 2020;6(6):591–608.

22. Santoro F, Di Biase L, Hranitzky P, et al. Ventricular fibrillation triggered by PVCs from papillary muscles: clinical features and ablation. J Cardiovasc Electrophysiol 2014;25(11):1158–64.

23. Sadek MM, Benhayon D, Sureddi R, et al. Idiopathic ventricular arrhythmias originating from the moderator band: electrocardiographic characteristics and treatment by catheter ablation. Heart Rhythm 2015;12(1):67–75.

24. Surget E, Cheniti G, Ramirez FD, et al. Sex differences in the origin of Purkinje ectopy-initiated idiopathic ventricular fibrillation. Heart Rhythm 2021; 18(10):1647–54.

25. Kumar N, Aksoy I, Phan K, et al. Coronary spasm during cardiac electrophysiological study following isoproterenol infusion. Interv Med Appl Sci 2014; 6(4):183–6.

26. Tadros R, Nannenberg EA, Lieve KV, et al. Yield and pitfalls of ajmaline testing in the evaluation of unexplained cardiac arrest and sudden unexplained death: single-center experience with 482 families. JACC Clin Electrophysiol 2017;3(12):1400–8.

27. Zehender M, Brugada P, Geibel A, et al. Programmed electrical stimulation in healed myocardial infarction using a standardized ventricular stimulation protocol. Am J Cardiol 1987;59(6):578–85.

28. Cheniti G, Vlachos K, Meo M, et al. Mapping and ablation of idiopathic ventricular fibrillation. Front Cardiovasc Med 2018;5:123.

29. Bogun F, Taj M, Ting M, et al. Spatial resolution of pace mapping of idiopathic ventricular tachycardia/ectopy originating in the right ventricular outflow tract. Heart Rhythm 2008;5(3):339–44.

30. Hillsley RE, Bollacker KD, Simpson EV, et al. Alteration of ventricular fibrillation by propranolol and isoproterenol detected by epicardial mapping with 506 electrodes. J Cardiovasc Electrophysiol 1995; 6(6):471–85.

31. Xanthos T, Pantazopoulos I, Demestiha T, et al. Epinephrine in ventricular fibrillation: friend or foe? A review for the Emergency Nurse. J Emerg Nurs 2011;37(4):408–12 [quiz: 25–6].

32. Kohl P, Nesbitt AD, Cooper PJ, et al. Sudden cardiac death by Commotio cordis: role of mechano-electric feedback. Cardiovasc Res 2001;50(2):280–9.

33. Trayanova NA, Constantino J, Gurev V. Models of stretch-activated ventricular arrhythmias. J Electrocardiol 2010;43(6):479–85.

34. Bode F, Franz MR, Wilke I, et al. Ventricular fibrillation induced by stretch pulse: implications for sudden death due to commotio cordis. J Cardiovasc Electrophysiol 2006;17(9):1011–7.

35. Quinn TA, Jin H, Lee P, et al. Mechanically induced ectopy via stretch-activated cation-nonselective channels is caused by local tissue deformation and results in ventricular fibrillation if triggered on the repolarization wave edge (commotio cordis). Circ Arrhythm Electrophysiol 2017;10(8): e004777.

36. Riemer TL, Sobie EA, Tung L. Stretch-induced changes in arrhythmogenesis and excitability in experimentally based heart cell models. Am J Physiol 1998;275(2):H431–42.

37. Maor E, Sugrue A, Witt C, et al. Pulsed electric fields for cardiac ablation and beyond: a state-of-the-art review. Heart Rhythm 2019;16(7):1112–20.

38. Sugrue A, Vaidya V, Witt C, et al. Irreversible electroporation for catheter-based cardiac ablation: a systematic review of the preclinical experience. J Interv Card Electrophysiol 2019;55(3): 251–65.

39. Livia C, Sugrue A, Witt T, et al. Elimination of Purkinje fibers by electroporation reduces ventricular fibrillation vulnerability. J Am Heart Assoc 2018;7(15): e009070.

40. Sugrue A, Vaidya VR, Livia C, et al. Feasibility of selective cardiac ventricular electroporation. PLoS One 2020;15(2):e0229214.

41. DeSimone CV, Asirvatham SJ. Purkinje tissue modification and ventricular fibrillation. Pacing Clin Electrophysiol 2019;42(10):1291–3.

42. Berenfeld O, Jalife J. Purkinje-muscle reentry as a mechanism of polymorphic ventricular arrhythmias in a 3-dimensional model of the ventricles. Circ Res 1998;82(10):1063–77.

43. Worley SJ, Swain JL, Colavita PG, et al. Development of an endocardial-epicardial gradient of activation rate during electrically induced, sustained ventricular fibrillation in dogs. Am J Cardiol 1985; 55(6):813–20.

44. Newton JC, Smith WM, Ideker RE. Estimated global transmural distribution of activation rate and conduction block during porcine and canine ventricular fibrillation. Circ Res 2004;94(6): 836–42.

45. Huang J, Dosdall DJ, Cheng KA, et al. The importance of Purkinje activation in long duration ventricular fibrillation. J Am Heart Assoc 2014;3(1):e000495.

46. Li L, Jin Q, Dosdall DJ, et al. Activation becomes highly organized during long-duration ventricular fibrillation in canine hearts. Am J Physiol Heart Circ Physiol 2010;298(6):H2046–53.

47. Tabereaux PB, Walcott GP, Rogers JM, et al. Activation patterns of Purkinje fibers during long-duration ventricular fibrillation in an isolated canine heart model. Circulation 2007;116(10):1113–9.

48. Lin C, Jin Q, Zhang N, et al. Endocardial focal activation originating from Purkinje fibers plays a role in the maintenance of long duration ventricular fibrillation. Croat Med J 2014;55(2):121–7.

49. Wu TJ, Lin SF, Hsieh YC, et al. Repetitive endocardial focal discharges during ventricular fibrillation with prolonged global ischemia in isolated rabbit hearts. Circ J 2009;73(10):1803–11.

50. Panitchob N, Li L, Huang J, et al. Endocardial activation Drives activation patterns during long-duration ventricular fibrillation and defibrillation. Circ Arrhythm Electrophysiol 2017;10(12):e005562.

51. Li L, Zheng X, Dosdall DJ, et al. Long-duration ventricular fibrillation exhibits 2 distinct organized states. Circ Arrhythm Electrophysiol 2013;6(6): 1192–9.

52. Dosdall DJ, Osorio J, Robichaux RP, et al. Purkinje activation precedes myocardial activation following defibrillation after long-duration ventricular fibrillation. Heart Rhythm 2010;7(3):405–12.

53. Tri J, Asirvatham R, DeSimone CV, et al. Intramural conduction system gradients and electrogram regularity during ventricular fibrillation. Indian Pacing Electrophysiol J 2018;18(6):195–200.

54. Tabereaux PB, Dosdall DJ, Ideker RE. Mechanisms of VF maintenance: wandering wavelets, mother rotors, or foci. Heart Rhythm 2009;6(3):405–15.

55. Filgueiras-Rama D, Jalife J. Structural and functional bases OF cardiac fibrillation. Differences and similarities between atria and ventricles. JACC Clin Electrophysiol 2016;2(1):1–3.

56. Zaitsev AV, Guha PK, Sarmast F, et al. Wavebreak formation during ventricular fibrillation in the isolated, regionally ischemic pig heart. Circ Res 2003; 92(5):546–53.

57. Davidenko JM, Pertsov AV, Salomonsz R, et al. Stationary and drifting spiral waves of excitation in isolated cardiac muscle. Nature 1992;355(6358): 349–51.

58. Nair K, Umapathy K, Farid T, et al. Intramural activation during early human ventricular fibrillation. Circ Arrhythm Electrophysiol 2011;4(5):692–703.

59. Samie FH, Berenfeld O, Anumonwo J, et al. Rectification of the background potassium current: a determinant of rotor dynamics in ventricular fibrillation. Circ Res 2001;89(12):1216–23.

60. Warren M, Guha PK, Berenfeld O, et al. Blockade of the inward rectifying potassium current terminates ventricular fibrillation in the Guinea pig heart. J Cardiovasc Electrophysiol 2003;14(6):621–31.

61. Krummen DE, Hayase J, Morris DJ, et al. Rotor stability separates sustained ventricular fibrillation from self-terminating episodes in humans. J Am Coll Cardiol 2014;63(24):2712–21.

62. Damiano RJ Jr, Smith PK, Tripp HF Jr, et al. The effect of chemical ablation of the endocardium on ventricular fibrillation threshold. Circulation 1986;74(3):645–52.

63. Dosdall DJ, Tabereaux PB, Kim JJ, et al. Chemical ablation of the Purkinje system causes early termination and activation rate slowing of long-duration ventricular fibrillation in dogs. Am J Physiol Heart Circ Physiol 2008;295(2):H883–9.

64. Kim YH, Xie F, Yashima M, et al. Role of papillary muscle in the generation and maintenance of reentry during ventricular tachycardia and fibrillation in isolated swine right ventricle. Circulation 1999; 100(13):1450–9.

65. Pak HN, Kim GI, Lim HE, et al. Both Purkinje cells and left ventricular posteroseptal reentry contribute to the maintenance of ventricular fibrillation in open-chest dogs and swine: effects of catheter ablation and the ventricular cut-and-sew operation. Circ J 2008;72(7):1185–92.

66. Krummen DE, Hayase J, Vampola SP, et al. Modifying ventricular fibrillation by targeted rotor substrate ablation: proof-of-concept from experimental studies to clinical VF. J Cardiovasc Electrophysiol 2015;26(10):1117–26.

67. Maury P, Duchateau J, Rollin A, et al. Long-lasting ventricular fibrillation in humans ECG characteristics and effect of radiofrequency ablation. Circ Arrhythm Electrophysiol 2020;13(10):e008639.

68. Tan NY, Christopoulos G, Ladas TP, et al. Regional and temporal variation of ventricular and conduction tissue activity during ventricular fibrillation in canines. Circ Arrhythm Electrophysiol 2021;14(10): e010281.

69. Shen MJ, Zipes DP. Role of the autonomic nervous system in modulating cardiac arrhythmias. Circ Res 2014;114(6):1004–21.

70. Chiou CW, Eble JN, Zipes DP. Efferent vagal innervation of the canine atria and sinus and atrioventricular nodes. The third fat pad. Circulation 1997; 95(11):2573–84.

71. Armour JA, Murphy DA, Yuan BX, et al. Gross and microscopic anatomy of the human intrinsic cardiac nervous system. Anat Rec 1997;247(2):289–98.

72. Manolis AA, Manolis TA, Apostolopoulos EJ, et al. The role of the autonomic nervous system in cardiac arrhythmias: the neuro-cardiac axis, more foe than friend? Trends Cardiovasc Med 2021;31(5): 290–302.

73. Frontera A, Vlachos K, Kitamura T, et al. Long-term follow-up of idiopathic ventricular fibrillation in a pediatric population: clinical characteristics, management, and complications. J Am Heart Assoc 2019; 8(9):e011172.

74. Kasanuki H, Ohnishi S, Ohtuka M, et al. Idiopathic ventricular fibrillation induced with vagal activity in patients without obvious heart disease. Circulation 1997;95(9):2277–85.

75. Opthof T, Misier AR, Coronel R, et al. Dispersion of refractoriness in canine ventricular myocardium. Effects of sympathetic stimulation. Circ Res 1991; 68(5):1204–15.

76. Ng GA, Brack KE, Patel VH, et al. Autonomic modulation of electrical restitution, alternans and ventricular fibrillation initiation in the isolated heart. Cardiovasc Res 2007;73(4):750–60.

77. Tomaselli GF, Zipes DP. What causes sudden death in heart failure? Circ Res 2004;95(8):754–63.

78. Barber MJ, Mueller TM, Henry DP, et al. Transmural myocardial infarction in the dog produces sympathectomy in noninfarcted myocardium. Circulation 1983;67(4):787–96.

79. Scherf D, Blumenfeld S, Yildiz M. Experimental study on ventricular extrasystoles provoked by vagal stimulation. Am Heart J 1961;62:670–5.

80. Scherf D, Cohen J, Rafailzadeh M. Excitatory effects of carotid sinus pressure. Enhancement of ectopic impulse formation and of impulse conduction. Am J Cardiol 1966;17(2):240–52.

81. Amitzur G, Manoach M, Weinstock M. The influence of cardiac cholinergic activation on the induction and maintenance of ventricular fibrillation. Basic Res Cardiol 1984;79(6):690–7.

82. Meng L, Tseng CH, Shivkumar K, et al. Efficacy of stellate ganglion blockade in managing electrical storm: a systematic review. JACC Clin Electrophysiol 2017;3(9):942–9.

83. Odero A, Bozzani A, De Ferrari GM, et al. Left cardiac sympathetic denervation for the prevention of life-threatening arrhythmias: the surgical supraclavicular approach to cervicothoracic sympathectomy. Heart Rhythm 2010;7(8):1161–5.

84. Collura CA, Johnson JN, Moir C, et al. Left cardiac sympathetic denervation for the treatment of long QT syndrome and catecholaminergic polymorphic ventricular tachycardia using video-assisted thoracic surgery. Heart Rhythm 2009;6(6):752–9.

85. Schlaich MP, Sobotka PA, Krum H, et al. Renal sympathetic-nerve ablation for uncontrolled hypertension. N Engl J Med 2009;361(9):932–4.

86. Krum H, Schlaich MP, Sobotka PA, et al. Percutaneous renal denervation in patients with treatment-resistant hypertension: final 3-year report of the Symplicity HTN-1 study. Lancet 2014;383(9917): 622–9.

87. Ukena C, Bauer A, Mahfoud F, et al. Renal sympathetic denervation for treatment of electrical storm: first-in-man experience. Clin Res Cardiol 2012; 101(1):63–7.

88. Armaganijan LV, Staico R, Moreira DA, et al. 6-Month outcomes in patients with implantable cardioverter-Defibrillators undergoing renal sympathetic denervation for the treatment of refractory ventricular arrhythmias. JACC Cardiovasc Interv 2015;8(7): 984–90.

89. Zhu C, Hanna P, Rajendran PS, et al. Neuromodulation for ventricular tachycardia and atrial fibrillation: a clinical scenario-based review. JACC Clin Electrophysiol 2019;5(8):881–96.

# Chemical Ablation of Ventricular Tachycardia Using Coronary Arterial and Venous Systems

Thomas Flautt, DO, Miguel Valderrábano, MD*

## KEYWORDS

- Ventricular arrhythmia • Ventricular tachycardia • Transcoronary ethanol ablation
- Radiofrequency catheter ablation • Ethanol • VT ablation

## KEY POINTS

- Radiofrequency catheter ablation is the first-line treatment of ventricular arrhythmias; however, difficult anatomic locations or proximity to coronary vessels may limit its efficacy.
- Transcoronary ethanol ablation (TCEA) has been used as an adjunctive ablation technique but has been plagued by complications including atrioventricular block, coronary arterial dissection, thrombosis, and myocardial infarction.
- Retrograde coronary venous ethanol ablation (RCVEA) has multiple advantages to TCEA including less risk with cannulation, unobstructed access to the coronary bed in patients with severe coronary artery disease, less risk of coronary collateral damage, and redundant venous anatomy.
- RCVEA provides access to the epicardium, targeting notoriously difficult areas to reach such as the left ventricular summit.

## INTRODUCTION

Ventricular arrhythmias (VAs) are an important cause of morbidity and mortality. VAs range from single premature ventricular complexes to sustained ventricular tachycardia (VT) and ventricular fibrillation.[1] For decades, surgeons, interventional cardiologists, and cardiac electrophysiologists have sought the safest and most efficacious treatment of VAs. Currently, radiofrequency catheter ablation (RFCA) is the undisputed first-line therapy for treatment of drug-refractory VAs.[2] The success of catheter ablation depends on the ability to reach the anatomic location of the VT substrate. VTs arising from deep intramural regions or near coronary vessels can have limited RFCA success.[3] It has proven to be 81% effective in the acute abolition of VT,[4] but only about 49% of patients will remain free of disease during medium-term follow-up.[5] In this article, the authors discuss the adjunctive techniques for targeting VAs, using chemical ablation of VAs in the coronary arterial and venous system.

## WHY ETHANOL?

Ethanol (CH3CH2OH) is a short-chain alcohol, water-soluble compound that rapidly crosses the cell membranes. When cells are exposed to high concentrations, ethanol solubilizes the cell membranes and alters the tertiary protein structures, leading to immediate cell destruction.[6,7] Most of the fluid membranes, including those that are low in cholesterol, are the most easily solubilized by ethanol. Ethanol interferes with the packing of molecules in the phospholipid bilayer of the cell

Division of Cardiac Electrophysiology, Department of Cardiology, Houston Methodist DeBakey Heart and Vascular Center, Houston Methodist Hospital, Houston, TX, USA
* Corresponding author. Division of Cardiac Electrophysiology, Department of Cardiology, Houston Methodist Hospital, 6550 Fannin Street, Suite 1801, Houston, TX 77030.
E-mail address: mvalderrabano@houstonmethodist.org

Card Electrophysiol Clin 14 (2022) 743–756
https://doi.org/10.1016/j.ccep.2022.08.002
1877-9182/22/© 2022 Elsevier Inc. All rights reserved.

membrane, thus increasing membrane fluidity. Additional subcellular effects have been reported, including biochemical alterations of mitochondria such as decreases in mitochondrial ATPase activity,[8] leading to mitochondrial dysfunction, as reported in ethanol-induced cardiomyopathy,[9] but it may not be significant in the acute setting.[10]

Intravascular ethanol infusion may have additional effects related to vascular damage with sclerosis of the injected vessel, which follows routinely after infusion. In intra-arterial infusions, tissue ischemia, and infarction of the injected territory are expected to play a role in ethanol's therapeutic effect.[11] Venous sclerosis is also to be expected.[12]

## HISTORY OF CHEMICAL ABLATION FOR VENTRICULAR ARRHYTHMIAS

The first successful VT ablation with ethanol (intramyocardial) was reported in dogs by Chilson and colleagues[13] in 1986 and by the transcoronary approach by Inoue and colleagues[14] in 1987, both in Zipes' animal laboratory. In their animal study, focal VT induced by intramyocardial injection of aconitine was suppressed by ethanol (at least 50% concentration) or phenol injection delivered into the artery supplying the aconitine-injected myocardial tissue. Successful VT elimination was correlated with myocardial necrosis and arterial thrombus formation, which were not achieved by lower (25%) ethanol concentrations. In 1988, Brugada and colleagues reported effective cure of VT by intracoronary arterial ethanol infusion in three patients who had remained in incessant VT refractory to multiple treatment modalities.[15] Kay and colleagues[16] prospectively evaluated the clinical utility of intra-arterial ethanol infusion for VT in 23 patients. They found that VT could be terminated by injections of saline solution or contrast medium in 11 of the 21 patients in whom the protocol could be completed. Ethanol was infused in 10 of these patients and led to acute elimination of VT inducibility in 90% of them.[16] After repeating the electrophysiology study, inducibility recovered in two other patients, yielding an overall success of 70%. Associated complications included complete atrioventricular block in four patients (40%) and pericarditis in one patient. Initial ethanol dose and concentration ("absolute" or 96%–98%) seemed to be arbitrarily selected. Haines and colleagues[17] performed a systematic study in dogs addressing these issues, testing different concentrations (0%, 10%, 25%, 50%, 75%, and 100%) as the ethanol concentration increased, the ablation vessels were more persistently occluded and the size of identifiable myocardial lesions increased significantly with increasing ethanol concentration, although there was significant variability within groups. **Table 1** summarizes the reported results of ethanol ablation of VT.[11]

## TRANSCORONARY ETHANOL ABLATION: CURRENT ROLE

Although RFCA with epicardial and endocardial mapping can successfully treat most refractory VTs, there remains a subset of patients whose VT is not amenable to RFCA. These are mainly VTs with deep midmyocardial origin in which radiofrequency energy cannot achieve sufficient therapeutic effect. Another group is patients with epicardial circuits and history of heart surgery, making epicardial access difficult if not impossible. In a large series of RF-refractory VTs, Kumar and colleagues showed transcoronary ethanol ablation (TCEA)'s value in rescuing these otherwise impossible to treat patients.[18]

Although TCEA is reasonably successful in treating RCFA-refractory VTs, there are technical difficulties and potential complications inherent to coronary artery instrumentation, such as coronary arterial dissection, thrombosis, and myocardial infarction. Other complications are related to spillage of ethanol to nontargeted myocardium resulting in interventricular conduction blocks and infarction of nonselected regions.[19,20]

## RETROGRADE CORONARY VENOUS ETHANOL ABLATION

Recognizing these limitations of intra-arterial delivery, Inoue and colleagues[14] originally described that coronary sinus (CS) phenol infusion in dogs led to "considerable" subendocardial necrosis, but there were no additional descriptions. Wright and colleagues[21] explored the retrograde venous approach in a canine model. Balloon occlusion of the distal anterior interventricular vein or the distal great cardiac vein (GCV) was performed, and then, ethanol was infused at 1.5, 3, and 5 mL. They found that transmural lesions could be achieved when infused ethanol volumes were at least 3 mL and hypothesized that for smaller volumes, collateral flow via thebesian veins into the left ventricular (LV) cavity could prevent ethanol from reaching the capillaries, where its ablative action would reach the myocardial cells.[11]

### Venous Versus Arterial Ethanol

Retrograde coronary venous ethanol ablation (RCVEA) is favored over TCEA for multiple reasons. With a venous approach, a relatively unobstructed access to the capillary bed is available

**Table 1**
Results of transcoronary arterial ethanol ablation of ventricular tachycardia

| Study Reference, Year | Study Design | Patients (n) | Age (Years) | Indications | Follow-up | Results | Complications | Observations |
|---|---|---|---|---|---|---|---|---|
| Brugada et al,[15] 1989 | Intracoronary 96% ethanol injection | 3 | 44,61,62 | Incessant tachycardia postmyocardial infarction | 2-9 months (mean 5,7) | Cease or arrhythmia in 100% (one recurrence at 1 month, repeating procedure successfully) | Short-lasting chest pain in all the patients <br><br><br><br><br> Temporary complete AV block with pacemaker implantation in 1 patient (33%) Small to moderate AST rise | Chemical abiation of the arrhythmogenic resulted in cure of the disorder. Size of the ablation should be as limited as possible. New collateral blood supply may lead to recurrence. |
| Kay et al,[16] 1992 | Intracoronary 96% ethanol injection | 23 (10 received ethanol) | 59±12 | Sustained nomomorphic ventricular tachycardia related to prior MI | 102-788 | Cease in 100%, with inducible VT in 3 patients (30%) Little or no change in LVEF | Complete AV block in 4 patients (40%) <br><br><br> Pericarditis (Dressler's syndrome) in 1 patient (10%) | Moderate degree of efficacy and potential for complications. Long-term control for particular patients.Limited by the frequent inability to localize the arrhythmia-related vessel. |

(continued on next page)

**Table 1**
*(continued)*

| Study Reference, Year | Study Design | Patients (n) | Age (Years) | Indications | Follow-up | Results | Complications | Observations |
|---|---|---|---|---|---|---|---|---|
| Tokuda et al,[20] 2011 | Intracoronary 96% ethanol injection | 27-out of these,22 received ethanol | 63 ± 13 | Symptomatic monomorphic VT refractory to RFA;structural heart disease | 20 ± 11 months | VT was no inducible after ablation in 18 patients (82%) VT recurrence in 14 patients (64%) Nine out of 11 were free from VT storm | Complete heat block in 5 patients (38 % of 13 patients with intact AV conduction) Temporary coronary spasm 1 patient (5%) Total mortality, 32%, early mortality (within 30 days) 14% and late mortality 18% CK,CK-MB and Trop I elevation | Important role for difficult VTs in high-risk patients. Prevents recurrences in 36% and improves arrhythmia control in an additional 27% |
| Sacher et al,[19] 2008 | Intracoronary 96% ethanol injection | 9 | 55 ± 9 | Refractory monomorphic VT due to scar-related re-entry; ischemic cardiomyopathy in 6 patients (67%) | 29 ± 23 | No VT recurrence in 67% No significant change in LVEF CK-MB and Trop I rise with injection | Transient ST-elevation during injection in 5 patients (55%) Immediate:transient severe hypotension in 2 patients (22%) and bilateral groin hematomas in 1 patient (11%) Three patients died in the follow -up from refractory HF (33%) | Applicable alternative espectially in cases of septal scar (VT circuits deep intramyocardial). TCEA rarely used (1.4%). |

*From* Schurmann P, Peñalver J, Valderrábano M. Ethanol for the treatment of cardiac arrhythmias. Curr Opin Cardiol. 2015;30(4):333-343. https://doi.org/10.1097/HCO. 0000000000000183; with permission.

even in patients with severe coronary artery disease. There is less risk associated with cannulation of the coronary veins than of the coronary arteries. There is also a less risk of damaging collateral arteries. RCVEA also remains a feasible option in patients in whom previous coronary artery bypass graft may limit access to the pericardium and to the coronary arteries for arterial ethanol ablation. However, there remain uncertainties regarding the safety and utility of RCVEA that this initial report cannot address. Although the size of the ventricular vein selected for ethanol infusion can be expected to correlate with the extent of tissue reached and ablated by ethanol, there is no control as to the extent of myocardial tissue ablated by ethanol, which may be excessive. In addition, the venous anatomy may not always provide access to the targeted myocardium.

The coronary venous anatomy is extremely redundant. Aside from venous return to the CS, thebesian veins can drain directly into the LV cavity.[21] Within the epicardial venous system, collateral veins abound, communicating epicardial veins with one another and the CS (**Fig. 1**). When targeting the myocardium with ethanol, it is important to use a vein with direct connection to capillaries to avoid ethanol shunting. Collateral veins may be present at baseline injection.

In some cases, collateral veins disappear after ethanol, whereas in others, they became more prominent. It has been hypothesized that ethanol obliterates capillaries. Collateral veins arising after the capillary territory obliterated by ethanol will disappear after ethanol, whereas those collateral veins arising before the capillaries may become more prominent. **Fig. 1** shows a schematic illustrating this concept.[22]

This is particularly true for VT originating from the LV summit (LVS), where an intramural origin, proximity to coronary vessels, and inaccessibility to the epicardial approach limit RFCA success.[23]

## VENOUS ETHANOL FOR LEFT VENTRICULAR SUMMIT
### Anatomy

Intramural branches of the coronary venous system offer a unique opportunity for reaching arrhythmogenic foci, and RCVEA can effectively treat VAs. [22,24,25] Successful VEA requires a comprehensive appreciation of the morphologic arrangement of cardiac veins, particularly of the LVS. The number and location of coronary tributaries vary, and their size and course are also notoriously diverse.[26] Previous studies have used computed tomography to describe the relationship between the coronary venous and arterial systems and the main tributaries of the CS[26,27]; however, the epicardial and intramural branches of LVS tributaries have not been studied in detail. LVS vein nomenclature often is imprecise and inconsistent, as LVS veins are referred to as "communicating veins" or "septal perforators,"[28–30] without discriminating their relationship

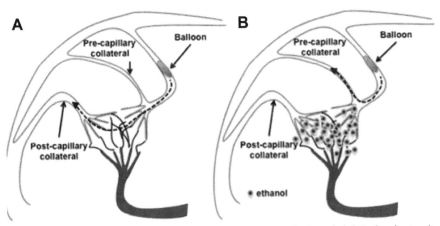

**Fig. 1.** Schematic of coronary venous flow and the proposed effects of ethanol. (*A*) Redundant epicardial coronary veins show vein branches followed by venules leading to capillaries. Precapillary collaterals and postcapillary collaterals exist. Not shown are thebesian veins draining into left ventricle (LV) and right ventricle (RV) cavity. Selective retrograde contrast injection shows flow into the capillaries (myocardial staining) and through postcapillary collaterals. (*B*) After ethanol infusion, capillaries are obliterated, and repeated retrograde contrast cannot reach postcapillary collaterals. If precapillary collaterals exist, flow through them is enhanced after ethanol. (*From* Kreidieh B, Rodríguez-Mañero M, Schurmann P, Ibarra-Cortez SH, Dave AS, Valderrábano M. Retrograde Coronary Venous Ethanol Infusion for Ablation of Refractory Ventricular Tachycardia. Circ Arrhythm Electrophysiol. 2016;9(7):10.1161/CIRCEP.116.004352 e004352. https://doi.org/10.1161/CIRCEP.116.004352; with permission.)

to neighboring structures such as the mitral annulus, aortic root, right ventricular (RV) outflow tract (RVOT), and LVOT.

Our group compiled 53 patients undergoing RCVEA for LVS VAs. We analyzed the angiographic anatomy of all 53 patients considered for LVS VEA and correlated vein location with the mapped geometry of the anterior intraventricular vein (AIV), LVOT, and RVOT on three-dimensional (3D) (CARTO) maps. Starting from the GCV, the LVS veins included the following (**Fig. 2**).

Below is a comprehensive review of the venous anatomy.

### Great cardiac vein –anterior intraventricular vein transition

Angulations in the GCV–AIV transition have previously been measured.[27] For the electrophysiologist attempting to reach the LVS area through the GCV or AIV, this is important because a steep angle at the GCV–AIV transition make difficult cannulation with large or stiff multipolar catheters. In our experience, sharply angled GCV–AIV transitions can make cannulation with a DecaNav (Biosense Webster) catheter difficult, and advancement of a subselector left internal mammary artery (LIMA) or JR4 into the proximal AIV

can be unstable and counterproductive when trying to direct their tip toward septal branches.[31]

### Left ventricular annular vein

Left ventricular annular vein: The LVA was present in 19 of 53 venograms (36%). Defined as a branch of the GCV arising before the GCV–AIV junction, in the mitral annulus and traveling toward the septum, ending in the aortomitral continuity (**Fig. 3**). The LVA communicated with atrial branches and with branches posterior to the aortic root. LVA communicated via collateral flow with the LVS septal veins in 11 of 19 patients (58%) (**Fig. 4**). In the LAO projection, the LVA vein coursed more septal than the AIV, toward the aortomitral continuity, giving posterior branches to the left atrium and anterior branches toward the AIV septal vein, which overlapped in this projection (see **Fig. 4F**). In the right anterior oblique (RAO) projection, the LVA was completely foreshortened (see **Fig. 4**) and overlapping the GCV, and only its retroaortic/atrial branches or collaterals to AIV septals were visible (see **Fig. 4G**). LVA cannulation with multielectrode catheters would typically contain atrial and ventricular signals (hence the "annular" denomination) (see **Fig. 4C**). The LVA contained arrhythmogenic substrate and was targeted for ethanol infusion in

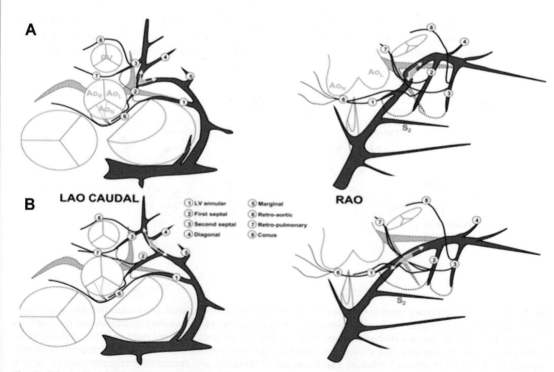

**Fig. 2.** Schematic of left ventricular (LV) summit (LVS) veins. (*A*) Angled great cardiac vein–anterior interventricular vein (GCV–AIV) junction. (*B*): Nonangled GCV–AIV junction. Left anterior oblique (LAO) caudal is best to display the sequence of LVS veins, whereas right anterior oblique (RAO) foreshortens the LV annular vein. LVS veins are labeled. Ao L, Ao R, Ao N, left, right, and noncoronary aortic cusp; PV, pulmonary valve.

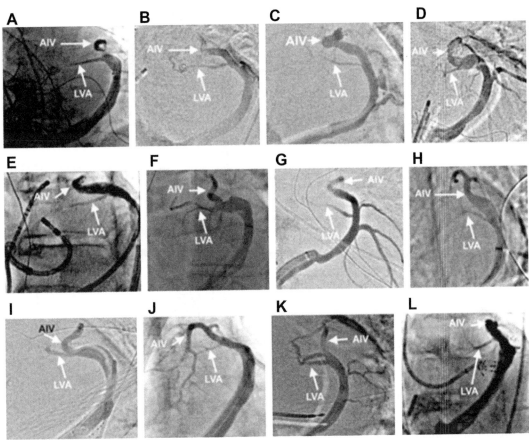

**Fig. 3.** Left ventricular annular (LVA) vein examples. (*A–L*) Examples of LVA shown in left anterior oblique, steep caudal projection. LVA arises from the GCV before the GCV–AIV transition, runs toward the septum, underneath the GCV–AIV junction, toward the aortomitral continuity (see aortic valve prosthesis in A).

a minority (6/53 [11%]) of cases, with acute success in all six cases.[31]

### Left ventricular septal veins

*Left ventricular summit septal veins:* Defined as branches of the AIV that ran rightward and intramural to the interventricular groove. LVS septal veins could arise as high as the GCV–AIV junction, and there typically were more than one. **Fig. 5** shows the examples of their variability. A previous report labeled some LVS septal as LVS "communicating vein," a denomination that also included LVA veins.[28] LVS septal veins run rightward and deep in the septum (true "perforators") (see **Fig. 4**F). LVS septal veins arising at the GCV–AIV junction could connect with retroaortic branches and contain atrial signals, analogous to LVA veins, or with branches posterior to the RV outflow between the RVOT and LVOT. **Fig. 6** shows the examples of two LVS septal veins illustrating their 3D relationships with neighboring structures. The first LVS septal had atrial and ventricular signals and was retroaortic (see **Fig. 6**A–E), whereas the

second LVS septal ran anterior to the aorta and posterior to the RVOT (see **Fig. 6**F–K). More commonly, all LVS septals were located anterior to the aortic root (**Fig. 7**) and not retroaortic (which was typical of LVA veins). LVS septals were present in all 53 venograms. The LVS septal was targeted for ethanol infusion in 38 of 53 cases, with success in 37 of 38 (97%).[31]

*Left ventricular summit diagonal veins:* Defined as branches of the AIV that ran leftward to the interventricular groove. Diagonals can arise as high as the GCV–AIV junction. Diagonal veins were present in 51 of 53 venograms (96%). Examples are shown in **Fig. 5**L, M. Despite the near-consistent presence of LVS diagonal veins, they seldom harbored signals targeted for VEA. LVS diagonal veins were targeted, with success for ethanol infusion in two cases.[31]

*Collateral flow:* LVS veins commonly had collaterals communicating one another. LVA communicated with LVS septal veins in 11 of 19 (58%). LVS septal veins 1 and 2 also communicated with each other in 25 of 53 (47%) (see **Figs. 4, 5**I, and **7**).[31]

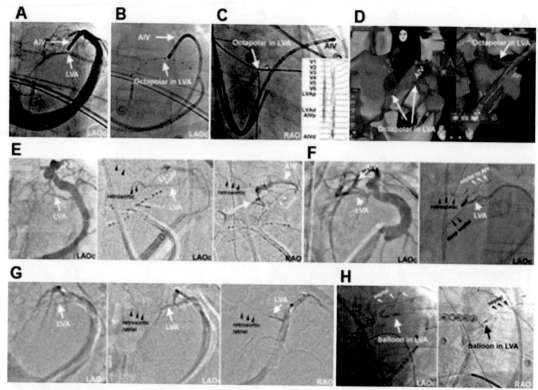

**Fig. 4.** Branching and 3-dimensional (3D) location of the LVA vein. (*A–D*). LVA cannulated with an octapolar cath-eter, in left anterior oblique steep caudal (LAOc) projection (*A, B*). (*C*) In right anterior oblique (RAO) projection, the LVA is foreshortened and basal and contains atrial and ventricular signals (inset). (*D*) Incorporating LVA to the 3D map, LVA wraps around the mitral valve in LAO (*left*) and posterior to the aorta in LAO cranial view (*right*) (*E–H*): Nonselective (e 1, f 1,g 1, h 1) versus selective LVA venograms. Selective LVA venograms show retroaortic branches and collaterals to septal branches of the AIV, both seen in LAOc (e 2, f 2, g 2) and RAO (e 3, g 3) projections.

*Branches beyond left ventricular summit:* Retro-aortic branches to right atrium and conus branches. Retroaortic branches of either LVA veins or proximal LVS septal veins arising close to the GCV–AIV junction could extend posterior to the aorta and connect with veins draining in the right atrium. Typically, LVS septal ran anterior to the aorta and posterior to the RVOT, but an RVOT conus vein, anterior to the RVOT, was seen in 7 of 53 cases.[31]

## Procedure

### Fluoroscopy
The veins are best visualized in left anterior oblique (LAO) (30°–45°), steep caudal (40°–50°) fluoro-scopic projection, analogous to the "spider view" used in coronary arteriography.

### Relevance of left anterior oblique caudal projection
Angiographic images of LVS veins are challenging due to foreshortening and overlap. Most previous reports contain RAO views, [28–30] which are adequate for LVS septal veins arising from the AIV, but RAO foreshortens the GCV as it wraps around the mitral annulus toward the LVS as well as LVA vein. Although RAO is useful to assess ret-roaortic versus retropulmonary vein courses, it has limited utility for vein selection. The LAO caudal is uniquely suited to display all LVS veins in their to-tality. The caudal angulation must be steep enough to display the AIV in an elongated fashion. Only then can the full spectrum of LVS veins be displayed at once.[31]

### Coronary sinus access and preliminary mapping
In all procedures, efforts should be made to localize VT substrate within an area amenable to RFA. Electroanatomical maps are constructed by using 3D mapping systems (NavX, St Jude Medi-cal, St Paul, MN) or Carto3 (Biosense-Webster, Diamond Bar, CA). Mapping strategies include substrate maps to localize low-bipolar voltage areas in the presence of structural heart disease,

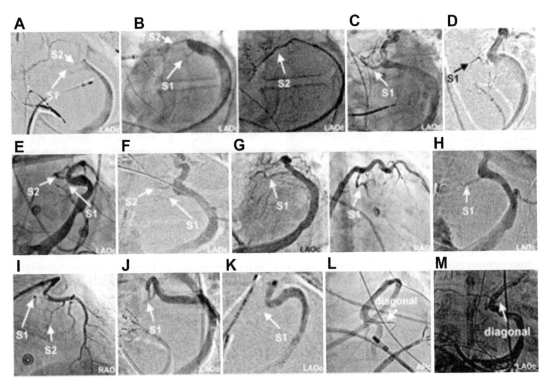

**Fig. 5.** LVS septal and diagonal veins. (*A–K*) Septal branches arise at the GCV–AIV junction (S1) and in the proximal AIV (S2). Typically, more than one septal branch exists with common collateral flow between them. In RAO (g 2), septal veins are foreshortened compared with LAO. (*L, M*) Diagonal veins arising from the proximal AIV (*L*: shown in anteroposterior cranial view [APc]) or from the GCV–AIV junction (*M*).

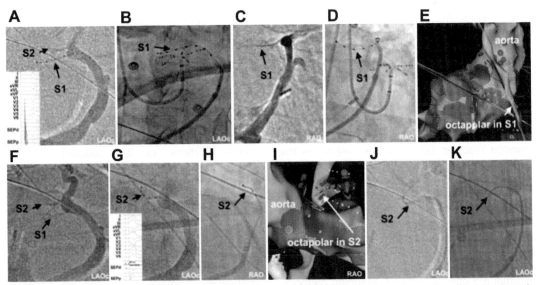

**Fig. 6.** Three-dimensional (3D) location of proximal GCV–AIV left ventricular summit septal veins. (*A*) Octapolar catheter in first septal (S1), showing atrial and ventricular signals (consecutive, proximal-to-distal septal bipolar signals SEPp-SEPd in the inset). (*B*) PentaRay catheter via retroaortic approach showing apparent overlap with octapolar. (*C–E*): Venogram and catheter positioning of S1 in RAO showing a posterior course relative to aorta, confirmed by 3D map from a left lateral view (*E*). (*F–K*): Cannulation of second septal (S2). Octapolar catheter in S2 (*G*) shows no atrial signals (inset) and an early signal in SEPd, which was targeted with ethanol. In RAO, octapolar catheter is foreshortened (*H*), but 3D map shows its course anterior to the aorta. (*J, K*) Selective venogram and balloon cannulation of S2.

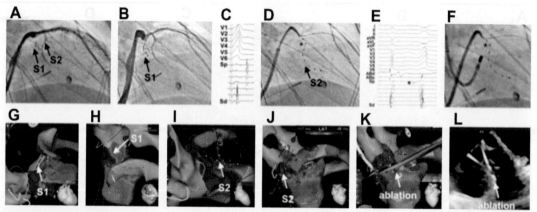

**Fig. 7.** Three-dimensional (3D) location of anterior interventricular vein (AIV) septal veins. (*A*) Right anterior oblique view of AIV venogram showing two septal branches with a collateral communication between them. (*B*) Octapolar catheter cannulation of the first septal (S1). (*C*) Consecutive proximal-to-distal bipolar signals from octapolar catheter (Sp to Sd) from S1 show atrial and ventricular electrograms. (*D*) Octapolar catheter cannulation of the second septal (S2). (*E*) Bipolar signals from S2 show earliest activation in the proximal electrodes (*asterisk*), not targeted with venous ethanol but by radiofrequency ablation by proximity, given that venous ethanol cannot be constrained to the proximal portion of a large vein. (*F*) Ablation catheter targeting endocardial site closest to earliest activation site. (*G, H*) S1 location relative to left ventricular outflow tract (LVOT) in 3D maps. (*I, J*) S2 location relative to LVOT in 3D maps. (*K, L*) Ablation catheter location in 3D map and intracardiac echocardiography.

activation maps, and pace-maps. Access to the epicardial space via a subxiphoid anterior puncture can be undertaken when suitable for epicardial mapping and ablation.[22]

RCVEA is considered (1) when RFA failed at the best endocardial sites as guided by the earliest activation or best pace-mapping (PM); (2) when feasible, epicardial RFA failed or was deemed not indicated due to proximity to coronary arteries or due to presence of the earliest activation site at a broad area; and (3) when optimal PM and/or earliest activation was obtained from within a coronary vein.[22]

Stable CS access is necessary. We perform coronary vein mapping by advancing a long 8F sheath in the CS via the right femoral vein (Preface, Biosense-Webster, Diamond Bar, CA) or via the right internal jugular vein (CPS sheath, St Jude Medical, Sylmar, CA). Coronary venograms are performed. A multipolar catheter is inserted in the CS and selected ventricular branches (4F quadripolar IBI, St Jude, or Deca-Nav, Biosense-Webster). A multipolar catheter is then inserted in the CS for local activation time and 3D electroanatomic maps (**Table 2**), although typically only the proximal AIV can be reached. Mapping methods used include activation or pace-map correlation maps using 3D mapping systems (CARTO, Biosense-Webster; or NavX, St Jude Medical). Most commonly, multielectrode catheters cannot penetrate small coronary veins, but they can indicate the earliest region around which to search penetrating intramyocardial branches. Mapping

and pacing from small coronary veins can also be performed by advancing an angioplasty wire (Balance Middleweight [BMW] 0.014″, Abbott), connected to an alligator clip in a unipolar configuration with reference electrode as a needle inserted in the thigh skin. This approach leads to significantly reduced noise compared with using Wilson's central terminal or an indifferent electrode in the inferior vena cava and provides exclusively local signals, compared with using a neighboring electrode. Selective wire cannulation of different targeted veins is achieved by introducing a LIMA angioplasty guide catheter and torqueing it in the desired direction, or simply by guiding the angioplasty wire with the help of a torqueing device. To obtain unipolar signals from selective portions of the targeted vein, an angioplasty balloon catheter or a microcatheter is advanced over the wire to cover it except for the most distal 3 to 5 mm, which acts as the active electrode.[3]

### Defining Target Venules

Once the earliest site in the GCV/AIV has been delineated, coronary venograms are performed to delineate the GCV, AIV, and small diagonal or septal tributaries to assess suitable target branches that provide access to the targeted VT substrate in the LVS. It is important to find the best fluoroscopic projection, which is highly variable. Balloon occlusion venograms are optimal, but not mandatory, for this purpose. For proximal

**Table 2**
**Procedural steps and required equipment used in retrograde coronary venous ethanol ablation of ventricular tachycardias.**

| Procedural Step | Device (Size, Manufacturer) | | |
|---|---|---|---|
| CS cannulation | Preface (Biosense Webster) | SL1 (Abbott) | Agilis (Abbott) |
| gcv/aiv mapping | DecaNav (7F, Biosense Webster) | INQUIRY (4-or 10- pole 4F,Abbott) | Map-iT (20-pole, 3.3F; APT EP) |
| Guide catheter | LIMA guide | LIMA guide | LIMA guide |
| Wire mapping | BMW (0.014 inch, abbott) | VisionWire (0.014 inch, Biotronik) | |
| Alligator clips Selective ethanol infusion | Threshold cable (Abbott) OTW Sprinter Legend (1.25−2.5 × 6mm; Medtronic) | Finecross (Terumo) | |

*Abbreviations:* AIV, anterior interventricular vein; BMW, balance middleweight; CS, coronary sinus; GCV, great cardiac vein; LIMA, left internal mammary artery; OTW, over the wire.

LVS diagonal branches of the AIV, we use the LAO caudal view and for septal AIV branches and use the RAO caudal view. Mapping, pacing, and selective cannulation of these branches are achieved by advancing an angioplasty guidewire (BMW 0.014 inch; Abbott, Santa Clara, CA) into the vessel with the help of a LIMA angioplasty guide catheter (Boston Scientific, Marlborough, MA) which adds stability and torqueability. An angioplasty balloon (typically 2 × 6 mm) is advanced over the wire except the most distal portion (approximately 3 mm of exposed angioplasty wire), which is configured as a unipolar electrode with an alligator clip. A specifically designed wire with an active distal electrode can be used (VisionWire, Biotronik, Berlin, Germany), otherwise any electrically conductive wire can be used. We use a needle inserted in the groin skin as the reference electrode, but the Wilson central terminal or an inferior vena cava electrode can be used as well. Unipolar signals and pace-maps can be used to confirm the candidacy of the targeted vein for ethanol ablation. If the targeted venule is tortuous, a Finecross microguide catheter (Finecross MG catheter, Terumo, Tokyo, Japan) can be used instead of the angioplasty balloon because it can follow the wire more readily.[3]

### Ethanol Delivery

If wire signals support the adequacy of the cannulated vein as target, the wire is then retracted, the angioplasty balloon is inflated, and contrast is injected in the targeted venule to assess its size and the extent of myocardial staining, which would indicate the tissue reached. It is important to recognize that no therapeutic effect is to be expected if the vein injected has collaterals back to the CS, bypassing myocardium, or if a large vein is injected and targeted signals are only present proximally in the vein. Initially, 1 cc of 96%–98% ethanol (American Regent Inc, Shirley, NY; or Akorn Inc, Lake Forest, IL) is delivered. The angioplasty balloon remains inflated after ethanol infusion until therapeutic response is assessed. A complete seal is not required because leaked ethanol is safely diluted by CS flow in the right atrium. Indeed, if the Finecross catheter is used, no venule occlusion ever occurs because it lacks a balloon.

After contrast is injected in the targeted vessel and myocardial staining is verified, repeat 1 cc injection (up to 4) of ethanol over 2 minutes each. Myocardial staining is observed, and intracardiac echocardiograms show an area of increased echogenicity. In our experience, repeated injections are necessary to consolidate a therapeutic effect because myocardial tissue reached by retrograde venous ethanol may be compromised by competing anterograde arterial flow.[3]

### Determinants of Ethanol Success

For therapeutic success, ethanol must reach the targeted myocardium. Failures are to be expected if (1) ethanol is delivered to the inappropriate target or (2) ethanol does not reach the target. Meticulous mapping is required to select the appropriate vein located in the myocardium where VAs come from. Technical difficulties reaching the targeted vein with a stable catheter for ethanol delivery can be significant because of the complex 3D architecture of the ventricular venous vasculature. Once cannulated, myocardial reach depends on the size of the injected vein, the extent of the capillary network associated with it, and the absence of collaterals that could shunt ethanol away from myocardium.[22] If the ablated vein allows, we typically will recannulate the targeted vein with a multipolar catheter. After cannulation, signals pre and post ethanol ablation are compared along with proof that the epicardium can no longer be captured with pacing.[25]

### Beyond Left Ventricular Summit: Substrate Ablation by Double Balloon Technique

VA in the setting of structural heart disease is most commonly the result of reentrant circuits originating in scar tissue (VT substrates), either from prior myocardial infarction or inflammatory processes. In these cases, VT ablation entails the elimination of areas of compromised conduction within the scar. It has been shown that aggressive substrate ablation improves results.[32–34] However, midmyocardial substrate reach may be difficult and overall success remains suboptimal.

Ablation success can be as low as 56% in non-ischemic cardiomyopathy, versus 60% in ischemic cardiomyopathy, and 79% in the absence of structural heart disease, with even lower long-term success rates.[35]

We have developed a double-balloon technique for large substate ablation.[36] **Fig. 8** shows an example.

The overall procedure strategy includes the following steps, after identifying the targeted vein: (1) inflation of both balloons; (2) injection of contrast; (3) injection of 1 cc ethanol over 1 minute; (4) injection of contrast to assess myocardial staining; (5) repeat injection of 1 cc ethanol (up to 4 per balloon positioning); and (6) balloon deflation, repositioning, and repeat injection as needed.[36]

Once early signals identify the optimal vein, contrast venography is again performed to assess collaterals. The wire is preloaded with an angioplasty balloon. A second preloaded wire and balloon are advanced in the vein as well. The targeted region of the vein is divided into segments. For each segment, a distal balloon (Sprinter 2.5 × 6 mm; Medtronic, Minneapolis, MN) is positioned and inflated at one end to occlude flow, leaving the wire in. The proximal balloon (Sprinter 2.75 × 6 mm; Medtronic) is positioned at the beginning of the segment and inflated. The wire of the proximal balloon is removed, and contrast is injected via the proximal balloon to verify distal occlusion and demonstrate the extent of myocardial staining via small intramural vein branches between the two balloons. Then, two to four injections of 1 cc ethanol are delivered slowly over 2 minutes. Intracardiac echocardiography is used to monitor changes in myocardial local echogenicity, indicating ethanol penetration into the

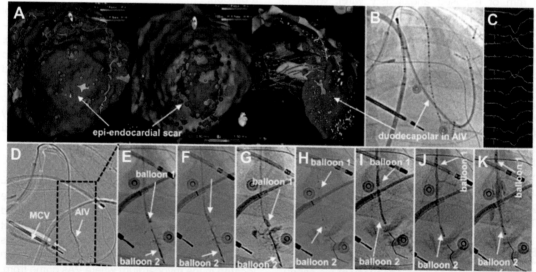

**Fig. 8.** Double-balloon technique for ethanol infusion in the anterior interventricular vein (AIV). (*A*) Scar maps of the epicardial surface (*left*), endocardial surface (*middle*), and location of the duodecapolar catheter in the AIV relative to the scar (*right*). (*B*) Fluoroscopic anteroposterior view of the duodecapolar catheter in the AIV. (*C*) Pacing from the apical scar reproduces QRS morphology of the ventricular tachycardia (VT). (*D*) AIV venogram showing AIV to middle cardiac vein (MCV) collateral flow. (*E–G*) Two balloons were inserted in the AIV: one for ethanol infusion (balloon 1) and one for prevention of flow into MCV (balloon 2). Repeated injections led to the increased staining of the myocardium. (*H–K*) Consecutive balloon repositioning for ethanol delivery in more proximal locations of the AIV. VT became uninducible.

tissue. Contrast injection after ethanol shows increased tissue staining compared with initial injection. The proximal balloon is then flushed, and the balloons are deflated and moved into more proximal portions of the vein. Sequentially, multiple positionings are used to deliver ethanol along the targeted portion of the vein (see **Fig. 8**)[36]

## SUMMARY

Chemical ablation using the transcoronary arterial system has a lengthy but arduous history. Although it has shown to be efficacious in controlling VAs, safety concerns from cannulation of the coronary arterial system to unwanted ethanol downstream effects have limited TCEAs use. RCVEA has shown the promising results. Although it seems to be in its infancy, RCVEA seems to be the future of chemical ablation in comparison with TCEA due to its increased safety and efficacy. The prospective randomized trial data are needed for this adjunctive treatment to RFCA.

## CLINICS CARE POINT

- Operators should be aware that venous ethanol ablation can be of help in radiofrequency-refractory VTs.

## DISCLOSURE

This study was supported by the Charles Burnett III and Lois and Carl Davis Centennial Chair endowments (Houston, Texas, USA).

## REFERENCES

1. Cronin EM, Bogun FM, Maury P, et al. 2019 HRS/EHRA/APHRS/LAHRS expert consensus statement on catheter ablation of ventricular arrhythmias. Heart Rhythm 2020;17:e2–154.
2. Pedersen CT, Kay GN, Kalman J, et al. EHRA/HRS/APHRS expert consensus on ventricular arrhythmias. Heart Rhythm 2014;11:e166–96.
3. Tavares L, Valderrabano M. Retrograde venous ethanol ablation for ventricular tachycardia. Heart Rhythm 2019;16:478–83.
4. Haqqani HM, Roberts-Thomson KC. Radiofrequency catheter ablation for ventricular tachycardia. Heart Lung Circ 2012;21:402–12.
5. Stevenson WG, Wilber DJ, Natale A, et al, Multicenter Thermocool VTATI. Irrigated radiofrequency catheter ablation guided by electroanatomic mapping for recurrent ventricular tachycardia after myocardial infarction: the multicenter thermocool ventricular tachycardia ablation trial. Circulation 2008;118:2773–82.
6. Baker RC, Kramer RE. Cytotoxicity of short-chain alcohols. Annu Rev Pharmacol Toxicol 1999;39:127–50.
7. Lasner M, Roth LG, Chen CH. Structure-functional effects of a series of alcohols on acetylcholinesterase-associated membrane vesicles: elucidation of factors contributing to the alcohol action. Arch Biochem Biophys 1995;317:391–6.
8. Lenaz G, Parenti-Castelli G, Sechi AM. Lipid-protein interactions in mitochondria. Changes in mitochondrial adenosine triphosphatase activity induced by n-butyl alcohol. Arch Biochem Biophys 1975;167:72–9.
9. Das AM, Harris DA. Regulation of the mitochondrial ATP synthase is defective in rat heart during alcohol-induced cardiomyopathy. Biochim Biophys Acta 1993;1181:295–9.
10. Auffermann W, Camacho SA, Wu S, et al. 31P and 1H magnetic resonance spectroscopy of acute alcohol cardiac depression in rats. Magn Reson Med 1988;8:58–69.
11. Schurmann P, Penalver J, Valderrabano M. Ethanol for the treatment of cardiac arrhythmias. Curr Opin Cardiol 2015;30:333–43.
12. Hammer FD, Boon LM, Mathurin P, et al. Ethanol sclerotherapy of venous malformations: evaluation of systemic ethanol contamination. J Vasc Interv Radiol 2001;12:595–600.
13. Chilson DA, Peigh PS, Mahomed Y, et al. Chemical ablation of ventricular tachycardia in the dog. Am Heart J 1986;111:1113–8.
14. Inoue H, Waller BF, Zipes DP. Intracoronary ethyl alcohol or phenol injection ablates aconitine-induced ventricular tachycardia in dogs. J Am Coll Cardiol 1987;10:1342–9.
15. Brugada P, de Swart H, Smeets JL, et al. Transcoronary chemical ablation of ventricular tachycardia. Circulation 1989;79:475–82.
16. Kay GN, Epstein AE, Bubien RS, et al. Intracoronary ethanol ablation for the treatment of recurrent sustained ventricular tachycardia. J Am Coll Cardiol 1992;19:159–68.
17. Haines DE, Whayne JG, DiMarco JP. Intracoronary ethanol ablation in swine: effects of ethanol concentration on lesion formation and response to programmed ventricular stimulation. J Cardiovasc Electrophysiol 1994;5:422–31.
18. Kumar S, Barbhaiya CR, Sobieszczyk P, et al. Role of alternative interventional procedures when endo- and epicardial catheter ablation attempts for ventricular arrhythmias fail. Circ Arrhythm Electrophysiol 2015;8:606–15.

19. Sacher F, Sobieszczyk P, Tedrow U, et al. Transcoronary ethanol ventricular tachycardia ablation in the modern electrophysiology era. Heart Rhythm 2008; 5:62–8.

20. Tokuda M, Sobieszczyk P, Eisenhauer AC, et al. Transcoronary ethanol ablation for recurrent ventricular tachycardia after failed catheter ablation: an update. Circ Arrhythm Electrophysiol 2011;4: 889–96.

21. Wright KN, Morley T, Bicknell J, et al. Retrograde coronary venous infusion of ethanol for ablation of canine ventricular myocardium. J Cardiovasc Electrophysiol 1998;9:976–84.

22. Kreidieh B, Rodriguez-Manero M, P AS, et al. Retrograde coronary venous ethanol infusion for ablation of refractory ventricular tachycardia. Circ Arrhythm Electrophysiol 2016;9:e004352.

23. Baldinger SH, Kumar S, Barbhaiya CR, et al. Epicardial radiofrequency ablation failure during ablation procedures for ventricular arrhythmias: reasons and implications for outcomes. Circ Arrhythm Electrophysiol 2015;8:1422–32.

24. Baher A, Shah DJ, Valderrabano M. Coronary venous ethanol infusion for the treatment of refractory ventricular tachycardia. Heart Rhythm 2012;9: 1637–9.

25. Tavares L, Lador A, Fuentes S, et al. Intramural venous ethanol infusion for refractory ventricular arrhythmias. Outcomes of a multicenter experience. J Am Coll Cardiol EP 2020;6(11):1420–31.

26. Loukas M, Bilinsky S, Bilinsky E, et al. Cardiac veins: a review of the literature. Clin Anat 2009;22:129–45.

27. Bai W, Xu X, Ma H, et al. Assessment of the relationship between the coronary venous and arterial systems using 256-slice computed tomography. J Comput Assist Tomogr 2020;44:1–6.

28. Komatsu Y, Nogami A, Shinoda Y, et al. Idiopathic ventricular arrhythmias originating from the vicinity of the communicating vein of cardiac venous systems at the left ventricular summit. Circ Arrhythm Electrophysiol 2018;11:e005386.

29. Yokokawa M, Good E, Chugh A, et al. Intramural idiopathic ventricular arrhythmias originating in the intraventricular septum: mapping and ablation. Circ Arrhythm Electrophysiol 2012;5:258–63.

30. Briceno DF, Enriquez A, Liang JJ, et al. Septal coronary venous mapping to guide substrate characterization and ablation of intramural septal ventricular arrhythmia. JACC Clin Electrophysiol 2019;5: 789–800.

31. Tavares L, Fuentes S, Lador A, et al. Venous anatomy of the left ventricular summit: therapeutic implications for ethanol infusion. Heart Rhythm 2021;18: 1557–65.

32. Soejima K, Stevenson WG, Maisel WH, et al. Electrically unexcitable scar mapping based on pacing threshold for identification of the reentry circuit isthmus: feasibility for guiding ventricular tachycardia ablation. Circulation 2002;106:1678–83.

33. Berruezo A, Fernandez-Armenta J, Andreu D, et al. Scar dechanneling: new method for scar-related left ventricular tachycardia substrate ablation. Circ Arrhythm Electrophysiol 2015;8:326–36.

34. Tzou WS, Frankel DS, Hegeman T, et al. Core isolation of critical arrhythmia elements for treatment of multiple scar-based ventricular tachycardias. Circ Arrhythm Electrophysiol 2015;8:353–61.

35. Kumar S, Romero J, Mehta NK, et al. Long-term outcomes after catheter ablation of ventricular tachycardia in patients with and without structural heart disease. Heart Rhythm 2016;13:1957–63.

36. Da-Wariboko A, Lador A, Tavares L, et al. Double-balloon technique for retrograde venous ethanol ablation of ventricular arrhythmias in the absence of suitable intramural veins. Heart Rhythm 2020;17: 2126–34.

# Improvement in Lesion Formation with Radiofrequency Energy and Utilization of Alternate Energy Sources (Cryoablation and Pulsed Field Ablation) for Ventricular Arrhythmia Ablation

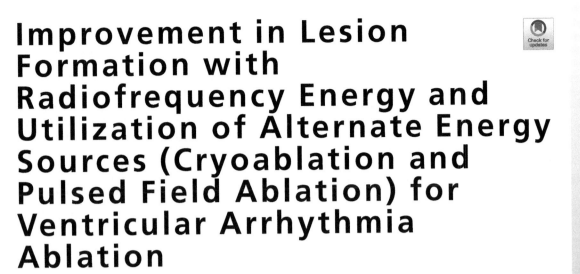

Hiroshi Nakagawa, MD, PhD[a],*, Atsushi Ikeda, MD, PhD[b],
Katsuaki Yokoyama, MD[b], Yoshimori An, MD[a], Ayman A. Hussein, MD[a],
Walid I. Saliba, MD[a], Oussama M. Wazni, MD[a], Quim Castellvi, PhD[c]

**KEYWORDS**

- Catheter ablation • Radiofrequency • Cryothermia • Pulsed electric field • Electroporation
- Ventricular tachycardia • Contact force

## INTRODUCTION

Various techniques and energy sources have been developed for catheter ablation of ventricular arrhythmias[1-3] Radiofrequency (RF) energy has been most commonly used for ablation with good safety and efficacy. However, there are several limitations to RF ablation: (1) relatively long procedural times; (2) high recurrence rate of ventricular arrhythmias; and (3) excessive tissue heating potentially leading to serious complications, including thrombo-embolism, steam pop (resulting in cardiac perforation), and coronary arterial injury.[1-6]

In this article, we describe several technologies to improve ablation lesion formation using RF current configurations, cryo-thermia, and pulsed electric field ablation systems.

## RADIOFREQUENCY ABLATION SYSTEMS
### Contact Force Sensing Catheter

During RF ablation, the electrode-tissue contact force is one of the major determinants of lesion size.[7-23] Although no effective lesion is formed without electrode-tissue contact, excessive contact may result in excessive tissue heating and an increased risk of deep steam pop (perforation) and collateral injury.[11,12,15,16,21]

Several RF ablation systems have been used clinically to measure real-time electrode contact force during mapping and ablation. One system uses three optical fibers to measure the micro-deformation of a deformable body in the catheter tip (TactiCath, Endosense SA/Abbott, Inc), which correlates well with catheter-tip contact force.[12,13,16-19] The other system uses a small

a Department of Cardiovascular Medicine, Cleveland Clinic, Cleveland, OH, USA; b Department of Medicine, Nihon University School of Medicine, Tokyo, Japan; c Department of Information and Communications Technologies, Pompeu Fabra University, Barcelona, Spain
* Corresponding author. Department of Cardiovascular Medicine, Cleveland Clinic, 9500 Euclid Avenue/J2-232, Cleveland, OH 44195.
E-mail address: hiroshinakagawa1@gmail.com

Card Electrophysiol Clin 14 (2022) 757–767
https://doi.org/10.1016/j.ccep.2022.08.003

spring between the ablation tip-electrode and catheter shaft combined with a tiny magnetic transmitter embedded in the tip and magnetic location sensors proximal to the tip to measure micro-deflection of the spring (ThermoCool Smart-Touch, Biosense Webster, Inc), corresponding well to catheter-tip force.[20–26] Both systems have high resolution (<1 g) in bench testing with an accurate display of the direction of contact force.[12,20] Many preclinical and clinical studies using these contact force sensing catheter with saline irrigation have confirmed the improved safety and efficacy of RF ablation.[17–20,23–26]

We performed a canine thigh muscle preparation to examine the relationship between contact force and RF lesion size in a controlled environment.[12] The ablation catheter containing the optical fiber contact sensor (TactiCath) was held perpendicular to the thigh muscle at contact force of 2, 10, 20, 30, and 40 g. RF energy was delivered at constant power (30 or 50 W) for 60 s. Increasing contact force progressively increased median lesion depth from 6.2 mm to 9.9 mm for 30 W and from 7.1 mm to 11.2 mm for 50 W (**Fig. 1A**). Importantly, lesion depth was significantly greater at 30 W and high contact force of 40 g than at 50 W and lower contact force of 10 g (median depth 9.9 mm vs 8.5 mm depth, $P<.01$).[12] Lesion diameter also increased significantly with increasing contact force (2 to 40 g) from 8.6 mm to 13.7 mm for 30W and from 10.2 mm to 15.2 mm for 50 W (**Fig. 1B**). These findings indicate that contact force had as much influence on lesion size as RF power. Excessive contact force also significantly increased the incidence of steam pop and thrombus formation during RF ablation (**Fig. 2**).[12]

We performed another study using the same contact force catheter with the addition of dynamic contact to simulate the beating heart. RF energy (20 W or 40 W) was delivered for 60 s to bovine skeletal muscles with a 20 g peak (systolic) and 10 g nadir (diastolic) at 50 and 100 catheter movements/min, or intermittent contact with a 20 g peak and 0 g nadir (loss of contact). Lesion depth and volume correlated linearly with the area under the contact force curve, described as the force–time integral (FTI).[13]

Using an ablation catheter equipped with a small spring and magnetic location sensors (ThermoCool SmartTouch), we performed preclinical animal studies to determine whether simultaneous measurements of contact force, RF power, and application time predict RF lesion size. Based on the study evaluating lesion depth with various combinations of contact force, power, and RF time, we developed a logarithmic formula (force–power–time index, Ablation Index) to predict lesion depth during RF ablation. This formula was then tested prospectively to predict lesion depth in the beating canine heart. The formula was able to indicate when to terminate RF application to obtain target lesion depths of 3, 5, 7, and 9 mm within a ±1 mm accuracy in the beating canine ventricles.[20,27,28] The incidence of steam pop increased significantly with increasing target lesion depth (no steam pop for 3 mm and 5 mm target depths, 7/40 RF applications [18%] for 7 mm target depth, and 15/40 RF applications [38%] for 9 mm target depth). This supports the use of contact force sensing catheter combined with Force-Power-Time Index (Ablation Index) to control RF lesion depth while reducing the incidence of tissue overheating (steam pop and collateral injury).

## Needle Radiofrequency Ablation System to Produce Deep Lesions

Catheter ablation of ventricular tachycardia (VT) can be challenging when the arrhythmogenic substrates are located deep within the myocardium. Active electrode cooling by saline irrigation allows the use of higher RF power and longer application time to produce deeper lesions, without increasing the risk of thrombus formation and also prevents a rise in impedance.[29,30] However, RF current density falls rapidly with the fourth power of distance from the ablation electrode, resulting in the active heating ("resistive heating") of tissue only adjacent to the electrode, whereas the tissue located at further distance is heated primarily by passive conduction of heat ("conductive heating").[30] Conductive tissue heating is a relatively slow process and may result in uneven distribution of heat within the tissue. During RF ablation, when the tissue temperature becomes excessive (>95–100°C), the tissue desiccates, with increased tissue resistivity (impedance rise). This limits effective RF current delivery within the tissue and prevents proper lesion formation. Tissue overheating is also associated with steam formation within the tissue, followed by steam expulsion and tissue disruption (ie, "steam pop"). Steam pop may result in tissue perforation and pericardial tamponade.[29,30] These fundamental limitations of RF ablation limit deep lesion formation and increase the risk of ablation.

Retractable needle ablation electrodes have been developed to deliver RF current deep within the myocardium to produce deep intramural lesions.[31,32] We performed a canine thigh muscle preparation using a 7.5 Fr catheter with a 4 mm tip electrode (not used for RF delivery) and a retractable 26-gauge 5 mm needle electrode

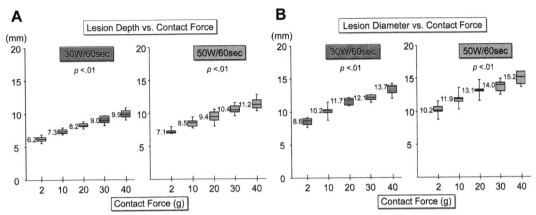

**Fig. 1.** Relationship between contact force and radiofrequency (RF) lesion size in a canine thigh muscle preparation. Lesion depth (*A*) and diameter (*B*) significantly increased by increasing contact force (2, 10, 20, 30, and 40 g) for both 30 W/60 s (left panel) and 50 W/60 s (right panel) RF applications (*P*<.01).

(Biosense Webster, Inc; **Fig. 3**). The ablation catheter was held perpendicular to the thigh muscle and the needle was advanced 5 mm into the muscle. RF current was applied between the needle and skin patch during needle irrigation (room temperature saline and contrast mixture at 2 mL/min). RF current was delivered for 60 sec using temperature control at 55°C (*n* = 16), 60°C (*n* = 18), or 65°C (*n* = 29), based on whichever temperature was higher, tip electrode or needle electrode. With increasing target temperature (55, 60, and 65°C), the median delivered RF power, lesion depth, and diameter significantly increased: RF power—7.9 W, 12.0 W, and 13.6 W; lesion depth: 6.8 mm, 8.3 mm and 8.5 mm; and lesion diameter: 8.0 mm, 10.6 mm and 13.0 mm, respectively). There was no thrombus formation in any RF

applications. Steam pop was not observed in any of the 16 RF application with target temperature of 55°C. However, steam pop occurred in 2/18 (11%) RF applications and 7/29 (24%) RF applications with target temperatures of 60°C and 65°C, respectively.

Berte and colleagues compared the ablation lesion size produced by a needle catheter to conventionally irrigated RF lesions using a sheep model. The needle was deployed from 3 to 8 mm in all seven animals (a mean length of 6 ± 1 mm). The needle ablation catheter (RF: 25–35 W for 60 s with room temperature saline injection through the needle: 2 mL/min) created significantly deeper (depth: 9.9 ± 2.7 mm) and larger (width: 8.5 ± 2.5 mm and volume: 1030 ± 362 mm³, *P*<.001) RF lesions in the sheep left ventricle (LV),

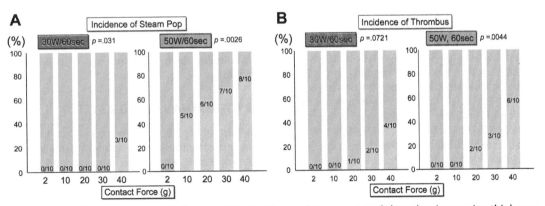

**Fig. 2.** Relationship between contact force and the incidence of steam pop and thrombus in a canine thigh muscle preparation. (*A*) The incidence of steam pop increased significantly by increasing contact force at 30 W/60 s (left panel) and 50 W/60 s (right panel) RF applications (*P* = .031 and *P* = .0026, respectively). (*B*) The incidence of thrombus formation increased significantly by increasing contact force at 50 W/60 s applications (right panel, *P* = .0044). At 30 W/60 s applications (left panel), there was a trend between the incidence of thrombus and contact force (*P* = .0721).

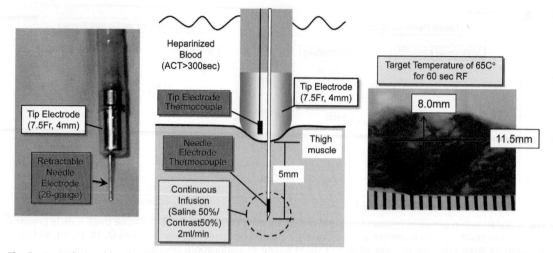

**Fig. 3.** An RF lesion (depth of 8 mm and diameter of 11.5 mm) produced by RF needle ablation in a thigh muscle preparation. The needle electrode was deployed 5 mm into the muscle and RF current was delivered between the needle electrode and a skin patch using electrode temperature control of 65°C for 60 s during needle irrigation (room temperature saline 50% and contrast 50% at 2 mL/min). There was no steam pop or thrombus formation.

compared with the lesions (depth: 5.2 ± 2.4 mm, width: 5.2 ± 1.7 mm and volume: 488 ± 384 mm³) produced by the conventional ablation catheter (RF: 30–35 W for 60 sec with saline irrigation of 30 mL/min).[32] Transmural lesions were observed more frequently with needle ablation (62.5% vs 17%, P<.01). No steam pop occurred in any of 60 RF applications using the needle ablation catheter, whereas steam pops were observed in 3 of 60 RF applications using the conventional catheter.[32]

Sapp and colleagues performed a clinical study using the needle ablation catheter in 8 patients (nonischemic cardiomyopathy in 6 patients and ischemic heart disease in 2 patients) with recurrent VT despite 1 to 4 prior failed ablation procedures (including a failed epicardial procedure).[33] After the needle electrode was inserted into the myocardium (7–9 mm deep), a median of 19 (range 3–48) RF applications were delivered per patient. The duration of RF application ranged from 131 to 2686 sec (median 1316 sec), with power ranging between 8 to 20 W during room temperature saline infusion at 2 mL/min. Among these 8 patients with multiple VTs, at least one of the VTs terminated or became noninducible after the procedure. During follow-up (median 12 months), 4 patients were free of recurrent VT, and 3 patients had improved but had a recurrence of a new VT. Two patients died due to the progression of preexisting heart failure. Complications included tamponade (resolved with percutaneous pericardial drainage) in 1 patient and anticipated heart block resulting from RF delivery at the LV basal septum in 2 patients.[33] These data suggest that needle catheter

RF ablation is feasible and allows successful ablation of some VTs that have been otherwise refractory to conventional ablation therapy. Saline irrigation (at room temperature) has the potential of acting as a heat sink for RF energy that may result in suboptimal thermal conduction, limiting the size of the ablation lesion. A novel RF ablation system using a needle electrode combined with heated saline injection has been developed to improve thermal conduction within the tissue for deeper RF lesion formation.[34] Normal saline is warmed (up to 60°C) by a heater integrated within the proximal portion of the needle electrode (**Fig. 4**A). Heated saline is injected into the myocardium via multiple radial outlets within the needle and RF current is delivered between the needle and the distal electrode. This system produces "thermal convection" within the tissue and creates full-thickness lesions in left ventricular (LV) myocardium with a lower risk of steam pop (**Fig. 4**B).[34]

## CRYOTHERMIA ABLATION SYSTEM

The size of cryo-ablation lesions is determined by a variety of factors, including freezing temperature, electrode size, application duration, and number of freeze/thaw cycles as well as contact force. For a given application time, lower temperatures create progressively larger lesions. However, after approximately 5 to 6 min at a given temperature, the lesion size plateaus.[35-37] Repetitive freeze/thaw cycles may enlarge cryo-lesions beyond those obtained with prolonged freezing at a given temperature.[38–40]

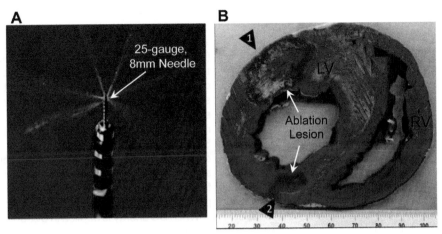

**Fig. 4.** Left ventricular lesions produced by an RF ablation system using a needle electrode combined with heated saline injection. (*A*) An 8-F quadripolar ablation catheter has a 4 mm-tip electrode with a 25 gauge needle, which is deployable up to 8 mm from the tip electrode. The needle has 24 radial side holes for heated saline injection. (*B*) Left ventricular lesions (*arrows*) are created using RF power of 15 to 45 W for 25 to 75 s during heated (60°C) saline injection through the needle (10 mL/min). (*From* Suzuki A, Lehmann HI, Wang S, et al. Monahan KH, Parker KD, Rettmann ME, Curley MG, Packer DL. Impact of myocardial fiber orientation on lesions created by a novel heated saline enhanced radiofrequency needle-tip catheter: an MRI lesion validation study. Heart Rhythm.2021;18:443-452; with permission.)

Current percutaneous cryoablation systems have limited freezing power and are primarily designed for the ablation of thinner tissue, such as atrial myocardium.[41] Surgical cryoablation using argon (Cardioblate CryoFlex, Medtronic, Inc) or liquefied nitrous oxide (cryoICE; Atricure, Inc) has previously been used successfully for the treatment of VT when RF catheter ablation procedures have been unsuccessful.[42,43]

Recently, cryoprobes cooled by liquid nitrogen have been developed, allowing significantly lower temperatures (up to −160°C) and generation of larger lesions for a given duration of exposure.[44] Berte and colleagues performed a preclinical study using this system in a sheep model. They performed epicardial (via a surgical sternotomy) and endocardial (via right atrial appendage for right ventricular (RV) ablation and via LV apex for LV ablation) cryo-probe ablation using the Ice-Sense cryoablation platform (IceCure Medical, Inc), which consists of a rigid probe with a freezing element (3.4 mm in diameter, 30 mm in length) and target freezing temperatures of −160°C. After obtaining adequate probe contact, 3 min freezes were performed in the RV. In the LV, 6 min freezes or two 4 min freezes (with 2 min waiting between freezes) were performed. A total of 45 cryoablation lesions were created: (1) Epicardial ablation—3 min freezes in RV ($n = 12$), 6 min freezes in LV ($n = 10$), and two 4 min freezes in LV ($n = 8$); and (2) Endocardial ablation—RV ($n = 7$) and LV ($n = 8$). A total of 28/45 (62%) lesions

were transmural and 35/45 (78%) had a lesion depth of greater than 10 mm with a mean lesion volume of 5055 ± 92 mm$^3$ (length 32 ± 4.6 mm, width 16.0 ± 6.4 mm and depth 11.2 ± 4.4 mm). There was a trend toward larger lesions with single 6 min freezing, compared with two 4 min freezing (6790 ± 44 mm$^3$ vs 5595 ± 63 mm$^3$, $P = .44$). Mean endocardial ablation lesion volume was larger than epicardial ablation lesion volume in the RV (4287 ± 610 mm$^3$ vs 2840 ± 916 mm$^3$, $P = .028$), but no significant differences were noted in the LV (endocardial ablation 7580 ± 3970 mm$^3$ vs epicardial ablation 6629 ± 2588 mm$^3$).[44]

## Effects of Contact Force for Cryoablation Lesion

Contact force is a major determinant of lesion size during RF ablation. However, the role of contact force in lesion size has not been well established for cryo-ablation. Some studies have proposed that ice ball contact (without direct electrode-tissue coupling) is sufficient for effective lesion formation.[45] We examined the relationship between electrode contact force and lesion size for catheter cryo-ablation using a canine thigh muscle preparation. A 10 French catheter with an 8.5 mm cryo-electrode was held perpendicular to the thigh muscle with three levels of contact force of 10 g and 30 g, or no electrode contact (1–2 mm above the muscle with ice ball formation at the electrode-tissue interface during freezing). The skin cradle over the thigh muscle was filled with heparinized canine blood at 37°C, circulating blood with a peak flow velocity of 0.5 m/s at the ablation site. Cryo-application was delivered for 120 s at target electrode temperature of −90°C.

Increasing contact force from 10 g to 30 g significantly increased lesion depth (median depth: 8.1 mm vs 10.0 mm, $P<.05$). Without direct electrode-tissue contact (1–2 mm above the muscle), cryo-application produced ice ball at the electrode-tissue interface, resulting in "ice ball contact." However, no lesion was detected in 3 of the 6 ablation sites and very shallow lesions (median depth of only 2.5 mm) were identified in the remaining three ablation sites. These findings indicate that contact force is one of the major determinants of lesion size for cryo-ablation. Importantly, no direct electrode-tissue contact before cryo-application would result in only Ice-ball contact, significantly limiting lesion formation. Catheter cryo-ablation systems that allow the measurement of real-time electrode contact force during mapping and ablation have not been developed yet.

## PULSED ELECTRIC FIELD ABLATION

The occurrence of complete atrioventricular (AV) conduction block caused by external direct current (DC) cardioversion during an electrophysiological study was reported in 1979.[46] It was assumed that the high-energy DC was accidently delivered through the mapping catheter positioned over the His bundle region. Several preclinical animal studies then showed that complete AV block can be produced by delivering of high-energy DC shock through a conventional diagnostic catheter positioned at the His bundle region.[47–49] Thus, the "closed-chest catheter ablation" procedure to produce complete AV block was developed for the treatment of drug-resistant supraventricular tachycardias,[50] and was explored for ablation of accessory AV pathways, atrial tachycardias, and life-threatening VT.[51,52]

However, it was abandoned shortly after RF ablation became available in the early 1990s, because DC ablation was associated with serious complications, including cardiac perforation, heart failure, lethal ventricular arrhythmias, and sudden cardiac death. In the international registry on DC ablation of VT, procedure-related deaths were noted, and on follow-up mortality was as high as 25%.[53] These complications were thought to be secondary to barotrauma resulting from the use of high-energy DC and a small ablation electrode of the conventional diagnostic catheter (such as

a 6 Fr, 2 mm electrode).[54,55] Barotrauma is caused by a high-pressure shock wave resulting from an electrically isolating vapor globe, leading to arcing (spark) and explosion.[54] To overcome these limitations, low-energy DC ablation without arcing was developed.[56] A newly designed capacitive power source was able to deliver less energy in a very short time (60–100 μs), preventing high peak current and high peak voltage (no barotrauma).[57,58] Several clinical studies showed that a lower energy level without a high-pressure shock wave is sufficient to create effective myocardial lesions for ablation, such as ablation of accessory AV pathways.[59]

When DC energy is applied in a short and pulsed fashion, the myocyte is exposed to an electric field, resulting in cell membrane permeabilization due to the formation of nanometric pores in the cell membrane (ie, electroporation, **Fig. 5**).[60–62] Depending upon the electric field applied (eg, voltage and pulse duration), the effect of electroporation can be transient and result in repair of cell membranes (viable cell) after electric field exposure. In this condition, the term of "reversible electroporation" is applied (upper panel in **Fig. 5**). However, greater electric field application leads to irreversible cell death by apoptosis (due to permanent permeabilization leading to cell lysis or severe disruption of cell homeostasis, including damage of mitochondria) and necrosis, resulting in "irreversible electroporation" (lower panel in **Fig. 5**).[60–62]

Pulsed electric field is a unique energy source for ablation because lesion formation does not result from tissue heating (such as RF, laser or ultrasound) or cooling (cryo-thermia). Major limitations of thermal ablation are the nonspecific damage of both cells and extra-cellular structures through heat-induced protein denaturation, the risk of complications such as cardiac perforation and tamponade (due to steam pop resulting from tissue overheating), pulmonary vein stenosis, phrenic nerve palsy, atrio-esophageal fistula and stroke due to thrombus formation.[1–6,55–57] Relatively large myocardial lesions can be created in a more controlled manner with pulsed electric field energy delivery, where lesion formation by nonthermal electroporation is not affected by local blood flow.

### Preclinical Studies of Pulsed Electric Field Ventricular Ablation

Recent preclinical studies suggest that pulsed field ablation (PFA)/irreversible electroporation (IRE) might be effective and safe for the treatment of cardiac arrhythmias.[63–72]

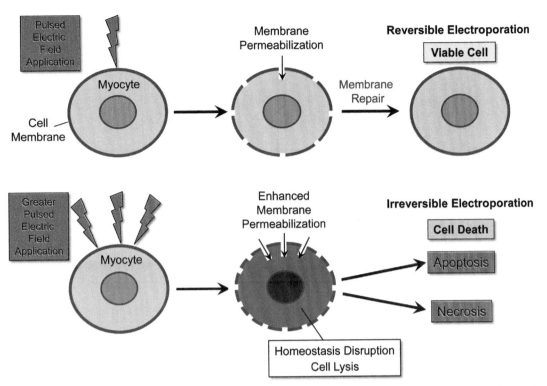

**Fig. 5.** Effects of pulsed electric field (PEF) applications on the myocyte with increasing PEF energy. See the text in detail.

Wittkampf and colleagues performed epicardial ventricular PFA in a porcine model using a monophasic external defibrillator (Lifepak 9, Physio-Control, Inc) and a custom-made 7 Fr, 20 mm circular catheter with 10 ablation electrodes (2 mm electrode length each, **Fig. 6**).[66] In order to investigate the effects of epicardial PFA on the coronary artery and lesion formation, ablation was targeted directly over the left anterior descending and circumflex coronary arteries with single cathodal DC applications of 200 J (between all 10 electrodes and a large skin patch, 20 J per electrode without arcing and a pressure wave). Coronary angiography directly after ablation showed short-lasting (<30 min) luminal narrowing in the targeted area with subsequent normalization, suggesting coronary spasm. Coronary angiography performed 3 months later, did not reveal significant arterial narrowing at the ablation site. Histology showed some intimal hyperplasia in 66 of 154 arteries inside the area of the ablation lesion, with only 8% ± 5% of luminal stenosis of the affected arteries. The myocardial lesion depth was 6.4 ± 2.6 mm (range 0 to 10.4 mm) and 4 of the 13 LV lesions were transmural (see **Fig. 6**).[66] Because the mechanism of lesion formation in PFA is unrelated to temperature, there was no

difference in myocardial injury surrounding arteries. Sparing of myocardium around an artery is frequently observed in RF or cryoablation lesions because, the arterial blood flow either cools or warms the surrounding myocardium, respectively.[30,73]

RF ablation within 2 mm of a coronary artery is associated with a significant risk of arterial stenosis or occlusion.[5,6] Tissue heating due to RF produces coagulation necrosis of the media and intima of the coronary artery and shrinkage of the collagen fibers, resulting in stenosis.[5] Epicardial cryoablation has a relatively low risk of arterial injury,[44] but lesion size may be limited, especially below areas of epicardial fat.

Pulsed electric field is a unique energy source for ablation because lesion formation does not result from tissue heating (such as RF, ultrasound, and laser ablation) or cooling (cryothermia). The relatively low risk of arterial injury suggests that myocardium is more sensitive to PFA injury than coronary arteries.[66] A preclinical study performed by the same authors suggests that the phrenic nerve also has a low susceptibility to injury by PFA.[67] These observations suggest that PFA may emerge as a preferred approach for epicardial ablation. The potential applications for epicardial

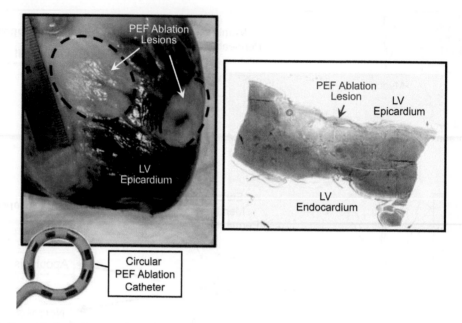

**Fig. 6.** Left ventricular lesions produced by epicardial pulsed electric field (PEF) applications using a circular electrode catheter. Left panel: A custom-made circular octopolar device (12 mm in diameter) with 2-mm-long electrodes is placed in the pericardial space through, and a single non-arcing, non-barotraumatic DC application (200 J) is delivered. The epicardial lesions in 3 weeks after ablation show pale regions (30 mm in diameter, delineated by black dashed *lines*). Right panel: Histologic section (elastic van Gieson staining) through the center of the lesion shows a transmural, continuous circumferential lesion (stained in pink). (*From* Wittkampf FHM, Van Es R and Neven K. Electroporation and its Relevance for Cardiac Catheter Ablation. J Am Coll Cardiol EP 2018;4:977–86; with permission.)

PFA include ablation of epicardial VT, atrial fibrillation (completion of the linear mitral isthmus lesion through the coronary sinus),[4] and epicardial accessory pathways (ablation within the coronary sinus or middle cardiac vein),[5,6] decreasing the risk of coronary arterial injury.

Many experimental studies were performed by several different groups using different electric field intensity, pulse duration and number, and electrode configurations.[60–72] However, preclinical data on optimal PFA/IRE protocols for clinical use of PFA are still lacking, including the use of optimized monophasic/biphasic waveforms which remains undisclosed by the industry.

### Effects of Contact Force for Pulsed Electric Field Ablation Lesion

Contact force has been shown to be a major determinant of lesion size during RF and cryo-ablation. In contrast, it has been reported that pulsed electric field does not require electrode contact to achieve effective ablation lesions.[74] However, the effects of electrode-tissue contact on lesion formation during PFA have not been well validated.

Using a beating swine heart model, we examined the relationship between average contact force and lesion size during PFA. A 7Fr catheter with a 3.5 mm saline irrigated ablation electrode and contact force sensor (TactiCath SE, Abbott, Inc) was positioned in RV and LV under a three-dimensional mapping system (EnSite, Abbott, Inc) and fluoroscopic guidance in two closed chest pigs (body weight 66 kg).

During constant atrial pacing at 90 beat/min, biphasic pulsed electric field current was delivered between the ablation electrode and a skin patch at 13 separate sites in RV (28 A and total duration of 1.4 ms) and 19 separate sites in LV (35 A and total duration of 1.6 ms) at average contact force: 1) low (4–12 g, median 8 g); 2) moderate (16–30 g, median 20 g); or 3) high (33–55 g, median 40 g). Ablation was also performed without electrode contact (1–2 mm away from the endocardium, confirmed by intracardiac echocardiography, n = 5). Pigs were sacrificed 2 h after ablation and lesion size was measured using triphenyl tetrazolium chloride (TTC) staining. Ablation lesions were clearly identified with TTC staining, showing dark central zones surrounded by pale boundaries. At constant pulsed electric field current and pulse duration, lesion depth increased significantly with increasing contact force (RV lesion depth—range 2.9 to 7.2 mm and LV lesion depth—range 2.6 to 8.0 mm). There were no detectable lesions resulting from ablation without electrode contact. These data indicate that, at the same pulsed electric field dose intensity, lesion depth increases significantly with increasing contact force. Therefore, electrode-tissue contact is required for effective lesion formation with PFA.

## SUMMARY

Current approaches to catheter ablation for ventricular arrhythmias rely on thermal energy to create lesions (heating: RF, laser, ultrasound, and cooling: cryothermia). Although thermal ablation has been proven to be effective, there are several limitations, including the risk of collateral injury (to phrenic nerve and esophagus), tissue overheating (steam pop/perforation), and narrowing/occlusion of blood vessels as well as thrombus formation. PFA/IRE offers a unique nonthermal ablation strategy that has the potential to overcome these limitations. However, further preclinical and clinical studies are required to optimize PFA/IRE strategies including pulsed electric field generator and ablation catheter configurations.

## FUNDING

This study was supported, in part, by a grant from Biosese Webster, Inc, Endosense SA, CryoCore, Inc and Galaxy Medical, Inc.

## REFERENCES

1. Cronin EM, Bogun FM, Maury P, et al. 2019 HRS/EHRA/APHRS/LAHRS expert consensus statement on catheter ablation of ventricular arrhythmias. Europace 2019;21:1143–4.

2. Al-Khatib SM, Stevenson WG, Ackerman MJ, et al. 2017 AHA/ACC/HR guideline for management of patients with ventricular arrhythmias and the prevention of sudden cardiac death: a report of the American College of Cardiology/American Heart Association Task force on clinical Practice Guidelines and the Heart Rhythm Society. Heart Rhythm 2018;15:e73–189.

3. Stevenson WG, Wilber DJ, Natale A, et al. Multicenter Thermocool VT Ablation Trial Investigators. Irrigated radiofrequency catheter ablation guided by electroanatomic mapping for recurrent ventricular tachycardia after myocardial infarction: the multicenter thermocool ventricular tachycardia ablation trial. Circulation 2008;118:2773–82.

4. Roberts-Thomson KC, Steven D, Seiler J, et al. Coronary artery injury due to catheter ablation in adults: presentations and outcomes. Circulation 2009;120:1465–73.

5. Aoyama H, Nakagawa H, Pitha JV, et al. Comparison of cryothermia and radiofrequency current in safety and efficacy of catheter ablation within the canine coronary sinus close to the left circumflex coronary artery. J Cardiovasc Electrophysiol 2005;16:1218–26.

6. Stavrakis S, Jackman WM, Nakagawa H, et al. Risk of coronary artery injury with radiofrequency ablation and cryoablation of epicardial posteroseptal accessory pathways within the coronary venous system. Circ Arrhythm Electrophysiol 2014;7:113–9.

7. Avitall B, Mughal K, Hare J, et al. The effects of electrode-tissue contact on radiofrequency lesion generation. PACE 1997;20:2899–910.

8. Haines DE. Determinants of lesion size during radiofrequency catheter ablation: the role of electrode-tissue contact force and duration of energy delivery. J Cardiovasc Electrophysiol 1991;2:509–15.

9. Strickberger SA, Vorperian VR, Man KC, et al. Relation between impedance and endocardial contact during radiofrequency catheter ablation. Am Heart J 1994;128:226–9.

10. Zheng X, Walcott GP, Hall JA, et al. Electrode impedance: an indicator of electrode-tissue contact and lesion dimensions during linear ablation. J Interv Card Electrophysiol 2000;4:645–54.

11. Biase LD, Natale A, Barrerr C, et al. Relationship between contact forces, lesion characteristics, "popping," and char formation: Experience with robotic navigation system. J Cardiovasc Electrophysiol 2009;20:436–40.

12. Yokoyama K, Nakagawa H, Shah DC, et al. Novel contact force sensor incorporated in irrigated radiofrequency ablation catheter predicts lesion size and incidence of steam pop and thrombus. Circ Arrhythmia Electrophysiol 2008;1:354–62.

13. Shah DC, Lambert H, Nakagawa H, et al. Area under the real-time contact force curve (force-time integral) predicts radiofrequency lesion size in an in vitro contractile model. J Cardiovasc Electrophysiol 2010;21:1038–43.

14. Thiagalingam A, d'Avila A, Foley L, et al. Importance of catheter contact force during irrigated radiofrequency ablation: evaluation in a porcine ex vivo model using a force-sensing catheter. J Cardiovasc Electrophysiol 2010;21:806–11.

15. Shah DS, Lambert H, Langenkamp A, et al. Catheter tip force required for mechanical perforation of porcine cardiac chambers. Europcae 2010;13:277–83.

16. Ikeda A, Nakagawa H, Lambert H, et al. Relationship between catheter contact force and radiofrequency lesion size and incidence of steam pop in the beating canine heart: electrogram amplitude, impedance, and electrode temperature are poor

predictors of electrode-tissue contact force and lesion size. Circ Arrhythm Electrophysiol 2014;7: 1174–80.

17. Kuck KH, Reddy VY, Schmidt B, et al. A novel radiofrequency ablation catheter using contact force sensing: Toccata study. Heart Rhythm 2012;9:18–23.

18. Reddy VY, Shah D, Kautzner J, et al. The relationsip between contact force and clinical outcome during radiofrequency catheter ablation of atrial fibrillation in the TOCCATA study. Heart Rhythm 2012;9:1789–95.

19. Neuzil P, Reddy VY, Kautzner J, et al. Electrical reconnection after pulmonary vein isolation is contingent on contact force during initial treatment: results from the EFFICAS I study. Circ Arrhytm Electrophysiol 2013;6:327–33.

20. Nakagawa H, Kautzner J, Natale A, et al. Locations of high contact force during left atrial mapping in atrial fibrillation patients: electrogram amplitude and impedance are poor predictors of electrode-tissue contact force for ablation of atrial fibrillation. Circ Arrhythm Electrophysiol 2013;6:746–53.

21. Nakagawa H, Jackman WM. The role of contact force in atrial fibrillation ablation. J Atr Fibrillation 2014;7(1):1027.

22. Perna F, Heist EK, Danik SB, et al. Assessment of catheter tip contact force resulting in cardiac perforation in swine atria using force sensing technology. Circ Arrhythm Electrophysiol 2011;4:218–24.

23. Martinek M, Lemes C, Sigmund E, et al. Clinical impact of an open-irrigated radiofrequency catheter with direct force measurement on atrial fibrillation ablation. 2012. Pacing Clin Electrophysiol 2012;35: 1312–8.

24. Kumar S, Haqqani HM, Chan M, et al. Predictive value of impedance changes for real-time contact force measurements during catheter ablation of atrial arrhythmias in human. Heart Rhythm 2013;10: 962–9.

25. Natale A, Reddy VY, Monir G, et al. Paroxysmal AF catheter ablation with a contact force sensing catheter. J Am Coll Cardiol 2014;64(7):647–56.

26. Jarman JWE, Panikker S, Das M, et al. Relationship between contact force sensing technology and Medium-term outcome of atrial fibrillation ablation : a multicenter study of 600 patients. J Cardiovasc Electrophysiol 2015;26:378–84.

27. El Haddad M, Taghji P, Phlips T, et al. Determinants of acute and late pulmonary vein reconnection in contact force - guided pulmonary vein isolation. Identifying the weakest link in the ablation chain. Circ Arrhythmia Electrophysiol 2017;10:e004867.

28. Taghji P, El Haddad M, Phlips T, et al. Evaluation of a strategy Aiming to Enclose the pulmonary veins with Contiguous and optimized radiofrequency lesions in Paroxysmal atrial fibrillation: a Pilot study. JACC Clin Electrophysiol 2018;4(1):99–108.

29. Nakagawa H, Yamanashi WS, Pitha JV, et al. Comparison of in vivo tissue temperature profile and lesion geometry for radiofrequency ablation with a saline-irrigated electrode versus temperature control in a canine thigh muscle preparation. Circulation 1995;91:2264–73.

30. Wittkampf FH, Nakagawa H. RF catheter ablation: lessons on lesions. Pacing Clin Electrophysiol 2006;29:1285–97.

31. Sapp JL, Cooper JM, Zei P, et al. Large radiofrequency ablation lesions can be created with a retractable infusion-needle catheter. J Cardiovasc Electrophysiol 2006;17:657–61.

32. Berte B, Cochet H, Magat J, et al. Irrigated needle ablation creates larger and more transmural ventricular lesions compared with standard unipolar ablation in an ovine model. Circ Arrhythm Electrophysiol 2015;8:1498–506.

33. Sapp JL, Beeckler C, Pike R, et al. Initial human feasibility of infusion needle catheter ablation for refractory ventricular tachycardia. Circulation 2013; 128:2289–95.

34. Suzuki A, Lehmann HI, Wang S, et al. Impact of myocardial fiber orientation on lesions created by a novel heated saline enhanced radiofrequency needle-tip catheter: an MRI lesion validation study. Heart Rhythm 2021;18:443–52.

35. Gill W, Fraser J, Carter DC. Repeated freeze-thaw cycles in cryosurgery. Nature 1968;219:410–3.

36. Mazur M. Causes of injury in frozen and thawed cells. Fed Proc 1965;24:5175–82.

37. Mazur P. Cryobiology: The freezing of biological systems. Science 1970;168:939–49.

38. McGrath JJ. Low temperature injury processes, in Advances in Bioheat and Mass Transfer: Microscale Analysis of thermal injury Processes, Instrumentation, modeling, and clinical applications. Am Soc mech Engin 1993;268:125–32.

39. Stewart GJ, Preketes A, Horton M, et al. Hepatic cryotherapy: Double-freeze cycles achieve greater hepatocellular injury in man. Cryobiology 1995;32: 215–9.

40. Gage AA, Guest K, Montes M, et al. Effect of varying freezing and thawing rates in experimental cryosurgery. Cryobiology 1985;22:175–82.

41. Kuck KH, Brugada J, Alexander A, et al. Radiofrequency ablation for Paroxysmal atrial fibrillation. N Engl J Med 2016;374(23):2235–45.

42. Pojar M, Harrer J, Omran N, et al. Surgical cryoablation of drug resistant ventricular tachycardia and aneurysmectomy of postinfarction left ventricular aneurysm. Case Rep Med 2014;2014:207851.

43. Spina R, Granger E, Walker B, et al. Ventricular tachycardia in hypertrophic cardiomyopathy with apical aneurysm successfully treated with left ventricular aneurysmectomy and cryoablation. Eur Heart J 2013;34:3631.7–1.

44. Berte B, Sacher F, Wielandts JY, et al. A new cryoenergy for ventricular tachycardia ablation: a proof-of-concept study. Europace 2017;19:1401–7.

45. Collins NJ, Barlow M, Paul Varghese P, et al. Cryoablation versus radiofrequency ablation in the treatment of atrial Flutter trial (CRAAFT). J Interv Card Electrophysiol 2006;16:1–5.

46. Vedel J, Frank R, Fontaine G, et al. [permanent intrahisian atrioventricular block induced during right intraventricular exploration]. Arch des maladies du coeur des vaisseaux 1979;72:107–12.

47. Gonzalez R, Scheinman M, Margaretten W, et al. Closed-chest electrode-catheter technique for his bundle ablation in dogs. Am J Physiol 1981;241:H283–7.

48. Bardy GH, Ideker RE, Kasell J, et al. Transvenous ablation of the atrioventricular conduction system in dogs: Electrophysiologic and histologic observations. Am J Cardiol 1983;51:1775–82.

49. Gallagher JJ, Svenson RH, Kasell JH, et al. Catheter technique for closed-chest ablation of the atrioventricular conduction system. N Engl J Med 1982;306:194–200.

50. Scheinman MM, Evans-Bell T. Catheter ablation of the atrioventricular junction: a report of the percutaneous mapping and ablation registry. Circulation 1984;70:1024–9.

51. Morady F, Scheinman MM, Winston SA, et al. Efficacy and safety of transcatheter ablation of posteroseptal accessory pathways. Circulation 1985;72:170–7.

52. Fontaine G, Tonet JL, Frank R, et al. [emergency treatment of chronic ventricular tachycardia after myocardial infarction by endocavitary fulguration]. Arch des maladies du coeur des vaisseaux 1985;78:1037–43.

53. Evans GT Jr, Scheinman MM, Zipes DP, et al. Catheter ablation for control of ventricular tachycardia: a report of the percutaneous cardiac mapping and ablation registry. PACE 1986;9:1391–5, 53.

54. Bardy GH, Coltorti F, Stewart RB, et al. Catheter-mediated electrical ablation: the relation between current and pulse width on voltage breakdown and shock-wave generation. Circ Res 1988;63:409–14.

55. Hauer RN, Robles de Medina EO, Borst C. Proarrhythmic effects of ventricular electrical catheter ablation in dogs. J Am Coll Cardiol 1987;10:1350–6.

56. Ahsan AJ, Cunningham D, Rowland E, et al. Catheter ablation without fulguration: design and performance of a new system. Pacing Clin Electrophysiol 1989;12:1557–61.

57. Lemery R, Lavallee E, Girard A, et al. Physical and dynamic characteristics of dc ablation in relation to the type of energy delivery and catheter design. Pacing Clin Electrophysiol 1991;14:1158–1168 34.

58. Lemery R, Leung TK, Lavallee E, et al. In vitro and in vivo effects within the coronary sinus of nonarcing and arcing shocks using a new system of low-energy dc ablation. Circulation 1991;83:279–93.

59. Lemery R, Talajic M, Roy D, et al. Success, safety, and late electrophysiological outcome of low-energy direct-current ablation in patients with the Wolff-Parkinson-White syndrome. Circulation 1992;85:957–62.

60. Weaver JC, Chizmadzhev YA. Theory of electroporation: a review. Bioelectrochem Bioenergetics 1996;41:135–60.

61. Tovar O, Tung L. Electroporation of cardiac cell membranes wit monophasic or biphasic rectangular pulses. Pacing Clin Electrophysiol 1991;14:1887–92.

62. Lee RC, Zhang D, Hannig J. Biophysical injury mechanisms in electrical shock trauma. Annu Rev Biomed Eng 2000;2:47–509.

63. Wittkampf FH, van Driel VJ, van Wessel H, et al. Feasibility of electroporation for the creation of pulmonary vein ostial lesions. J Cardiovasc Electrophysiol 2011;22:302–9.

64. Wittkampf FHM, Van Driel V, Van Wessel H, et al. Myocardial lesion depth with circular electroporation ablation. Circ Arrhythm Electrophysiol 2012;5:581–6.

65. Van Driel VJHM, Neven KGEJ, Van Wessel H, et al. Pulmonary vein stenosis after catheter ablation electroporation versus radiofrequency. Circ Arrhythmia Electrophysiol 2014;7:734–8.

66. Neven K, van Driel V, van Wessel H, et al. Safety and feasibility of closed chest epicardial catheter ablation using Electroporation. Circ Arrhythm Electrophysiol 2014;7:913–9.

67. van Driel VJ, Neven K, van Wessel H, et al. Low vulnerability of the right phrenic nerve to electroporation ablation. Heart Rhythm 2015;12:1838–44.

68. Neven K, Van Es R, Van Driel V, et al. Acute and long-term effects of full-power electroporation ablation directly on the porcine esophagus. Circ Arrhythmia Electrophysiol 2017;10:e004672.

69. Koruth J, Kuroki K, Iwasawa J, et al. Preclinical evaluation of pulsed field ablation: electrophysiological and histological assessment of thoracic vein isolation. Circ Arrhythm Electrophysiol 2019;12:e007781.

70. Loh P, Van Es R, Groen MHA, et al. Pulmonary vein isolation with single pulse irreversible electroporation. Circ Arrhythm Electrophysiol 2020;13:e008192.

71. Reddy VY, Anic A, Koruth J, et al. Pulsed field ablation in Patients with persistent atrial fibrillation. J Am Coll Cardiol 2020;76:1068–80.

72. Wittkampf FHM, Van Es R, Neven K. Electroporation and its Relevance for cardiac catheter ablation. J Am Coll Cardiol 2018;4:977–86.

73. Lustgarten D, Bell S, Hardin N, et al. Safety and efficacy of epicardial cryoablation in a canine model. Heart Rhythm 2005;2:82–90.

74. Witt C, Livia C, Witt T, et al. Electroporative myocardial ablation utilizing a non-contact, Virtual electrode: proof of concept in ex-vivo and in-vivo canine hearts heart Rhythm 2017;14(5):S144–234.

# Adjunctive Therapies for Ventricular Arrhythmia Management
## Autonomic Neuromodulation—Established and Emerging Therapies

Justin Hayase, MD, Jason S. Bradfield, MD*

## KEYWORDS

- Ventricular arrhythmias • Electrical storm • Autonomic modulation

## KEY POINTS

- The autonomic nervous system is a key contributor to ventricular arrhythmogenesis and provides numerous therapeutic targets in arrhythmia management.
- Mounting clinical data support the application of various autonomic modulation therapies for ventricular arrhythmias including beta blockade, sedation, thoracic epidural anesthesia, stellate ganglion blockade, surgical cardiac sympathetic denervation, and renal artery denervation.
- Emerging therapies in autonomic modulation that require more data include stellate ganglion ablation, transcutaneous stellate ganglion modulation, tragus nerve stimulation, deep plexus blockade, and ganglionated plexus ablation.

## INTRODUCTION

Ventricular arrhythmias are an important cause of sudden cardiac death and often require a multimodal approach for management.[1] Therapeutic options include recognition and correction of underlying causes (eg, electrolyte derangements, ischemia, toxins, and so forth), an implantable cardioverter defibrillator for secondary prevention, goal-directed medical therapy for associated cardiomyopathy, antiarrhythmic medications, and catheter ablation. Autonomic modulation is a cornerstone of management of ventricular arrhythmias that can often be underappreciated. The authors review the established and emerging autonomic modulation therapies in this article (**Fig. 1**). At the outset, they present a case that highlights the value of autonomic modulation in the management of ventricular arrhythmias.

## Case Presentation

The patient was a 45-year-old man with history of coronary artery disease and reduced ejection fraction of 30% to 35% with single-chamber VDD implantable cardioverter-defibrillator (ICD) implantation who presented to the hospital with 5 ICD shocks for ventricular fibrillation (VF) over a 24-hour period. Coronary angiography demonstrated no targets for revascularization. His medications included metoprolol succinate 200 mg daily and ranolazine 500 mg twice daily in addition to maximally tolerated goal-directed medical therapy for ischemic cardiomyopathy. ICD interrogation demonstrated multiple episodes of premature ventricular contraction (PVC)-initiated VF, with similar far-field PVC morphology for the episodes (**Fig. 2**). A prior exercise treadmill test had showed exercise-induced PVCs as well as runs of nonsustained polymorphic ventricular tachycardia. He

UCLA Cardiac Arrhythmia Center, David Geffen School of Medicine at UCLA, 100 Medical Plaza, Suite 660, Los Angeles, CA, USA
* Corresponding author.
E-mail address: JBradfield@mednet.ucla.edu

Card Electrophysiol Clin 14 (2022) 769–778
https://doi.org/10.1016/j.ccep.2022.06.004
1877-9182/22/© 2022 Elsevier Inc. All rights reserved.

cardiacEP.theclinics.com

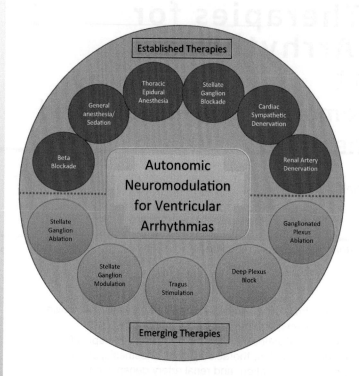

**Fig. 1.** Central illustration. Established and emerging autonomic modulation therapies.

was admitted to the hospital and telemetry monitoring showed occasional PVCs with similar morphology, suggesting upper septal, fascicular origin. He was taken to the electrophysiology laboratory for attempt at PVC ablation; however, this procedure was complicated by repetitive episodes of VF during diagnostic catheter placement and prolonged hemodynamic instability, so ablation could not be performed. He was subsequently referred for bilateral surgical stellate ganglionectomy for cardiac sympathetic denervation (CSD), which was successfully performed via video-assisted thoracoscopic surgery. He was able to be discharged from the hospital with no changes to his cardiac medications, and he has done well with no ICD shocks for more than 1 year.

## AUTONOMIC NEUROMODULATION
### Established Therapies

#### Medications
In a study by Nademanee and colleagues, published in 2000, the key role of the autonomic nervous system in ventricular arrhythmias was demonstrated.[2] In 49 patients presenting with electrical storm (ES), patients were either managed by sympathetic blockade with either β-blocker or left stellate ganglion blockade (group 1) or with antiarrhythmic medications (group 2). At the time, antiarrhythmic medications such as lidocaine, procainamide, and bretylium were

standard recommendations in accordance with Advanced Cardiac Life Support guidelines. In their study, patients in group 1 had a significantly reduced mortality rate at 1 week compared with group 2 (22% vs 82%, $P$ = .0001). The use of β-blockers currently carries a class I indication for patients with ventricular arrhythmias with structural heart disease and a class IIa recommendation for patients with ventricular arrhythmias and no structural abnormalities[1]; this highlights the importance of the autonomic nervous system and its modulation for management of ventricular arrhythmias.

#### Sedation
Deep sedation with intubation can be considered for patients presenting with ES refractory to antiarrhythmic medications as a means of suppressing the sympathetic overdrive that often accompanies recurrent arrhythmias as well as the repetitive ICD therapies required to terminate them. In a multicenter study of 116 patients with ongoing ventricular arrhythmias in spite of a median of 2.0 antiarrhythmic medications, 47.4% of patients had acute termination of ventricular arrhythmias within 15 minutes of sedation.[3] In another observational study of 46 patients with ES, there were 15 patients who remained refractory in spite of usual care, and 80% of those had abatement of arrhythmias with the use of deep sedation.[4]

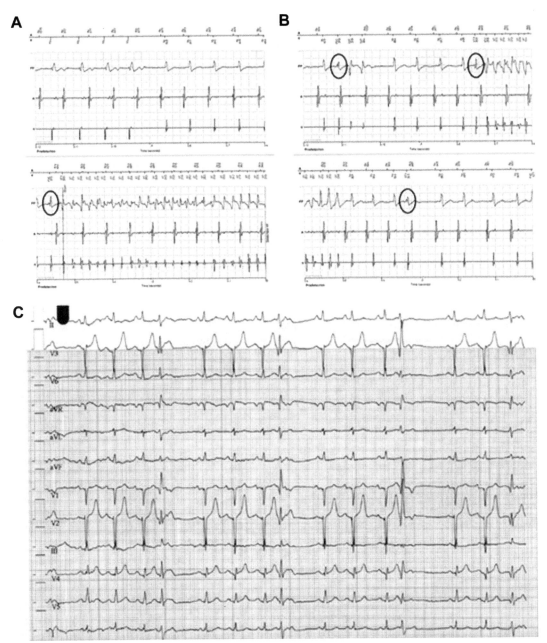

**Fig. 2.** ICD interrogation and 12-lead ECG. (*A*) ICD interrogation showing episode of sustained ventricular fibrillation initiated with PVC. (*B*) ICD electrograms of PVCs and nonsustained VF initiated by PVCs with similar morphology (*red circles*) as PVC-triggered sustained VF episodes. (*C*) 12-lead ECG from prior exercise treadmill test showing frequent exercise-induced PVCs with narrow QRS, qR morphology in V1, lead V2 pattern break, and AVL/AVR discordance that suggests upper septal origin. ECG, electrocardiogram.

Sedation remains a universally available technique for autonomic modulation.

### Thoracic epidural anesthesia

Thoracic epidural anesthesia (TEA) provides a rapid means of bilateral, sympathetic modulation that can be performed at the bedside by experienced providers. TEA can be performed via epidural needle placement at the T1-T2 or T2-T3 interspace and epidural catheter advancement beyond the needle tip. Infusion of 0.25% bupivacaine or 0.20% ropivacaine can then be administered and titrated to arrhythmic response. In a multicenter series of 11 patients presenting

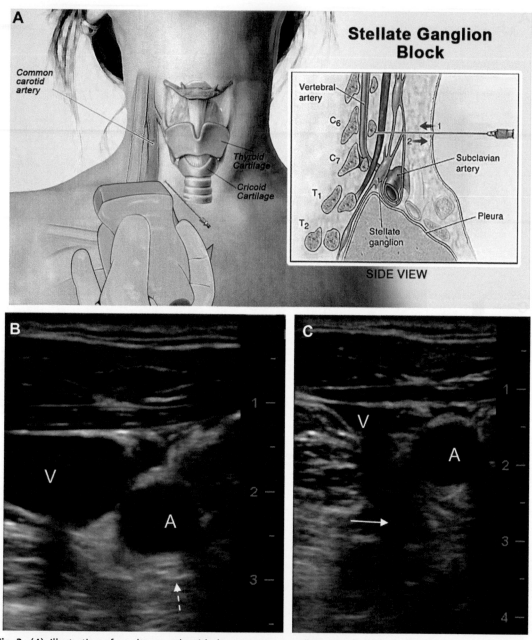

**Fig. 3.** (*A*): Illustration of an ultrasound-guided percutaneous stellate ganglion block. (*B–C*) Ultrasound images of the percutaneous approach on the right side. (*B*) Taken before needle insertion. Dashed arrow indicates the sympathetic ganglion. (*C*) Taken during needle insertion (*arrow*) and anesthetic infusion. Letter A marks the carotid artery and letter V the jugular vein. (FUDIM, M., BOORTZ-MARX, R., PATEL, C.B., SUN, A.Y. and PICCINI, J.P. (2017), Autonomic Modulation for the Treatment of Ventricular Arrhythmias: Therapeutic Use of Percutaneous Stellate Ganglion Blocks. J Cardiovasc Electrophysiol, 28: 446-449. https://doi.org/10.1111/jce.13152.)

with ES, 5 (45%) had a complete response with cessation of arrhythmias following TEA and dose titration.[5] This therapeutic option can provide a bridge to more durable treatment with either catheter ablation or surgical CSD.

**Stellate ganglion blockade**
Numerous case reports and case series have illustrated the benefits of percutaneous stellate ganglion blockade (SGB) in the management of refractory ventricular arrhythmias.[6–8] This

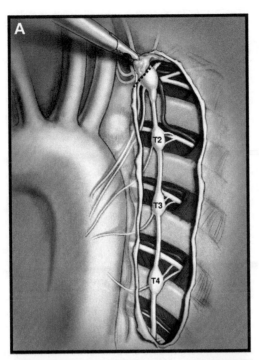

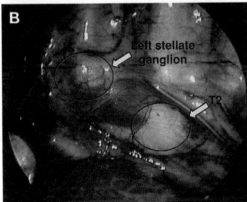

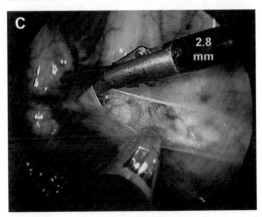

**Fig. 4.** Anatomy of left cardiac sympathetic denervation (LCSD). (*A*) An anatomic drawing of the left cardiac sympathetic chain after exposure through the pleura that is resected during VATS-LCSD. The stellate ganglion is located under the superior edge of the incision. The dashed line indicates the resection of the lower half of the left stellate ganglion occurring just above the major lower branches. (*B*, *C*) Videoscopic still frames of

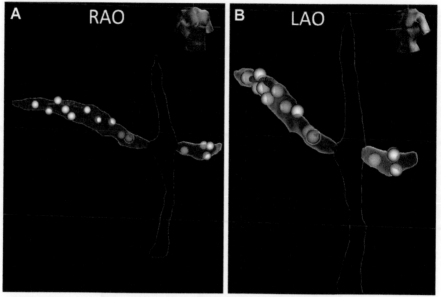

**Fig. 5.** Representative anatomic geometry from a renal artery denervation procedure using the EnSite (Abbott Medical, Minneapolis, MN) mapping system. (*A*) Right anterior oblique view (RAO). (*B*) Left anterior oblique (LAO) view. Ablation lesions are represented as white dots. (*From* Bradfield JS, Hayase J, Liu K, Moriarty J, Kee ST, Do D, Ajijola OA, Vaseghi M, Gima J, Sorg J, Cote S, Pavez G, Buch E, Khakpour H, Krokhaleva Y, Macias C, Fujimura O, Boyle NG and Shivkumar K. Renal denervation as adjunctive therapy to cardiac sympathetic denervation for ablation refractory ventricular tachycardia. Heart Rhythm. 2019; with permission.)

procedure can be performed under either fluoroscopic[6] or ultrasound guidance (**Fig. 3**).[7] SGB is commonly performed with injection of 0.25% bupivacaine, with meta-analysis data demonstrating significant reduction in ventricular arrhythmia burden.[9] In a later single-center study of 30 consecutive patients with ES, there was a 92% reduction in ventricular arrhythmias over the 72 hours following SGB.[10] This treatment can result in acute arrhythmia reduction with duration of effect depending on the anesthetic agent used and, similar to TEA, may provide a means of bridging to more definitive intervention.

### Surgical cardiac sympathetic denervation

Surgical CSD has long been an effective therapy for certain channelopathies such as long QT syndrome or catecholaminergic polymorphic ventricular tachycardia (**Fig. 4**).[11] Mounting clinical evidence now support CSD via resection of the stellate ganglion in the management of refractory ventricular arrhythmias including monomorphic ventricular tachycardia (VT). Multicenter data have shown the efficacy of this procedure for management of refractory ventricular arrhythmias.[12] Greater benefit may be derived in patients undergoing bilateral CSD (vs left-sided only), patients with faster ventricular arrhythmias, and those with less severe New York Heart Association functional status. Surgical CSD now carries a class IIb guideline recommendation for patients with ventricular arrhythmias refractory to conventional therapies.[1]

### Renal artery denervation

Renal artery denervation (RDN) may provide an alternative target for autonomic modulation by decreasing renal afferent signals and thus reducing sympathetic input to the heart (**Fig. 5**).[13] In a retrospective, propensity-matched study of 32 patients with refractory ventricular arrhythmias, patients who underwent catheter ablation plus RDN had greater arrhythmia reduction compared with those receiving catheter ablation alone.[14] In a case series of 10 patients who underwent RDN following CSD, ventricular arrhythmias and ICD shocks were significantly reduced following RDN.[15] This effect was driven primarily by patients

VATS-LCSD before (*B*) and after (*C*) dissection of the pleura. VATS, video-assisted thoracic surgery. (*From* Collura CA, Johnson JN, Moir C and Ackerman MJ. Left cardiac sympathetic denervation for the treatment of long QT syndrome and catecholaminergic polymorphic ventricular tachycardia using video-assisted thoracic surgery. Heart Rhythm. 2009;6:752-9; with permission.)

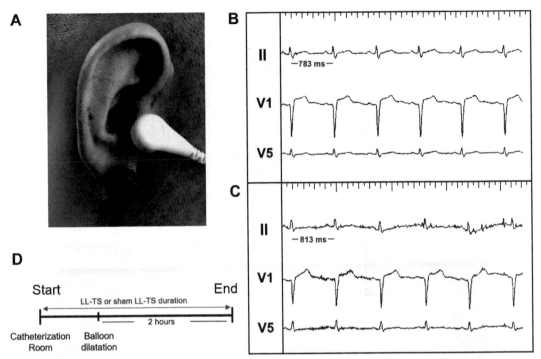

**Fig. 6.** (*A*) The positioning of the electrode for stimulation of the right tragus. (*B*) Before stimulation, sinus cycle length is 783 ms. (*C*) During stimulation at 5 mA, there is an increase in the sinus cycle length to 813 ms. (*D*) Low-level tragus stimulation (LL-TS) or sham LL-TS was started once the patient arrived in the catheterization room and lasted for 2 h after balloon dilatation (reperfusion). (*From Yu L, Huang B, Po SS, Tan T, Wang M, Zhou L, Meng G, Yuan S, Zhou X, Li X, Wang Z, Wang S and Jiang H. Low-Level Tragus Stimulation for the Treatment of Ischemia and Reperfusion Injury in Patients With ST-Segment Elevation Myocardial Infarction: A Proof-of-Concept Study. JACC Cardiovasc Interv. 2017;10:1511-1520; with permission.*)

who had an observed effect after CSD, with RDN resulting in incremental arrhythmia suppression. If patients did not have benefit from CSD, then less benefit was observed with RDN as well.

## Emerging Therapies

### Stellate ganglion ablation and transcutaneous modulation

As discussed earlier, SGB can provide acute relief for ventricular arrhythmias, especially in the throes of ES. Based on case report data, more durable effect might be achieved with percutaneous stellate ganglion ablation using either radiofrequency energy[16] or cryoablation[17]; however, these methods require further study. Alternative means of noninvasive stellate ganglion modulation are also being investigated. In a pilot study involving healthy volunteers, the application of phototherapy using a low-level laser resulted in reduction in serum adrenaline levels. In a follow-up of 11 patients with ES, complete arrhythmia suppression was achieved in 7 patients using phototherapy.[18] In a double-blind, sham-controlled randomized controlled trial of 26 patients, transcutaneous

magnetic stimulation resulted in significantly fewer ventricular arrhythmia episodes compared with sham control (4.5 vs 10.7, *P* < .001).[19] Should these treatment options prove effective in future studies, these therapies could become life-saving tools to use at the bedside of critically ill patients.

### Tragus stimulation

The auricular branch of the vagus nerve courses through the tragus and offers a potential noninvasive target for autonomic modulation. Animal model data have shown the impact of intermittent low-level tragus nerve stimulation in a postinfarction canine study[20]; this was further evaluated in a proof-of-concept randomized trial of patients undergoing percutaneous coronary intervention for acute ST elevation myocardial infarctions, which resulted in significant reduction in reperfusion ventricular arrhythmias in the treatment arm (**Fig. 6**).[21]

### Deep plexus block

The deep plexus represents a convergence of sympathetic nerves from bilateral stellate ganglia

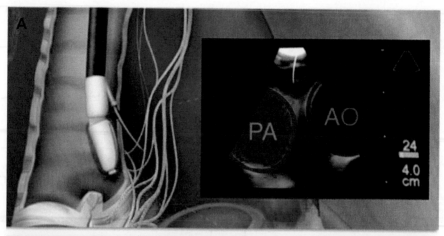

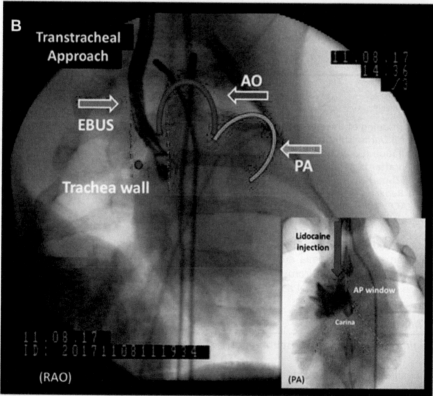

**Fig. 7.** EBUS-guided transtracheal blockade of cardiac plexus. (*A*) Ultrasound real-time imaging of the aortopulmonary (AP) window allows for safe positioning of injection needle into the pretracheal space (illustration). (*B*) EBUS needle is advanced through the trachea anterior wall into the space between the aortic arch and pulmonary artery. Injection of a contrast-lidocaine solution into the site of block (AP window) demonstrates the absence of either systemic (intravascular) or intrapericardial inadvertent assessment (lower right). Stellate ganglia stimulation catheters are shown in the background. AO, aorta (arch); EBUS, endobronchial ultrasound; PA, pulmonary artery; (PA), posteroanterior projection; (RAO), right anterior oblique projection; red circle, right paratracheal space. (*From* Assis FR, Yu DH, Zhou X, Sidhu S, Bapna A, Engelman ZJ, Misra S, Okada DR, Chrispin J, Berger R, Mandal K, Lee H and Tandri H. Minimally invasive transtracheal cardiac plexus block for sympathetic neuromodulation. Heart Rhythm. 2019;16:117-124; with permission.)

in the aortopulmonary window anterior to the trachea. Transtracheal lidocaine injection into the deep plexus was able to inhibit sympathetic

response to either right or left stellate ganglia in a porcine model (**Fig. 7**).[22] In a case report of a single patient with incessant VT, endobronchial ultrasound-guided deep plexus lidocaine and botulinum toxin injection resulted in acute termination of VT.[23] VT ultimately recurred and the patient succumbed to their arrhythmias, but this nonetheless serves as an illustration of feasibility of the procedure.

### Ganglionated plexus ablation

The ganglionated plexi (GP) are epicardial structures that facilitate afferent and efferent autonomic nervous system effects on cardiac electrophysiological and mechanical properties. The GPs have been implicated in the pathogenesis of atrial fibrillation[24] and in neurocardiogenic syncope,[25] but their role in ventricular arrhythmias is less understood. In general, GP ablation has aimed primarily at decreasing parasympathetic effects on the heart; however, in a canine study, ablation of the GP at the ligament of Marshall had similar effects as ablation of the left stellate ganglion in modulation of ventricular effective refractory period, markers of sympathetic tone, and in postinfarction ventricular arrhythmias.[26] However, ES following atrial fibrillation cryoablation has also been reported,[27] and given the primary focus of ablation of GPs as a means for parasympathetic inhibition, tremendous caution is warranted for the study of GPs as a therapeutic target for ventricular arrhythmias.

## SUMMARY

Modulation of the autonomic nervous system represents an essential component in the management of ventricular arrhythmias. There are now numerous treatment modalities available to the clinician, which has helped to improve patient outcomes with these life-threatening arrhythmias. In addition, many new therapies are in development and show promise. Neurocardiac intervention has a bright future.

## CLINICS CARE POINTS

- The autonomic nervous system is a key player in the pathogenesis of ventricular arrhythmias
- Autonomic modulation plays a key therapeutic role in the management of patients with ventricular arrhythmias
- Autonomic targets for ventricular arrhythmia management primarily aim to decrease sympathetic or increase parasympathetic tone

## DISCLOSURE

J. Hayase: consultant (NeuCures).

## REFERENCES

1. Al-Khatib SM, Stevenson WG, Ackerman MJ, et al. AHA/ACC/HRS guideline for management of patients with ventricular arrhythmias and the prevention of sudden cardiac death: executive summary: a report of the american college of cardiology/american heart association task force on clinical practice guidelines and the heart rhythm society. J Am Coll Cardiol 2017;72(14):1677–749.
2. Nademanee K, Taylor R, Bailey WE, et al. Treating electrical storm : sympathetic blockade versus advanced cardiac life support-guided therapy. Circulation 2000;102:742–7.
3. Martins RP, Urien JM, Barbarot N, et al. Effectiveness of deep sedation for patients with Intractable electrical storm refractory to antiarrhythmic Drugs. Circulation 2020;142:1599–601.
4. Bundgaard JS, Jacobsen PK, Grand J, et al. Deep sedation as temporary bridge to definitive treatment of ventricular arrhythmia storm. Eur Heart J Acute Cardiovasc Care 2020;9:657–64.
5. Do DH, Bradfield J, Ajijola OA, et al. Thoracic epidural anesthesia can Be effective for the Short-Term management of ventricular tachycardia storm. J Am Heart Assoc 2017;6.
6. Hayase J, Patel J, Narayan SM, et al. Percutaneous stellate ganglion block suppressing VT and VF in a patient refractory to VT ablation. J Cardiovasc Electrophysiol 2013;24(8):926–8.
7. Fudim M, Boortz-Marx R, Patel CB, et al. Autonomic modulation for the treatment of ventricular arrhythmias: therapeutic Use of percutaneous stellate ganglion blocks. J Cardiovasc Electrophysiol 2017;28: 446–9.
8. Cardona-Guarache R, Padala SK, Velazco-Davila L, et al. Stellate ganglion blockade and bilateral cardiac sympathetic denervation in patients with life-threatening ventricular arrhythmias. J Cardiovasc Electrophysiol 2017;28:903–8.
9. Meng L, Tseng CH, Shivkumar K, et al. Efficacy of stellate ganglion blockade in managing electrical storm: a Systematic review. JACC Clin Electrophysiol 2017;3:942–9.
10. Tian Y, Wittwer ED, Kapa S, et al. Effective use of percutaneous stellate ganglion blockade in patients with electrical storm. Circ Arrhythm Electrophysiol 2019;12:e007118.
11. Schwartz PJ. Cardiac sympathetic denervation to prevent life-threatening arrhythmias. Nat Rev Cardiol 2014;11:346–53.
12. Vaseghi M, Barwad P, Malavassi Corrales FJ, et al. Cardiac sympathetic denervation for refractory

ventricular arrhythmias. J Am Coll Cardiol 2017;69: 3070–80.

13. Bradfield JS, Vaseghi M, Shivkumar K. Renal denervation for refractory ventricular arrhythmias. Trends Cardiovasc Med 2014;24:206–13.

14. Evranos B, Canpolat U, Kocyigit D, et al. Role of adjuvant renal sympathetic denervation in the treatment of ventricular arrhythmias. Am J Cardiol 2016; 118:1207–10.

15. Bradfield JS, Hayase J, Liu K, et al. Renal denervation as an adjunctive therapy to cardiac sympathetic denervation for ablation refractory ventricular tachycardia. Heart Rhythm 2019;17(2):220–7.

16. Hayase J, Vampola S, Ahadian F, et al. Comparative efficacy of stellate ganglion block with bupivacaine vs pulsed radiofrequency in a patient with refractory ventricular arrhythmias. J Clin Anesth 2016;31: 162–5.

17. Chatzidou S, Kontogiannis C, Tampakis K, et al. Cryoablation of stellate ganglion for the management of electrical storm: the first reported case. Europace 2021;23:1105.

18. Nonoguchi NM, Adachi M, Nogami A, et al. Stellate ganglion phototherapy using low-level laser: a novel rescue therapy for patients with refractory ventricular arrhythmias. JACC Clin Electrophysiol 2021;7: 1297–308.

19. Markman TM, Pothineni NVK, Zghaib T, et al. Effect of transcutaneous magnetic stimulation in patients with ventricular tachycardia storm: a randomized clinical trial. JAMA Cardiol 2022;7(4):445–9.

20. Yu L, Wang S, Zhou X, et al. Chronic intermittent low-level stimulation of tragus reduces cardiac autonomic remodeling and ventricular arrhythmia inducibility in a post-infarction canine model. JACC Clin Electrophysiol 2016;2:330–9.

21. Yu L, Huang B, Po SS, et al. Low-level tragus stimulation for the treatment of ischemia and reperfusion Injury in patients with ST-Segment elevation myocardial infarction: a proof-of-concept study. JACC Cardiovasc Interv 2017;10:1511–20.

22. Assis FR, Yu DH, Zhou X, et al. Minimally invasive transtracheal cardiac plexus block for sympathetic neuromodulation. Heart Rhythm 2019;16:117–24.

23. Yu DH, Assis FR, Lerner AD, et al. Endobronchial ultrasound-guided transtracheal cardiac plexus neuromodulation for refractory ventricular tachycardia. HeartRhythm Case Rep 2020;(6):370–4.

24. Stavrakis S, Po S. Ganglionated plexi ablation: Physiology and clinical applications. Arrhythm Electrophysiol Rev 2017;6:186–90.

25. Pachon JC, Pachon EI, Pachon JC, et al. Cardioneuroablation"–new treatment for neurocardiogenic syncope, functional AV block and sinus dysfunction using catheter RF-ablation. Europace 2005;7:1–13.

26. Liu S, Yu X, Luo D, et al. Ablation of the ligament of Marshall and left stellate ganglion similarly reduces ventricular arrhythmias during acute myocardial infarction. Circ Arrhythm Electrophysiol 2018;11: e005945.

27. Munkler P, Wutzler A, Attanasio P, et al. Ventricular tachycardia (VT) storm after cryoballoon-based pulmonary vein isolation. Am J Case Rep 2018;19: 1078–82.

# Stereotactic Radiotherapy in the Management of Ventricular Tachycardias
## More Questions than Answers?

Jana Haskova, MD[a,*], Marek Sramko, MD, PhD[a], Jakub Cvek, MD, Ing, PhD[b],
Josef Kautzner, MD, PhD[a,c]

## KEYWORDS

- Ventricular tachycardia • Catheter ablation • Stereotactic body radiotherapy
- Stereotactic arrhythmia radiotherapy

## KEY POINTS

- Stereotactic body radiotherapy (SBRT) is an attractive alternative treatment method for ventricular tachycardias recurring despite previous catheter ablation(s).
- Initial clinical experience showed that cardiac SBRT using a single radiation dose of 25 Gy is feasible and may prevent or decrease the risk of ventricular tachycardia recurrences.
- Although acute toxicity of SBRT is generally low, delayed side effects may limit wider acceptance of this strategy.
- Many unanswered questions remain, including unknown mechanism of action, variable time to effect, the optimal method of substrate targeting, long-term safety, and definition of an optimal candidate for this treatment.

## INTRODUCTION

Patients with structural heart disease of different etiology, especially with left ventricular dysfunction, have an increased risk of ventricular arrhythmias and sudden cardiac death. The mechanism of these arrhythmias is predominantly re-entrant, related to the presence of fibrosis or scar tissue (eg, after previous myocardial infarction). At present, the best strategy to prevent sudden cardiac death is the implantation of an implantable cardioverter-defibrillator (ICD).[1,2] However, ICD does not prevent recurrences of ventricular arrhythmias. Besides antiarrhythmic drugs, the treatment strategy includes catheter ablation, preferably performed at an expert center. Current approaches of catheter ablation allow extensive substrate modification in a majority of cases,

regardless of hemodynamic tolerability of ventricular tachycardia (VT). Catheter ablation has become a preferred method for the management of electrical storms and in some cases, it may be a life-saving procedure.[3–7]

However, catheter ablation can be sometimes limited by the large size of the substrate and/or by the inability to reach its critical region for various reasons, such as deep intramyocardial location, presence of left ventricular thrombus, or adhesions within the pericardial sac precluding epicardial mapping and ablation. Published literature suggests that this may happen in up to 10% of cases.[8] Alternate approaches include bipolar ablation, alcohol ablation, and/or hybrid procedure with a surgical window to enable epicardial ablation after freeing the adhesions. Targeted radiotherapy was explored as an

[a] Department of Cardiology, IKEM, Vídeňská 1958/9, Prague 140 21, Czech Republic; [b] Department of Oncology, University Hospital Ostrava and Ostrava University Medical School, 17 listopadu 1790/5, Ostrava-Poruba 708 00 Czech Republic; [c] Palacky University Medical School, Olomouc, Czech Republic
* Corresponding author. Department of Cardiology, IKEM, Vídeňská 1958/9, Prague, 140 21, Czech Republic.
E-mail address: hasj@ikem.cz

Card Electrophysiol Clin 14 (2022) 779–792
https://doi.org/10.1016/j.ccep.2022.06.010
1877-9182/22/© 2022 Elsevier Inc. All rights reserved.

alternative therapeutic modality. Less than 10 years ago, the first reports on the therapeutic use of stereotactic radiotherapy in cases of failed catheter ablation were published.[9,10] Since then, many groups around the globe published their first experience with the strategy called stereotactic body radiotherapy (SBRT), stereotactic ablative radiotherapy (SABR) or stereotactic arrhythmia radiotherapy (STAR). The initial experience created a wave of enthusiasm, and many started to believe that SBRT may even replace catheter ablation. The goal of this review is to briefly summarize available evidence, discuss different aspects of this treatment strategy, and highlight the unanswered questions.

## History

### How Did it all Start?

Several research groups have experimented with cardiac SBRT since the beginning of this century. Initial concepts focused on functional change in the electrophysiological properties of the myocardium. One group identified upregulation of connexin 43 (Cx43) after lower dose radiation (15 Gy), resulting in a reduction of the vulnerability to ventricular arrhythmias.[11] This was observed without serious tissue injury and the effect was noticeable for at least 1 year after SBRT.[12] Soon after, the concept of cardiac SBRT changed toward the creation of cardiac lesions that should modify the arrhythmogenic substrate.[13] Using photons, the dose of 25 Gy or higher was needed to produce an electrophysiologic effect, such as atrioventricular block or cavotricuspid isthmus block, in experimental animals. The electrophysiologic effect was caused by fibrosis and observed with a delay, but consistently by 90 days. Subsequent experimental studies confirmed the accuracy of dose delivery to the desired target.[14] Even higher doses were tested to achieve pulmonary vein isolation in animal models (>32.5 Gy).[15]

In summary, although the initial concept of SBRT for VT focused on modification of electrophysiological properties without causing fibrosis, the paradigm rapidly shifted toward the quest for a radioablative effect with the creation of fibrotic lesions. Early preclinical studies have helped to determine the therapeutic radiation dose for VT management.

## The First Clinical Experience

The first clinical case of SBRT for cardiac arrhythmia was performed in 2012 at Stanford University Medical Center on a 71-year-old man with severe ischemic cardiomyopathy (left ventricular ejection fraction, LVEF, 24%) and drug-refractory VT.[9] The patient received multiple ICD shocks and was not considered to be a candidate for catheter ablation. The morphology of the VT was suggestive of inferior wall exit, which correlated with inferior wall scar on imaging. Radioablation of this region was performed (CyberKnife; Accuray Inc, Sunnyvale, CA) with a maximum dose of 33 Gy. The patient tolerated the procedure well and his monthly number of VT episodes declined from 562 episodes per month (averaged over 2 months before ablation) to 52 episodes per month (averaged over 2–9 months after ablation). The cycle length of the VT was slower and repeat imaging showed consolidation of the pre-existing scar with only mild extension. This patient died 9 months later due to respiratory failure. This case report was published in 2015.

However, the first publication of the clinical effect of SBRT in the management of intractable VT came from Ostrava University Hospital in the Czech Republic in 2014.[10] SBRT was performed in a 72-year-old woman with dilated cardiomyopathy (LVEF 25%) and recurrent VTs after a failure of endo- and epicardial catheter ablation. Robotic system CyberKnife (Accuray Inc, Sunnyvale, CA) was used. The posterolateral region of the left ventricle was irradiated with 25 Gy with a relatively rapid decrease in the number of ectopy and no recurrences of VT. No adverse effects were observed except for a mild increase in high-sensitivity troponin. She died 4 years later due to the progression of heart failure.

The first case series of five patients who underwent SBRT for VT was published by Cuculich and colleagues.[16] Patients with at least three episodes of ICD-treated VT, and failed catheter ablation (or with a contraindication to ablation) were recruited. Planning of SBRT was performed using a combination of scar imaging and body surface mapping during VT to identify exit sites for a given VT. In one patient, no VT was inducible from the ICD, and results of previous invasive electroanatomic mapping and 12 lead electrocardiograms (ECGs) were employed. A linear accelerator (TrueBeam, Varian Medical Systems, Palo Alto) was used for SBRT. Importantly, the first 6 weeks after SBRT was not taken into consideration for evaluation of the efficacy, constituting a "blanking period," during which 680 VT episodes occurred. After the 6-week blanking period, there were 4 episodes of VT during the next 46 patient months, which represented a relative reduction of 99.9% from baseline. Four surviving patients could stop antiarrhythmics several weeks after treatment. One patient died because of a fatal stroke 3 weeks after SBRT, the other restarted amiodarone for a recurrence of VT, and another patient underwent catheter ablation after SBRT.

This initial experience showed that cardiac SBRT using a single radiation dose of 25 Gy is feasible and may prevent or decrease the risk of VT recurrences. However, as in preclinical studies, data from the first case series also suggested that the effect may not be immediate.

### More Advanced Clinical Experience

The Washington University group that published the first case series subsequently presented the first prospective (phase I/II) and by far the largest such study, on a total of 19 patients with refractory VT and/or ventricular ectopy causing cardiomyopathy (ENCORE VT study).[17] Three patients did not have previous catheter ablation for various reasons. More than half of the patients were on more than one antiarrhythmic drug. Target delineation was performed again using imaging strategies, such as computed tomography (CT), cardiac magnetic resonance, or Positron emission tomography (PET), in a combination with body surface mapping. The aim was to target all areas of ventricular scar approximating the VT exit site and harboring related circuits. As in the early series, a linear accelerator (TrueBeam, Varian Medical Systems, Palo Alto) was used for SBRT. The primary efficacy endpoint was defined as the number of subjects with any reduction in the number of ICD treatments for VT, or 24 hour burden of premature ventricular beats, comparing the 6-month period before and after SBRT. Again, a 6-week blanking period was used to allow for treatment effect. The median follow-up was 13 months. A significant reduction of VT episodes or ectopic burden was observed in 17 of 18 patients (94%). In 16 VT patients, 94% total VT episode reduction was observed outside of the 6-week blanking period. This allowed a decrease in antiarrhythmic medication. In two patients with premature beats, the burden was reduced from 24% to 2% and 26% to 9%. Although VT burden was reduced in nearly all, many (11 of 16, 69%) had some recurrence of VT during the 6 months following the blanking period. In terms of safety, the authors reported that significant toxicity (grade 3) was observed only in two patients (10.5%)—heart failure and pericarditis. Two more patients had radiation pneumonitis (grade 2) (11.1%) that resolved with steroids.

The second prospective study was published by our consortium and included 10 subjects with structural heart disease and recurrent VT despite previous catheter ablation.[18] Compared with the ENCORE VT study, we used a different source for SBRT, a robotic radiation therapy system (CyberKnife, Accuray Inc, Sunnyvale, CA). This allows for more inhomogeneous dose distribution while preserving safety due to better compensation for respiratory movements. The planned target volume (PTV) was based on the previous location of the substrate on electroanatomical maps and indirect comparison with a CT scan of the heart. The resulting PTV was visibly lower when compared with the ENCORE VT study (22.2 mL, range 14.2–29.6 mL vs. 98.9 mL, range 60.9–298.8 mL). We also observed a significant decrease in VT burden after SBRT (from 212 episodes to 26 ($P = 0.012$). However, the effect was slightly less profound than in the ENCORE VT study (from 119 to 3). The reasons for this difference could be several. First, we irradiated a smaller volume of the tissue to minimize the risk of collateral damage and future and unknown side effects. Second, all our patients were off antiarrhythmic drugs at the time of SBRT when compared with uninterrupted antiarrhythmic therapy in the ENCORE VT study. Third, the differences in the substrate itself (most of our patients had ischemic cardiomyopathy vs. 42% of patients with nonischemic cardiomyopathy in the ENCORE-VT study). Interestingly, in two subjects the effect was not significant and in the other two patients, the effect was delayed (3 and 6 months). Three patients died during the follow-up, none of them due to arrhythmic causes (one died of Alzheimer's disease and two due to progression of heart failure). Furthermore, the incidence of adverse effects in our series was low. Four patients had transient nausea and two other subjects presented with a progression of their mitral valve disease.

More recently, researchers from Emory University reported their experience with 10 patients with severe heart failure and refractory VTs who underwent SBRT.[19] A single dose of 25 Gy was used. Etiologies of heart failure were ischemic in 40% (4/10) and nonischemic in 60% (6/10). All patients had previous catheter ablation, three had left ventricular-assist devices, and one had intra-aortic balloon support. To normalize results for different times of the follow-up, the authors defined a total ventricular arrhythmia burden as VT seconds/30 days, anti-tachycardia pacing (ATP) sequences/30 days, and ICD shocks/30 days. Two patients were placed in hospice care, with de-escalation of medical care soon after SBRT. In the remaining eight patients, the mean follow-up was 176 days. Analysis of ICD data showed a total reduction in seconds of detected VT by 69% (pretreatment 1065 seconds/month vs. post-treatment 332 second/month). The total reduction in ATP sequences was 48% (17.3 pretreatment and 8.9 post-treatment). Reduction in total ICD shocks after SBRT was 68% (2.9 shocks/month pretreatment and 0.9 shocks/month post-treatment). One patient did not respond to SBRT at all and had worsening of VTs. With regard to safety, two patients presented with mild pneumonitis. One patient experienced slow VT during SBRT and had to be resuscitated. Three patients received a heart transplant after SBRT.

In 2021, several other groups presented their first experience with SBRT for VTs in small series of patients.[20–23] The results were similar to the initial studies, with relatively high mortality, reflecting the severity of heart disease in this high-risk population. Other studies showed less optimistic data. Gianni and colleagues reported the results of a pilot study on five patients with refractory VTs (80% ischemic cardiomyopathy).[24] During a mean follow-up of 12 ± 2 months, all patients experienced clinically significant mid-to-late-term ventricular arrhythmia recurrence; two patients died of complications associated with advanced heart failure. No radiation-related complications were documented within this time window. The UCLA group presented their single-center experience with SBRT in eight patients with refractory VTs.[24] Majority of patients had recurrences of VT during follow-up and no significant difference in VT burden was observed when comparing 3 months before and 3 months after SBRT. Only alternative analysis comparing subsequent 3-month periods throughout the follow-up showed a decrease in average total ICD therapies from a median of 69.5 [interquartile range (IQR) 43.5, 115.8] pre-SBRT to 13.3 (IQR 7.7, 35.8) post-SBRT (P = 0.036). The Brigham and Women's group from Boston reported their experience with six patients with ischemic cardiomyopathy and VT, refractory to catheter ablations, and anti-arrhythmic medications.[25] Device-treated or sustained VT episodes were not significantly reduced by radioablation (median 42 [IQR: 19–269] to 29 [IQR: 0–81]; P = 0.438). However, a reduction in device shocks was observed from 12 (IQR: 3–19) to 0 (IQR: 0–1) (P = 0.046). Over a follow-up period of 231 (IQR: 212–311) days, three patients died of end-stage heart failure and three of six patients had possible adverse events (heart failure exacerbation, pneumonia, and an asymptomatic pericardial effusion). Several other prospective trials focused on efficacy and safety are ongoing, such as the German multicenter RAV-ENTA (NCT03867747)[26] and Italian STRA-MI-VT (NCT04066517).[27]

Our recent experience with SBRT in patients with advanced heart failure, a higher proportion of nonischemic cardiomyopathy, and more catheter ablation sessions before SBRT also suggests that a significant percentage of patients have recurrences of VT after SBRT, and often need additional catheter ablations for frequent recurrences of VT. The effect of SBRT in a majority of cases appears to be delayed. Total nonarrhythmic mortality in this population with advanced heart failure is quite high. We expect a more definite answer after the completion of our randomized trial (NCT04612140).

In summary, available outcomes data demonstrate a clear decrease in the number of VT episodes following SBRT; however, it is important to emphasize that the studies differ in inclusion criteria, patient population, targeting strategy, SBRT equipment, and efficacy assessment. Because most patients treated with cardiac SBRT are elderly and/or with advanced heart disease, the current results are associated with a high mortality rate, and additionally have no control arm, which limits optimal analysis of the long-term comparative efficacy and safety of the technique.

## Discussion: The Unanswered Questions

### What are the Tissue Effects of Radiotherapy?

The tissue effect of SBRT for VT in humans remains largely unknown. We already discussed that a 25 Gy dose was determined in early experimental studies as appropriate for the development of fibrotic lesions. Later studies focused more on the mechanism of injury in the myocardium. Irradiation of rat myocardium revealed apoptosis within the first 5 months, leading to the subsequent replacement of myocardial cells by fibrous tissue.[28] Another study in irradiated pig hearts revealed inflammatory changes with cleaved caspase-3 (a marker of apoptosis) at 3 months and marked fibrosis at 6 months.[29] Our recent report analyzing three postmortem hearts after SBRT is in line with the earlier discussed experimental data on early apoptosis and delayed fibrosis.[30] We also reported on a redo SBRT case because of inaccuracy of substrate targeting and observed on an electroanatomical map development of a region of low voltage corresponding to the irradiated tissue.[31] Extension of low-voltage areas after SBRT was observed in other patients also who undergo remapping (**Fig. 1**).

Other researchers claim that the clinical effect is not necessarily related to the development of fibrosis and do not consider fibrosis as the main antiarrhythmic mechanism. Some have observed phenotypic changes such as vacuolar degeneration, interstitial and subsarcolemmal edema, cell junction disruption, immune cell infiltrates, and microvascular inflammatory responses.[32–34]

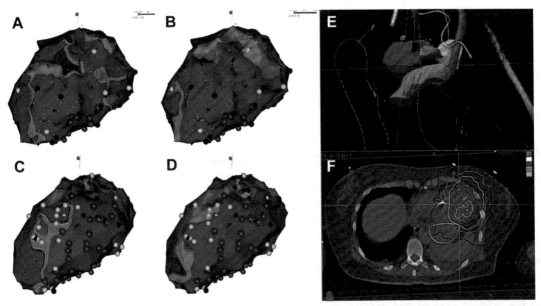

**Fig. 1.** Electroanatomical voltage maps from a female patient with burnt-out hypertrophic cardiomyopathy before (*A* and *B*) and after (*C* and *D*) SBRT of the substrate in the lateral wall, together with depiction of planned therapeutic volume as three-dimensional (3D) reconstruction (*E*) or in axial view (*F*). Explanation: *A* and *B*—bipolar and unipolar voltage maps showing large low voltage area in the lateral wall from the apex almost to the base; *C* and *D*—bipolar and unipolar voltage maps in corresponding projection depicting more homogeneous low-voltage area with large zone of noncapture (*gray dots*); *E*—3D reconstruction of the planned treatment volume in red on the lateral aspect of the left ventricle, corresponding to the region of dense scar on electroanatomical map; and *F*—radiosurgical treatment plan in axial view with red contours marking the planned therapeutic volume.

These changes may be a basis for functional ablation—disruption of cardiomyocyte electrical conduction without myocardial death. Indeed, some studies showed a slowing of intracardiac conduction on ECG.[34] More recently, an entirely different concept of functional ablation in the absence of transmural fibrosis has been proposed.[35] Based on experimental data, the authors suggest that the electrophysiological effect is due to enhanced electrical conduction in the irradiated tissue mediated by increases in components of the natrium channel and Cx43. This could be achieved even with a lower treatment dose than 25 Gy.

Therefore, it is not clear whether SBRT should aim primarily at the development of fibrosis or the modification of electrophysiological properties of the tissue without significant tissue injury and development of fibrosis. This is a fundamental question that remains without a clear answer.

## How Fast is the Clinical Effect?

This is another unanswered question that reflects uncertainty about the tissue effect of SBRT. Clinical studies with SBRT showed variable time frames for clinical effects. On one hand, we have reports of immediate results with SBRT. Anecdotal cases have shown acute termination of an electrical storm.[36,37] Such observations may be supported by the earlier discussed experimental studies that suggested a rapid mechanism of action unrelated to fibrosis.[33–35] On the other hand, many studies have observed a rather delayed effect. Even the ENCORE VT trial evaluated the effect after a 6-week blanking period because there were many recurrences immediately after SBRT.[17] Our experience supports a rather delayed effect. We observed the late abolition of VTs in some patients in our first series.[18] Similarly, in an earlier case report we witnessed the delayed disappearance of VT episodes within 6 months after SBRT in a patient with cardiac myxoma.[38] Later, we published a case of redo SBRT because of inaccuracy in planning, and the therapeutic effect after the second SBRT was noted only after 3 months.[31] A more recent postmortem analysis of three hearts after SBRT also reported delayed effects of radiotherapy in all subjects.[30] These observations are in line with animal studies showing the delayed effects of radiation therapy on the AV node and other tissues.[13,29,39]

Overall, although the clinical effect of SBRT may be immediate or early in some cases, predominantly it appears to be delayed. This may have important implications for the management of patients with electrical storms. The other question remains when to repeat catheter ablation or redo SBRT if VT recurs after radiotherapy because this is largely an unchartered territory.

### How Important is the Accuracy of Planning?

In SBRT, the accuracy of clinical target volume (CTV) determination might be of great importance for successful treatment. We have developed a strategy of accurate image integration, merging data from an electroanatomic mapping system with CT scans (**Fig. 2**). In a case report, we showed that this strategy allowed more precise delineation of the intended target during redo SBRT.[31] A detailed study on the accuracy and reproducibility of this method showed that detailed electroanatomical maps of at least three chambers allow very accurate and reproducible co-registration with preprocedural CT for SBRT.[40] We believe that such precise delineation of the electrophysiological substrate and co-registration with a pre-SBRT CT scan is important to ensure optimal targeting (**Fig. 3**). Alternatively, the American Heart Association 17-segment model was used by some groups to unite different imaging modalities and mapping data with standard orthogonal views obtained during radiation simulation.[41] However, no data on the reproducibility of this strategy have been published. Yet, reproducibility may be a crucial problem as shown by a recent German study in which patient data sets were sent to five university centers for independent CTV determination and subsequent structural analysis.[42] Remarkable differences regarding the degree of agreement of the CTV definition on the electroanatomical maps and the preprocedural CT were noted, indicating a loss of agreement during the transfer process.

Some other groups propose body surface mapping together with the imaging of the heart and scar tissue as a noninvasive strategy to determine PTV.[16,17] In principle, this noninvasive electrocardiographic imaging (ECGi) uses an array of ECG electrodes and inverse solution algorithms to project activation from the body surface on the heart model to determine the source of activation and/or exit of the re-entrant VT. Although this strategy appears to be attractive, it has several limitations. One of them is accuracy. Spatio-temporal variability of recovered electrograms limits the precise localization of arrhythmia circuits from the body surface.[43] The other reason is that the critical isthmus of re-entry or site of origin in focal arrhythmias may not correlate with the site of the earliest epicardial breakthrough.[44] The third reason is the inability to cover adequately the interventricular septum. Finally, patients with large substrates may have inducible several morphologies of VT only during electrophysiology study that enables recording and pacing from different sites in ventricles.

In summary, invasive electroanatomical mapping and pacing in sinus rhythm and/or during VT allow usually quite a reasonable prediction of critical parts of the substrate. Strategies of co-registration of the electrophysiological substrate and preprocedural CT should provide the most accurate CTV. This cannot be done with the same precision when inducing VT from the device and mapping only on the body surface. Therefore, the clinical utility of noninvasive ECGi with CT imaging needs to be evaluated further for efficacy and accuracy in future studies.

### How Safe is Cardiac SBRT?

An important question that remains to be answered is the safety of SBRT when the target organ is the heart. Oncology literature shows a wide variation in cardiac toxicity because of radiation therapy. A seminal phase 3 trial on an escalation of therapeutic dose in stage III lung cancer (RTOG 0617) reported worse survival in patients receiving higher doses.[45] Interestingly, it was the dose delivered to the heart that was contributing to the increased risk of death in these patients. Pooled analysis of dose escalation trials delivering 70 Gy –90 Gy for lung cancer described cardiac toxicity in 23% of patients.[46] Importantly, the median of the presentation was 26 months. Pericardial effusions, constrictive pericarditis, and/or myocardial infarctions were the most frequent manifestations of toxicity. A concise review of cardiac toxicity and its mechanisms was published by Banfill and colleagues and they refer to existing cardiac dose constraints for radiotherapy of thoracic organs that are based on the Qualitative Analyses of Normal Tissue Effects in the Clinic (QUANTEC).[47,48] QUANTEC recommended that the volume of heart receiving greater than or equal to 30 Gy (V30) should be kept below 46% and mean heart dose less than 15 Gy. In line with this recommendation, Darby and colleagues reported an increased risk of major adverse cardiac events (MACE; defined as myocardial infarction, coronary revascularization, or death from ischemic heart disease) in breast cancer survivors, with a linear relationship to cardiac radiation dose.[49] The rate of MACE increased by 7.4% per 1 Gy increase in mean heart dose in this cohort of patients. Another study showed that compliance with QUANTEC recommendation of V25 <10% and a mean heart

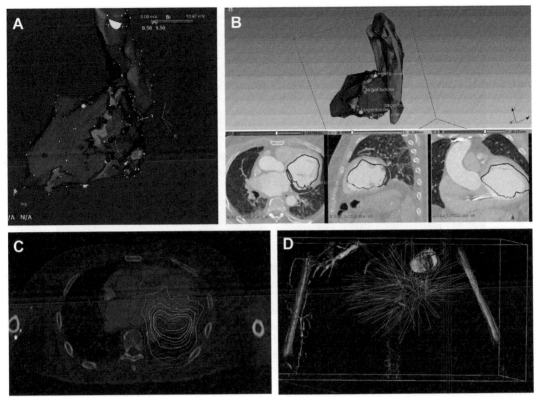

**Fig. 2.** An example of the process of co-registration of a substrate derived from an electroanatomical voltage map of a patient with the posterolateral scar. (*A*). Bipolar voltage map with the red zone of low voltage and ablation tags marking exits on superior and inferior aspect of the scar, (*B*). a three-dimensional (3D) reconstruction of the planned therapeutic volume (in red) and co-registration with CT scan, (*C*). Treatment plan in axial view with isodose lines, (*D*). The target for SBRT with prescribed radiotherapy doses.

dose of less than 4 Gy in breast cancer therapy can be achieved with a predicted risk of cardiac mortality of less than 1%.[50] However, since the probability of cardiac toxicity approached 1% even with a smaller value of V25, no single-dose volume cut-off value seems to ensure the lowest risk of cardiac toxicity. On top of that, QUANTEC recommendations deal with fractionated radiotherapy instead of single-shot irradiation as in cardiac SBRT.

More recently, several studies have been published exploring the relationship between the cardiac radiation dose, MACE, and mortality in patients with lung cancer. In a review by Zhang and colleagues,[51] four studies were identified that described SBRT treatment in younger patients. Heart V30 was associated with higher total mortality and mean heart dose was linked to a higher rate of cardiac events.[46,52]

Finally, an analysis of 64 studies on radiotherapy of surrounding organs showed that high doses reaching the heart (above 40 Gy) were associated with an increased rate of unexplained death.[53] Such a dose led to the occurrence of pericardial effusion. Therefore, the current guidelines

recommend limiting the dose to the heart and pericardium.[54]

Besides cardiac toxicity, thoracic SBRT can cause serious or life-threatening radiation-related side effects by damaging other thoracic organs at risk.[55,56] The risk of radiation pneumonitis and/or pulmonary fibrosis has been correlated with the size or location of the target. The majority of studies noted safe treatment with a rate of symptomatic lung toxicity below 10% after lung SBRT with a mean lung dose of the combined lungs of 8 Gy in 3–5 fractions. Mild esophageal toxicity, including esophagitis or stricture, is another well-known complication of radiotherapy involving the mediastinum.[57] Although many dose constraints have been reported, clinical estimates of risk are limited, whereas toxicity could be caused by other factors (eg, individual sensitivity or iatrogenic manipulations of the esophagus), and only five deaths in four centers because of bleeding ulcers or fistulas have been reported. An additional consideration is toxicity to gastric tissue. Doses to the stomach limit SBRT target coverage in case of pancreatic, liver,

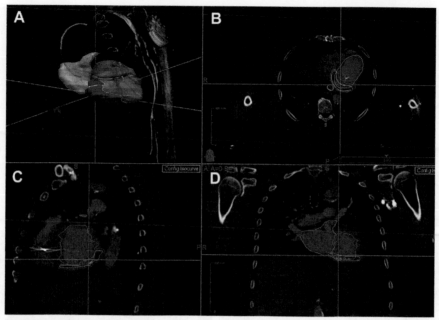

**Fig. 3.** An example of a radiosurgical plan in a patient with ischemic cardiomyopathy and a substrate for VT inferobasally. (*A*). a three-dimensional (3D) reconstruction of the planned therapeutic volume (red); (*B–D*). Treatment plan in sagittal, axial, and coronal orientation. Color lines delineate areas with the same dose (*isodose lines*).

or adrenal tumors often,[58] and the same dose reduction might be expected in cardiac SBRT, particularly when the substrate is located in the inferior wall. Moreover, uncertainties caused by stomach-filling should be considered when targeting the inferior wall of the heart.[59]

When viewed in the context of collateral cardiac damage (based on the evidence discussed), SBRT focused on the heart raises concerns about long-term damage. Yet, reviewing the published series of SBRT for VT, one gets the impression that the therapy is quite safe. In this respect, it is important to emphasize that the numbers of patients studied for therapeutic cardiac SBRT are still very small, and reported follow-up is short (usually up to 1 year) (**Table 1**). In our series of 33 cases, we observed one death due to esophagopericardial fistula that occurred 9 months after SBRT.[60] In addition, there were two cases of progression of mitral valve disease that required surgical replacement more than 2 years after SBRT. The second case of gastropericardial fistula at 2.4 years, requiring surgical repair, is mentioned in an abstract from the ENCORE VT study.[61] The same abstract reports on a case of pericardial effusion at 2.2 years.

In summary, although the acute toxicity of SBRT is generally low, delayed side effects may limit the wider acceptance of this strategy. Longer, vigilant follow-up is necessary to describe the true safety profile of SBRT for VT. Until a greater understanding of the long-term cardiac effect is achieved, SBRT remains a last resort for ventricular arrhythmia management, reserved for situations when catheter ablation fails.

### Who is an Optimal Candidate for SBRT?

Considering all the earlier discussed data, we feel that currently, SBRT should be offered only as a bail-out therapy when all other attempts fail. In our experience, repeated catheter ablations often achieve substantial substrate modification and noninducibility of VTs. However, the question remains: how many attempts should the patient undergo before the referral for SBRT? The volume of VT ablation and expertise of the ablation center is also an important consideration before referral for SBRT because currently there are no standardized guidelines for referral for SBRT. The quality and quantity of catheter ablation varies for patients referred to SBRT and contributes heavily to the heterogeneity in reported outcomes. Another reason for considering SBRT may be an absolute contraindication to catheter ablation. However, such cases are very rare.

Another controversial scenario is whether SBRT should be offered to patients with idiopathic VT or premature ventricular contraction-related cardiomyopathy. Because these are not life-threatening conditions, the myocardium is normal with no significant scar tissue on imaging, with younger patients,

**Table 1**
An overview of published complications of SBRT for VT

| First Author and Year of Publication | Number of Patients | Delivery System | Mean PTV (cm³) | Follow Up (month) | Adverse Events CTCAE (G3–G5) | Notes |
|---|---|---|---|---|---|---|
| Carbuciccho C et al,[20] 2021 | 7 | MLA | 183±53 | 8 (median) | No serious adverse events | 3x death unrelated to SBRT 1x Pulmonary fibrosis G1, 1x GIT disorder G2 |
| Chin R et al,[24] 2020 | 8 | MLA | 121±50 | 7.8 (median) | No serious adverse events | 3x death unrelated to SBRT |
| Cuculich P.S et al,[16] 2017 | 5 | MLA | 49±72 | 12 months | No serious adverse events | 1x death stroke 3 weeks after SBRT 3 moths after SBRT inflammatory changes in the adjacent lung tissue – resolution at 12 months |
| Gerard I.J et al,[67] 2021 | 2 | MLA | 103 (case1) 66 (case2) | 17 months 12 months | No serious adverse events | – |
| Gianni C 2020[23] | 5 | CK | 143±45 | 12±2 months | No serious adverse events | 2x death due to advanced HF |
| Haskova J et al,[38] 2018 (case report) | 1 | CK | 70 | 9 months | Deadly complication esophagopericardial fistula | – |
| Ho L et al,[21] 2021 | 7 | MLA | 55±29 | 14.5 (median) | No serious adverse events | 1x death due to hepatic failure 47 day after SBRT 1x epicardial effusion G1 6 months after SBRT |
| Lloyd M.S et al,[19] 2020 | 10 | MLA | 81±56 | 176 days (mean) | 2x pneumonitis (CTCAE class. unknown) | 2x excluded from follow-up due to terminal HF 5 days after SBRT 1 x slow VT under ICD detection limit |

(continued on next page)

**Table 1**
*(continued)*

| First Author and Year of Publication | Number of Patients | Delivery System | Mean PTV (cm³) | Follow Up (month) | Adverse Events CTCAE (G3-G5) | Notes |
|---|---|---|---|---|---|---|
| Neuwirth R et al,[18] 2019 | 10 | CK | 23±5 | 28 (median) | 1x progression of mitral regurgitation | – |
| Robinson C.G. et al,[17] 2018 | 19 | MLA | 99 (61±299) | 13 months | 1x HF, 1x pericarditis, 1x pericardial effusion, 1x pneumothorax | 1x gastric hemorrhage G2 2x pneumonitis G2 2x pleural effusion G1 |
| Robinson C.G. (Encore-VT Long term– unpublished text, abstract) | 19 | MLA | | 12.8–28.8 months | 1x pericardial effusion at 2.2 years 1x gastropericardial fistula at 2.4years | 8 x deaths in the whole group: 1x unrelated pancreatitis 3x unlikely (accident, amiodarone toxicity, VT recurrences) 2x possible due to VT and worsening cardiac status 2x possible due to HF |
| Yugo D et al,[22] 2021 | 3 | MLA | 83±18 | 13.5±2.8 months | No serious adverse events | – |

*Abbreviations:* CK, CyberKnife, CTCAE (G1-G5) - Common Terminology Criteria for Adverse Events https://www.uptodate.com/., 18.6.2022, 15:13, GIT, gastrointestinal, HF, Heart Failure; ICD, implantable cardioverter defibrillator; MLA, Medical Linear Accelerator; PTV, planned target volume; SBRT, stereotactic body radiation therapy; VT, ventricular tachycardia.

and a high success rate of catheter ablation, we feel that SBRT is not indicated in such a cohort.

Can new and improved catheter ablation technologies reduce the need for SBRT?

Recently, novel technologies have emerged that can radically improve the efficacy of catheter ablation. The most disruptive one is the irreversible electroporation or pulse-field ablation. This is a nonthermal energy source that consists of ultrashort pulses of direct current resulting in the creation of pores in the cell membranes of cardiomyocytes.[62,63] Preliminary results in patients with atrial fibrillation are exciting[64,65] and animal experiments for VT ablation have also shown encouraging results.[66]

In summary, the promising early experience with irreversible electroporation suggests that soon, catheter ablation of VT could be more efficacious and probably safer. Such improvement may heavily influence the refinement or the need for SBRT in VT management.

## SUMMARY

SBRT has emerged as a potentially attractive, less invasive strategy of refractory VT management. So far, clinical studies documented a rather modest efficacy in the suppression of refractory VTs. The major unanswered questions revolve around the mechanism of action, time to effect, and the long-term safety of this treatment. At this stage of development, it remains an experimental treatment. In our opinion, SBRT should be offered only as a bail-out strategy in cases of otherwise intractable VTs, after failed catheter ablation(s) at an expert center. Further studies, with comparative treatment arms, are needed to address these unanswered questions.

## CLINICS CARE POINTS

- Stereotactic body radiotherapy (SBRT) is an alternative treatment method for ventricular tachycardias (VT) after failed catheter ablation(s).

- Initial clinical experience with cardiac SBRT suggests reasonable efficacy in decreasing VT recurrences.

- Although the acute toxicity of SBRT targeting myocardial substrate is low, more information is needed on long-term safety.

- At this stage, SBRT should be offered primarily as a bail-out procedure when repeated catheter ablation for VT fails.

## FUNDING

This work was supported by the grant project AZV NU20-02-00244 from the Ministry of Health of the Czech Republic and by funding from theEuropean Union's Horizon 2020 research and innovation program under the grant agreement No. 945119.

## DISCLOSURE

The authors have nothing to disclose. However, outside of this article, J. Kautzner reports personal fees from Abbott, Bayer, Biosense Webster, Biotronik, Boehringer Ingelheim, CubeVision, Medtronic, Mylan, Pfizer, and ProMed CS for lectures, advisory boards, and consultancy.

## REFERENCES

1. Connolly SJ, Hallstrom AP, Cappato R, et al. Meta-analysis of the implantable cardioverter defibrillator secondary prevention trials. Eur Heart J 2000;21: 2071–8.
2. Nanthakumar K, Epstein AE, Kay GN, et al. Prophylactic implantable cardioverter-defibrillator therapy in patients with left ventricular systolic dysfunction: a pooled analysis of 10 primary prevention trials. J Am Coll Cardiol 2004;44:2166–72.
3. Mallidi J, Nadkarni GN, Berger RD, et al. Meta-analysis of catheter ablation as an adjunct to medical therapy for treatment of ventricular tachycardia in patients with structural heart disease. Heart Rhythm 2011;8:503–10.
4. Marchlinski FE, Haffajee CI, Beshai JF, et al. Long-term success of irrigated radiofrequency catheter ablation of sustained ventricular tachycardia: post-approval THERMOCOOL VT trial. J Am Coll Cardiol 2016;67:674–83.
5. Sapp JL, Wells GA, Parkash R, et al. Ventricular tachycardia ablation versus escalation of antiarrhythmic drugs. N Engl J Med 2016;375:111–21.
6. Aldhoon B, Wichterle D, Peichl P, et al. Outcomes of ventricular tachycardia ablation in patients with structural heart disease: the impact of electrical storm. PloS One 2017;12:e0171830.
7. Maskoun W, Saad M, Abualsuod A, et al. Outcome of catheter ablation for ventricular tachycardia in patients with ischemic cardiomyopathy: a systematic review and meta-analysis of randomized clinical trials. Int J Cardiol 2018;267:107–13.
8. Tokuda M, Kojodjojo P, Tung S, et al. Acute failure of catheter ablation for ventricular tachycardia due to structural heart disease: causes and significance. J Am Heart Assoc 2013;2:e000072.
9. Loo BW Jr, Soltys SG, Wang L, et al. Stereotactic ablative radiotherapy for the treatment of refractory cardiac ventricular arrhythmia. Circulation: Arrh Electrophysiol 2015;8:748–50.

10. Cvek J, Neuwirth R, Knybel L, et al. Cardiac radio-surgery for malignant ventricular tachycardia. Cureus 2014;6(7).

11. Amino M, Yoshioka K, Tanabe T, et al. Heavy ion radiation up-regulates Cx43 and ameliorates arrhythmogenic substrates in hearts after myocardial infarction. Cardiovasc Res 2006;72(3):412–21.

12. Amino M, Yoshioka K, Fujibayashi D, et al. Year-long upregulation of connexin43 in rabbit hearts by heavy ion irradiation. Am J Physiol Heart Circ Physiol 2010; 298(3):H1014–21.

13. Sharma A, Wong D, Weidlich G, et al. Noninvasive stereotactic radiosurgery (CyberHeart) for creation of ablation lesions in the atrium. Heart Rhythm 2010;7:802–10.

14. Gardner EA, Sumanaweera TS, Blanck O, et al. In Vivo dose measurement using TLDs and MOSFET dosimeters for cardiac radiosurgery. J Appl Clin Med Phys 2012;13(3):3745.

15. Blanck O, Bode F, Gebhard M, et al. Dose-escalation study for cardiac radiosurgery in a porcine model. Int J Radiat Oncol Biol Phys 2014;89(3): 590–8.

16. Cuculich PS, Schill MR, Kashani R, et al. Noninvasive cardiac radiation for ablation of ventricular tachycardia. N Engl J Med 2017;377: 2325–36.

17. Robinson CG, Samson PP, Moore KM, et al. Phase I/II trial of electrophysiology-guided noninvasive cardiac radioablation for ventricular tachycardia. Circulation 2019;139:313–21.

18. Neuwirth R, Cvek J, Knybel L, et al. Stereotactic radiosurgery for ablation of ventricular tachycardia. Europace 2019;21:1088–195.

19. Lloyd MS, Wight J, Schneider F, et al. Clinical experience of stereotactic body radiation for refractory ventricular tachycardia in advanced heart failure patients. Heart Rhythm 2020;17(3):415–22.

20. Carbucicchio C, Andreini D, Piperno G, et al. Stereotactic radioablation for the treatment of ventricular tachycardia: preliminary data and insights from the STRA-MI-VT phase Ib/II study. J Interv Card Electrophysiol 2021;62(2):427–39.

21. Ho LT, Chen JL, Chan HM, et al. First Asian population study of stereotactic body radiation therapy for ventricular arrhythmias. Sci Rep 2021;11(1): 10360.

22. Yugo D, Lo LW, Wu YH, et al. Case series on stereotactic body radiation therapy in non-ischemic cardiomyopathy patients with recurrent ventricular tachycardia. Pacing Clin Electrophysiol 2021;44(6): 1085–93.

23. Gianni C, Rivera D, Burkhardt JD, et al. Stereotactic arrhythmia radioablation for refractory scar-related ventricular tachycardia. Heart Rhythm 2020;17(8): 1241–8.

24. Chin R, Hayase J, Hu P, et al. Non-invasive stereotactic body radiation therapy for refractory ventricular arrhythmias: an institutional experience. J Interv Card Electrophysiol 2021;61(3): 535–43.

25. Qian PC, Quadros K, Aguilar M, et al. Substrate modification using stereotactic radioablation to treat refractory ventricular tachycardia in patients with ischemic cardiomyopathy. JACC Clin Electrophysiol 2022;8(1):49–58.

26. Blanck O, Buergy D, Vens M, et al. Radiosurgery for ventricular tachycardia: preclinical and clinical evidence and study design for a German multi-center multi-platform feasibility trial (RAVENTA). Clin Res Cardiol 2020;109(11):1319–32.

27. Carbucicchio C, Jereczek-Fossa BA, Andreini D, et al. STRA-MI-VT (STereotactic RadioAblation by Multimodal Imaging for Ventricular Tachycardia): rationale and design of an Italian experimental prospective study. J Interv Card Electrophysiol 2021; 61(3):583–93.

28. Salata C, Ferreira-Machado SC, De Andrade CBV, et al. Apoptosis induction of cardiomyocytes and subsequent fibrosis after irradiation and neoadjuvant chemotherapy. Int J Radiat Biol 2014;90(4): 284–90.

29. Lehmann HI, Graeff C, Simoniello P, et al. Feasibility study on cardiac arrhythmia ablation using high-energy heavy ion beams. Scientific Rep 2016;6: 38895.

30. Kautzner J, Jedlickova K, Sramko M, et al. Radiation-induced changes in ventricular myocardium after stereotactic body radiotherapy for recurrent ventricular tachycardia. JACC Clin Electrophysiol 2021;7(12):1487–92.

31. Peichl P, Sramko M, Cvek J, et al. A case report of successful elimination of recurrent ventricular tachycardia by repeated stereotactic radiotherapy: the importance of accurate target volume delineation. J Eur Heart J Case Rep 2020;5(2): ytaa516.

32. Rapp F, Simoniello P, Wiedemann J, et al. Biological cardiac tissue effects of high-energy heavy ions e investigation for myocardial ablation. Sci Rep 2019;9:5000.

33. Kiani S, Kutob L, Schneider F, et al. Histopathologic and ultrastructural findings in human myocardium after stereotactic body radiation therapy for recalcitrant ventricular tachycardia. Circ Arrhythm Electrophysiol 2020;13(11):e008753.

34. Cha MJ, Seo JW, Kim HJ, et al. Early changes in rat heart after high-dose irradiation: implications for antiarrhythmic effects of cardiac radioablation. J Am Heart Assoc 2021;10:e019072.

35. Zhang DM, Navara R, Yin T, et al. Cardiac radiotherapy induces electrical conduction reprogramming in the

absence of transmural fibrosis. Nat Commun 2021; 12(1):5558.

36. Scholz EP, Seidensaal K, Naumann P, et al. Risen from the dead: cardiac stereotactic ablative radiotherapy as last rescue in a patient with refractory ventricular fibrillation storm. Heartrhythm Case Rep 2019;5(6):329–32.

37. Jumeau R, Ozsahin M, Schwitter J, et al. Rescue procedure for an electrical storm using robotic non-invasive cardiac radio-ablation. Radiother Oncol 2018;128:189–91.

38. Haskova J, Peichl P, Pirk J, et al. Stereotactic radiosurgery as a treatment for recurrent ventricular tachycardia associated with cardiac fibroma. HeartRhythm Case Rep 2018;5:44–7.

39. Zei PC, Wong D, Gardner E, et al. Safety and efficacy of stereotactic radioablation targeting pulmonary vein tissues in an experimental model. Heart Rhythm 2018;15:1420–7.

40. Abdel-Kafi S, Sramko M, Omara S, et al. Accuracy of electroanatomical mapping-guided cardiac radiotherapy for ventricular tachycardia: pitfalls and solutions. Europace 2021;23(12):1989–97.

41. Brownstein J, Afzal M, Okabe T, et al. Method and atlas to enable targeting for cardiac radioablation employing the American Heart Association segmented model. Int J Radiat Oncol Biol Phys 2021;111(1):178–85.

42. Boda-Heggemann J, Blanck O, Mehrhof F, et al. Interdisciplinary clinical target volume generation for cardiac radioablation: multicenter benchmarking for the RAdiosurgery for VENtricular TAchycardia (RAVENTA) Trial. Int J Radiat Oncol Biol Phys 2021;110(3):745–56.

43. Bear LR, Huntjens PR, Walton RD, et al. Cardiac electrical dyssynchrony is accurately detected by noninvasive electrocardiographic imaging. Heart Rhythm 2018;15(7):1058–69.

44. Bhaskaran A, Downar E, Chauhan VS, et al. Electroanatomical mapping-guided stereotactic radiotherapy for right ventricular tachycardia storm. HeartRhythm. Case Rep 2019;5(12):590–2.

45. Bradley JD, Paulus R, Komaki R, et al. Standarddose versus high-dose conformal radiotherapy with concurrent and consolidation carboplatin plus paclitaxel with or without cetuximab for patients with stage IIIA or IIIB non-small-cell lung cancer (RTOG 0617): a randomised, two-by-two factorial phase 3 study. Lancet Oncol 2015;16(2):187–99.

46. Wang K, Eblan MJ, Deal AM, et al. Cardiac toxicity after radiotherapy for stage III non-small cell lung cancer: pooled analysis of dose escalation trials delivering 70 to 80 Gy. J Clin Oncol 2017;35:1387–94.

47. Banfill K, Giuliani M, Aznar M, et al. Cardiac toxicity of thoracic radiotherapy: existing evidence and future directions. J Thorac Oncol 2021;16(2):216–27.

48. Gagliardi G, Constine LS, Moiseenko V, et al. Radiation dose-volume effects in the heart. Int J Radiat Oncol Biol Phys 2010;76:S77–85.

49. Darby SC, Ewertz M, McGale P, et al. Risk of ischemic heart disease in women after radiotherapy for breast cancer. N Engl J Med 2013;368:987–98.

50. Moiseenko V, Einck J, Murphy J, et al. Clinical evaluation of QUANTEC guidelines to predict the risk of cardiac mortality in breast cancer patients. Acta Oncol 2016;55(12):1506–10.

51. Zhang TW, Snir J, Boldt RG, et al. Is the importance of heart dose overstated in the treatment of non-small cell lung cancer? A systematic review of the literature. Int J Radiat Oncol Biol Phys 2019;104:582–9.

52. Dess RT, Sun Y, Matuszak MM, et al. Cardiac events after radiation therapy: combined analysis of prospective multicenter trials for locally advanced non-small-cell lung cancer. J Clin Oncol 2017;35:1395–402.

53. Niska JR, Thorpe CS, Allen SM, et al. Radiation and the heart: systematic review of dosimetry and cardiac endpoints. Expert Rev Cardiovasc Ther 2018;16:931–50.

54. Nestle U, De Ruysscher D, Ricardi U, et al. ESTRO ACROP guidelines for target volume definition in the treatment of locally advanced non-small cell lung cancer. Radiother Oncol 2018;127:1–5.

55. Corradetti MN, Haas AR, Rengan R. Central-airway necrosis after stereotactic body-radiation therapy. N Engl J Med 2012;366:2327–9.

56. Kong FS, Moiseenko V, Zhao J, et al. Organs at risk considerations for thoracic stereotactic body radiation therapy: what is safe for lung parenchyma? Int J Radiat Oncol Biol Phys 2021;110(1):172–87.

57. Nuyttens JJ, Moiseenko V, McLaughlin M, et al. Esophageal dose tolerance in patients treated with stereotactic body radiation therapy. Semin Radiat Oncol 2016;26(2):140–8.

58. Mahadevan A, Moningi S, Grimm J, et al. Maximizing tumor control and limiting complications with stereotactic body radiation therapy for pancreatic cancer. Int J Radiat Oncol Biol Phys 2021;110(1):206–16.

59. Tanaka O, Taniguchi T, Ono K, et al. Adrenal stereotactic body radiation therapy: the effects of a full and empty stomach on radiation dose to organs at risk. Int J Radiat Oncol Biol Phys 2021;111(3):e481.

60. Haskova J, Jedlickova K, Cvek J, et al. Oesophagopericardial fistula as a late complication of stereotactic radiotherapy for recurrent ventricular tachycardia. Europace 2022;9:euab326.

61. Robinson CG, Samson P, Moore KMS, et al. Longer term results from a Phase I/II study of EP-guided noninvasive cardiac radioablation for treatment of

792          Haskova et al

ventricular tachycardia (ENCORE-VT). Int J Radiat Oncol 2019;105:682 (abstract).

62. Anic A, Breskovic T, Sikiric I, et al. Pulsed field ablation: a promise that came true. Curr Opin Cardiol 2021;36(1):5–9.

63. McBride S, Avazzadeh S, Wheatley AM, et al. Ablation modalities for therapeutic intervention in arrhythmia-related cardiovascular disease: focus on electroporation. J Clin Med 2021;10(12):2657.

64. Reddy VY, Anter E, Rackauskas G, et al. Lattice-tip focal ablation catheter that toggles between radiofrequency and pulsed field energy to treat atrial fibrillation: a first-in-human trial. Circ Arrhythm Electrophysiol 2020;13(6):e008718.

65. Reddy VY, Dukkipati SR, Neuzil P, et al. Pulsed field ablation of paroxysmal atrial fibrillation: 1-year outcomes of IMPULSE, PEFCAT, and PEFCAT II. JACC Clin Electrophysiol 2021;7(5):614–27.

66. Yavin HD, Higuchi K, Sroubek J, et al. Pulsed-field ablation in ventricular myocardium using a focal catheter: the impact of application repetition on lesion dimensions. Circ Arrhythm Electrophysiol 2021;14(9):e010375.

67. Gerard IJ, Bernier M, Hijal T, et al. Stereotactic Arrhythmia Radioablation for Ventricular Tachycardia: Single Center First Experiences. Advances in Radiation Oncology 2021;6. https://doi.org/10.1016/j.adro.2021.100702.

# Surgical Ablation of Ventricular Tachycardia

Takashi Nitta, MD, PhD[a,b]

## KEYWORDS

- Ventricular tachycardia • Surgery • Mapping • Ablation • Cryothermia • Surgical ablation

## KEY POINTS

- Surgery for ventricular tachycardia (VT) is indicated in patients in whom pharmacotherapy or catheter ablation is ineffective or frequent episodes of VT are not suppressed resulting in frequent activation of implantable cardioverter defibrillator.
- Resection of fibrous endocardium combined with encircling cryothermia at the border between the infarcted and normal myocardium is performed for ischemic VT.
- Intraoperative mapping is essential in surgery for VT associated with cardiomyopathy. Close collaboration between the physician and surgeon is important and intraoperative use of an electroanatomic mapping system is helpful.
- In addition to resection of tumors, cryothermia of the thinned subepicardial myocardium at the edge of tumor is recommended in VT associated with cardiac tumors.

## INTRODUCTION

Direct surgery was the only non-pharmacological therapy for ventricular tachycardia (VT) before the implantable cardioverter defibrillator (ICD) began to be widely used in the 1980s.[1–3] Thereafter, ICD implantation has become the first-line therapy for the prevention of sudden cardiac death because of ventricular tachyarrhythmias. For the cure of VT, catheter ablation has been shown to be effective in selective patients and several antiarrhythmic drugs have been used to suppress the VT occurrence and minimize ICD therapies. Despite these advances in cardiac electrophysiology, there are patients who require direct surgery for VT for various indications and conditions. In this article, we review indications for surgery, the underlying electrophysiology of ischemic and nonischemic VT, and describe surgical techniques used for the treatment of VT.

## INDICATION FOR SURGERY

The recommendations for surgical ablation of VT are shown in **Table 1**.[4] As a life-saving procedure, surgical ablation of VT is recommended in patients with monomorphic sustained VT for which pharmacotherapy or catheter ablation is ineffective, or in whom frequent VT episodes are not suppressed, or when there is frequent delivery of ICD therapies associated with the above condition.[5–7]

Surgery for VT is reasonable in patients with sustained monomorphic VT and heart failure or thromboembolism associated with left ventricular (LV) aneurysm or asynergy due to myocardial infarction. Surgery may be considered for sustained monomorphic VT in patients after myocardial infarction or for the VT originating from the ventricular insertion site of the left ventricular assist device (LVAD),[8] and reasonable for the VT associated with cardiac tumors.[9,10]

## ISCHEMIC VENTRICULAR TACHYCARDIA
### Endocardial Resection with Cryothermia

Reentry within scar tissue is the predominant mechanism in ischemic VT. Conduction is slowed within the surviving myocardium in the scarred tissue, and/or anisotropic conduction can occur within the thinned-out myocardium. Slow

[a] Hanyu General Hospital, Shimo-iwase 446, Hanyu City, Saitama 348-8505 Japan; [b] Nippon Medical School, Tokyo, Japan
E-mail address: nitta@nms.ac.jp

Card Electrophysiol Clin 14 (2022) 793–799
https://doi.org/10.1016/j.ccep.2022.06.005

**Table 1**
**Recommendations for surgical ablation of ventricular tachycardia**

| Recommendations | COR | LOE | GOR (Minds) | LOE (Minds) |
|---|---|---|---|---|
| In patients with recurrent sustained monomorphic VT or frequent ICD therapies for whom antiarrhythmic medications are ineffective or for whom catheter ablation is not successful, surgical ablation is recommended. | I | C | B | V |
| For patients with sustained monomorphic VT after MI who have heart failure or thromboembolism associated with LV aneurysm or asynergy, surgical ablation is reasonable. | IIa | C | B | V |
| For patients with sustained monomorphic VT after MI, surgical ablation may be considered. | IIb | C | C1 | V |
| For patients with sustained monomorphic VT originating from the insertion site of LVAD, surgical ablation may be considered. | IIb | C | B | IVb |
| For patients with sustained monomorphic VT associated with cardiac tumors, surgical ablation may be reasonable. | IIb | C | C1 | V |

*Abbreviations:* COR, class of recommendation; GOR, grades of recommendation; ICD, implantable cardioverter-defibrillator; LOE, level of evidence; LV, left ventricular; LVAD, left ventricular assist device; MI, myocardial infarction; Minds, Medical Information Network Distribution; VT: ventricular tachycardia.
*Data from* Nogami A, Kurita T, Abe H, et al. JCS/JHRS 2019 Guideline on Non-Pharmacotherapy of Cardiac Arrhythmias [published correction appears in Circ J. 2021;85(9):1692-1700]. Circ J. 2021;85(7):1104-1244.

conduction allows sufficient time for the myocardium to recover from its refractory period and reentrant activations to be sustained. In such patients with ischemic etiology of VT substrate, surgical endocardial resection of the scarred tissue (**Fig. 1**A), combined with encircling cryothermia at the border between the infarcted and normal myocardium (**Fig. 1**B), eradicates the substrates for reentrant activations and prevents VT occurrence.[1,2] In most patients, the opening of the LV is reduced by a purse-string suture to reform the LV shape in an attempt to improve the LV systolic performance (**Fig. 1**C).[11] The opening of the LV is closed directly or with a Dacron patch (**Fig. 1**D).

In the early period of surgery for ischemic VT, in the late 1970s, intraoperative mapping was performed to locate the earliest activation or the site of slow conduction.[3] Data from intraoperative mapping, including epicardial and endocardial electrograms and activation patterns during VT, provided deep understanding of the underlying electrophysiology and reentrant activation mechanisms. In addition, the technique of the intraoperative mapping has developed dramatically by advancements in automated mapping systems and use of multiple electrodes (**Fig. 2**), enabling simultaneous multichannel recording and analysis and three-dimensional dynamic display of activation patterns. Other analyses, such as the entrainment mapping technique have also demonstrated utility in planning surgical VT ablation.[12] Sequential map-guided

subendocardial resection is theoretically an ideal approach in surgery of VT and provides excellent results, including postoperative VT inducibility and a long-term freedom from VT recurrence.[13,14]

## Non-map-guided Endocardial Resection

Most patients with ischemic VT have anterior LV myocardial infarction and the substrate for VT locates in the patchy surviving myocardium in the scar tissue, forming a reentrant circuit for the sustenance of VT. The distribution of the substrate varies, therefore the earliest activation site of VT, which is the exit from the reentrant circuit, can change its location. In fact, many patients have multiple monomorphic VT sharing the same substrate, but exhibiting different activation patterns and VT morphologies by changing the exit site from the reentrant circuit.

Although intraoperative mapping study is useful in localizing the earliest activation site that directs the optimal site for surgical intervention, the reentrant circuit or the substrate of VT is not always defined by the study. Endocardial resection with or without cryothermia and without intraoperative mapping study has been shown to provide excellent clinical outcomes equivalent to those of the map-guided procedure.[11,15] Also from the perspective of prevention of nonclinical VT after ablative surgery, broad resection of the scarred endocardium with encircling cryothermia at the

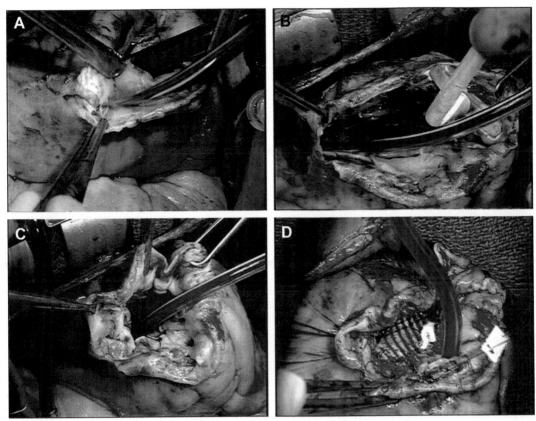

**Fig. 1.** Endocardial resection and encircling cryothermia. (*A*) After a ventriculotomy is placed in the anterior LV, the scarred endocardium with patchy surviving myocardium is resected circumferentially with scissors. (*B*) Cryothermia is applied at the border between the endocardial resection and normal endocardium. (*C*) The opening of the LV is reduced by a purse-string suture. (*D*) The LV is closed with a Dacron patch. LV, left ventricular.

border between the infarcted and normal myocardium is recommended in ischemic VT, irrespective of the results or execution of intraoperative mapping study.

## NONISCHEMIC VENTRICULAR TACHYCARDIA

VTs not associated with coronary artery disease or myocardial ischemia are classified as nonischemic VT. Nonischemic VT includes various underlying heart diseases, such as cardiomyopathy, infiltrative disorders, cardiac tumors, but may also include patients with no structural heart disease. A surgery for nonischemic VT preoperative and intraoperative mapping is essential, because the substrate for VT is not easily visible or demonstrable. Preoperative imaging with delayed enhancement of cardiac MRI may help identify scar tissue that may guide surgical ablation. Even in the VT associated with cardiac tumors that are usually clearly visualized or picturized, the location of the VT substrate is hardly defined.

### Cardiomyopathy

Both dilated and hypertrophic forms of cardiomyopathy are associated with ventricular tachyarrhythmias; however, patients referred for surgery for VT are more likely to have hypertrophic cardiomyopathy as deeply located scar tissue may not be amenable to catheter ablation. Myocardial fibrosis has been shown to be the substrate for ventricular tachyarrhythmias in the hypertrophied myocardium.[16] As the myocardial fibrosis can extend intramurally, the site of origin of VT may be in the mid myocardium, well below the epicardial adipose tissue, or near an epicardial coronary artery, which cannot be effectively and safely ablated by catheter technique either from the LV endocardium or epicardium.

As mentioned above, preoperative and intraoperative mapping of the endocardium and epicardium for identifying the origin of the tachycardia and the site of the reentrant circuit is essential, and close collaboration between the physician and surgeon is required. Intraoperative use of

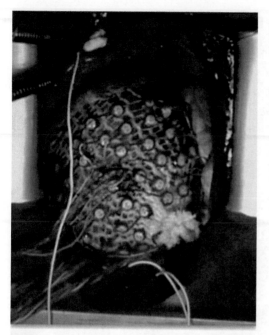

**Fig. 2.** Epicardial mapping of ventricles with a net-electrode. A total of 64 bipolar electrodes are mounted on an elastic net that covers the right and left ventricles to record epicardial electrograms.

electro-anatomic mapping system (**Fig. 3**) is helpful[17] in determining the substrate and the site of origin of VT in relation to the cardiac anatomic landmarks, such as the coronary vessels. Because not all of the precordial leads are properly recorded during open-chest procedures, QRS

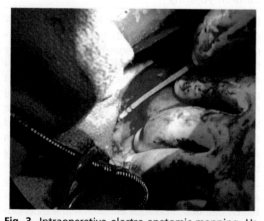

**Fig. 3.** Intraoperative electro-anatomic mapping. Using an electromagnetic navigation technology, a precise localization of the substrates of arrhythmias with high geometric accuracy is enabled. A location pad placed beneath the operating table and the local electrogram is recorded during VT by roving the electrode-magnetic catheter on the heart. VT, ventricular tachycardia.

morphologies of the induced VT or the paced rhythm are assessed only by the limb leads and the limited precordial leads, usually V5 and V6. After the chest is opened and the heart is elevated for intraoperative epicardial mapping, verification of the QRS morphologies during sinus rhythm, paced rhythm, or induced VT, is recommended to distinguish clinical VT from nonclinical VTs.

After the surgical target is determined by the intraoperative mapping, myocardial dissection or cryoablation is performed to ensure full-thickness necrosis at these sites. Cryothermia has some advantages over radiofrequency as an ablation energy in surgery for VT. Cryothermia can produce larger necrosis, thereby effectively ablating a widely and deeply distributed substrate of VT. Collagen fiber is preserved after cryothermia; this may be advantageous in preserving the function of the ventricle. In addition, thermal damage by cryothermia to neighboring tissues, such as coronal arteries, has been shown to be irreversible or minor.

## Midventricular hypertrophy with apical aneurysm

Midventricular hypertrophy of the LV is frequently complicated with an apical LV aneurysm[18] caused by persisting high pressure in the apical chamber of the LV. Stretch and distension of the aneurysm wall causes endocardial ischemia, fibrosis of the endocardium, and forms a substrate for VT. Catheter ablation is often not successful in patients with a narrow channel between the proximal and distal apical chambers of the LV, because of restricted manipulation of the catheter, myocardial hypertrophy, and intramural substrate.

Surgery is indicated in patients with unsuccessful catheter ablation or in those who are not suitable for the catheter ablation. The surgical procedure is similar to that of ischemic VT: aneurysm resection, endocardial resection, and cryothermia at the border between the fibrous and normal myocardium.[19]

## Left ventricular summit ventricular tachycardia

LV summit is the most superior anterior region of the LV, surrounded by the left anterior descending coronary artery, the left circumflex coronary artery, and the anterior interventricular vein.[20] Catheter ablation of the VT originating from this region (LV summit VT) frequently fails, because of the hypertrophic LV myocardium covered by a thick epicardial fat pad that hampers transmural ablation and the potential injury to the major coronary vessels. Even with a combined endocardial and epicardial approach, the results of catheter ablation are unsatisfactory.

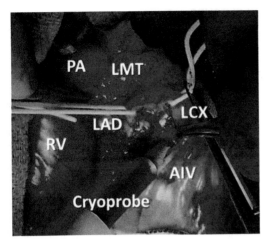

**Fig. 4.** Epicardial cryothermia for LV summit VT. Epicardial fat over the earliest activation site of VT was removed by using harmonic scalpel and the coronary vessels (LAD, LCX, and AIV) were carefully dissected and snared. Cryothermia was applied directly on the myocardium. AIV, anterior interventricular vein; LAD, left anterior descending coronary artery; LCX, left circumflex coronary artery; LMT, left main trunk of the left coronary artery; LV, left ventricular; PA, pulmonary artery; RV, right ventricle; VT, ventricular tachycardia.

Surgery for LV summit VT is a challenging therapeutic option. At the epicardium of the earliest activation site of VT, determined by intraoperative epicardial mapping, the coronary vessels are carefully dissected and snared, so that cryoprobe can be placed under the coronary vessels and avoid thermal injury to the vessels. Epicardial fat is removed by using harmonic scalpel to apply cryothermia directly on the myocardium (**Fig. 4**). Cryoablation of the LV endocardium beneath the epicardial earliest activation site is recommended to create a transmural lesion at the substrate of VT.

### Cardiac tumor

Arrhythmic events, including sudden cardiac arrest and VT, are the major complications in pediatric patients with cardiac tumors. Frequent pathologies of pediatric cardiac tumors are rhabdomyoma, followed by fibroma, myxoma, and others. Large fibromas manifest with VT in more than half of the patients.[9]

Surgical resection of tumors has been shown to eliminate or effectively suppress VT in patients with cardiac tumors.[9,10,21,22] Complete resection of tumors provides a highly curative outcome; however, there are some patients whose tumors are not completely resectable, because of the location or distribution of tumors.[22]

Even if the tumor is clearly recognized on the epicardial surface, intraoperative mapping is recommended to formulate the optimal surgical strategy.[21,22] In prior studies, epicardial voltage mapping during sinus rhythm showed low-voltage and fractionated electrograms or late potential recorded at the epicardium over the border of tumor, and activation mapping during VT showed that the earliest activation occurred close to the border of tumor. These data suggest that subepicardial myocardium over the tumor is displaced by tumors and the conduction is slowed at the thinned myocardium, leading to the reentrant mechanism of VT. From these findings, cryothermia of the thinned subepicardial myocardium at the edge of tumor is recommended to eradicate the substrate for VT (**Fig. 5**).

### Others

Arrhythmogenic right ventricular cardiomyopathy (ARVC) is a heritable cardiac disorder that causes progressive replacement of right ventricular myocardium by fibrofatty tissue.[23] ARVC is one of the leading causes of arrhythmic cardiac arrest in young people and athletes. ICD is indicated in ARVC patients to prevent sudden cardiac death. As the fibrofatty change is confined within the right ventricular free wall except in advanced-stage patients, surgical isolation of the entire right ventricular free wall prevents propagation of the abnormal activations to the remaining part of the heart.[24] Because the procedure poses a subtotal loss of right ventricular systolic function and the

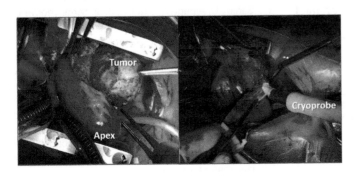

**Fig. 5.** Congenital cardiac fibroma with VT in 1.11-year-old girl. The tumor and arrhythmias were diagnosed prenatally. The tumor located at the lateral LV was completely removed by using an electrocautery and feeding arteries were ligated. Then, a series of cryothermia were applied at the thinned subepicardial myocardium at the edge of tumor. LV, left ventricular; VT, ventricular tachycardia.

postoperative pulmonary circulation depends on the pulmonary vascular resistance and LV systolic and diastolic function, the procedure is indicated only in selected patients.

Other scenarios in which surgical VT ablation include patients with LVADs who develop VT. This may be related to the LVAD inflow cannula site or at another site. Catheter ablation can only be considered if the potential site of ablation is far away from the LVAD inflow cannula. In patients with LVAD inflow cannula-related VT, cryothermia at the boundary between the scar and the normal myocardium to connect scar to fixed anatomic borders in the region has been shown to reduce the incidence of VT during and after LVAD support.[8]

## SUMMARY

Although catheter ablation for VT has gained acceptance as first-line therapy for recurrent VT over the years, there are several scenarios in which surgical VT ablation remains as an important treatment option. Cardiac electrophysiologists should consider surgical ablation as an option for patients with recurrent VT and failed catheter ablation (intramural substrate, proximity to coronary vessels, and large area of scar). Integration of electroanatomical mapping during surgical ablation allows for a targeted approach, which is essentially an extension of the catheter ablation technique and requires collaboration between electrophysiologists and arrhythmia surgeons. Specific scenarios where surgical ablation for VT may be considered a first-line option include VT arising from an LV apical aneurysm related to hypertrophic cardiomyopathy, LV summit VTs, and VTs associated with cardiac tumors.

## CLINICS CARE POINTS

Underlying pathologies of VT include patchy surviving myocardium with surrounding fibrosis due to myocardial infarction or cardiomyopathy, cardiac tumors, and others. Surgical ablation is recommended as a life-saving procedure in patients with monomorphic sustained VT for which pharmacotherapy or catheter ablation is ineffective, or in whom frequent VT episodes are not suppressed, or when there is frequent delivery of ICD therapies associated with the above condition. Surgical ablation is reasonable in patients with sustained monomorphic VT after myocardial infarction who have heart failure or thromboembolism associated with LV aneurysm or asynergy, or in patients with sustained monomorphic VT associated with cardiac tumors.

## DISCLOSURE

The author has nothing to disclose.

## REFERENCES

1. Harken AH, Josephson ME, Horowitz LN. Surgical endocardial resection for the treatment of malignant ventricular tachycardia. Ann Surg 1979;190:456–60.
2. Josephson ME, Harken AH, Horowitz LN. Endocardial excision: a new surgical technique for the treatment of recurrent ventricular tachycardia. Circulation 1979;60:1430–9.
3. Horowitz LN, Harken AH, Kastor JA, et al. Ventricular resection guided by epicardial and endocardial mapping for treatment of recurrent ventricular tachycardia. N Engl J Med 1980;302:589–93.
4. JCS/JHRS 2019 Guideline on non-pharmacotherapy of cardiac arrhythmias. Circ J 2021;85:1104–244.
5. Bhavani SS, Tchou P, Saliba W, et al. Surgical options for refractory ventricular tachycardia. J Card Surg 2007;22:533–4.
6. Anter E, Hutchinson MD, Deo R, et al. Surgical ablation of refractory ventricular tachycardia in patients with nonischemic cardiomyopathy. Circ Arrhythm Electrophysiol 2011;4:494–500.
7. Kumar S, Barbhaiya CR, Sobieszczyk P, et al. Role of alternative interventional procedures when endo- and epicardial catheter ablation attempts for ventricular arrhythmias fail. Circ Arrhythm Electrophysiol 2015;8:606–15.
8. Mulloy DP, Bhamidipati CM, Stone ML, et al. Cryoablation during left ventricular assist device implantation reduces postoperative ventricular tachyarrhythmias. J Thorac Cardiovasc Surg 2013;145:1207–13.
9. Miyake CY, Del Nido PJ, Alexander ME, et al. Cardiac tumors and associated arrhythmias in pediatric patients, with observations on surgical therapy for ventricular tachycardia. J Am Coll Cardiol 2011;58:190–9.
10. Nathan M, Fabozzo A, Geva T, et al. Successful surgical management of ventricular fibromas in children. J Thorac Cardiovasc Surg 2014;148:2602–8.
11. Sartipy U, Albage A, Straat E, et al. Surgery for ventricular tachycardia in patients undergoing left ventricular reconstruction by the Dor procedure. Ann Thorac Surg 2006;81:65–71.
12. Nitta T, Schuessler RB, Mitsuno M, et al. Return cycle mapping after entrainment of ventricular tachycardia. Circulation 1998;97:1164–75.
13. Haines DE, Lerman BB, Kron IL, et al. Surgical ablation of ventricular tachycardia with sequential map-guided subendocardial resection: electrophysiologic assessment and long-term follow-up. Circulation 1988;77:131–41.

14. Bakker PF, Hauer RN, Derksen R, et al. Sequential map-guided endocardial resection for ventricular tachycardia improves outcome. Eur J Cardiothorac Surg 2001;19:448–53.

15. Dor V, Sabatier M, Montiglio F, et al. Results of non-guided subtotal endocardiectomy associated with left ventricular reconstruction in patients with ischemic ventricular arrhythmias. J Thorac Cardiovasc Surg 1994;107:1301–7.

16. Maron BJ. Contemporary insights and strategies for risk stratification and prevention of sudden death in hypertrophic cardiomyopathy. Circulation 2010;121: 445–56.

17. Nitta T, Sakamoto S. Intraoperative mapping during surgical ablation procedures; interventional cardiac electrophysiology - a multidisciplinary approach. Minneapolis (MN): Cardiotext Publishing; 2015. p. 417–30.

18. Martin S, Maron MS, Finley JJ, Martijn Bos J, et al. Prevalence, clinical significance, and natural history of left ventricular apical aneurysms in hypertrophic cardiomyopathy. Circulation 2008;118:1541–9.

19. Osawa H, Fujimatsu T, Takai F, et al. Hypertrophic cardiomyopathy with apical aneurysm: left ventricular reconstruction and cryoablation for ventricular tachycardia. Gen Thorac Cardiovasc Surg 2011; 59:354–8.

20. Yamada T, McElderry HT, Doppalapudi H, et al. Idiopathic ventricular arrhythmias originating from the left ventricular summit: anatomic concepts relevant to ablation. Circ Arrhythm Electrophysiol 2010;3: 616–23.

21. Sakamoto S, Nitta T, Murata H, et al. Electroanatomical mapping-assisted surgical treatment of incessant ventricular tachycardia associated with an intramyocardial giant lipoma. J Interv Card Electrophysiol 2012;33:109–12.

22. Sakamoto S, Hiromoto A, Murata H, et al. Surgical procedure for targeting arrhythmogenic substrates in the treatment of ventricular tachycardia associated with cardiac tumors. Heart Rhythm 2020;17: 238–42.

23. Corrado D, Link MS, Calkins H. Arrhythmogenic right ventricular cardiomyopathy. N Engl J Med 2017;376:61–72.

24. Cox JL, Bardy GH, Damiano RJ Jr, et al. Right ventricular isolation procedures for nonischemic ventricular tachycardia. J Thorac Cardiovasc Surg 1985; 90:212–24.

# Moving?

## Make sure your subscription moves with you!

To notify us of your new address, find your **Clinics Account Number** (located on your mailing label above your name), and contact customer service at:

**Email: journalscustomerservice-usa@elsevier.com**

**800-654-2452** (subscribers in the U.S. & Canada)
**314-447-8871** (subscribers outside of the U.S. & Canada)

**Fax number: 314-447-8029**

**Elsevier Health Sciences Division**
**Subscription Customer Service**
**3251 Riverport Lane**
**Maryland Heights, MO 63043**

*To ensure uninterrupted delivery of your subscription, please notify us at least 4 weeks in advance of move.

ELSEVIER

Printed and bound by CPI Group (UK) Ltd, Croydon, CR0 4YY

03/10/2024

01040365-0007